PEER REJECTION

The Guilford Series on Social and Emotional Development

CLAIRE B. KOPP and STEVEN R. ASHER, *Editors*

Peer Rejection

Developmental Processes and Intervention Strategies

Karen L. Bierman

Foreword by John D. Coie

THE GUILFORD PRESS
New York   London

Library of Congress Cataloging-in-Publication Data

Bierman, Karen L.
  Peer rejection : developmental processes and intervention strategies /
by Karen L. Bierman.
      p.   cm. — (The Guilford series on social and emotional
  development)
Includes bibliographical references and index.
  ISBN 1-57230-923-7 (hc) ISBN 1-59385-243-6 (pbk)
  1. Rejection (Psychology) in children. 2. Social interaction in
children. 3. Behavioral assessment of children. 4. Child
psychotherapy. I. Title. II. Series.
  BF723.R44B54 2004
  155.4' 18—dc21
                                                    2003007554

About the Author

Karen L. Bierman, PhD, is Director of the Children, Youth, and Families Consortium (CYFC) at the Pennsylvania State University, and Distinguished Professor of Clinical Child Psychology. Her research has focused on understanding how peer relationships contribute to children's social–emotional development, social competence, and school adjustment. Dr. Bierman is particularly interested in the design and evaluation of programs that promote social competence and positive intergroup relations and that reduce aggression and violence. Currently, she is the director of the Pennsylvania site of the Fast Track project, a national, multisite prevention trial, funded by the National Institute of Mental Health (with additional funding from the National Institute on Drug Abuse and the U.S. Department of Education), which focuses on preventing antisocial behavior among high-risk youth. She is also coinvestigator of the newly funded PROSPER program, supported by the National Institute on Drug Abuse, which involves the diffusion of empirically supported prevention programs to schools through the use of cooperative-extension-facilitated university–community partnerships.

Foreword

Acts of seriously disturbing violence enacted on school grounds across the United States over the past decade have created widespread interest in the phenomenon of youth whose anger at peers is such that they bring weapons to their schools with the intention of killing large numbers of schoolmates, including many with whom they have little previous connection. These tragic acts highlight something that has existed in our schools long before this recent rash of violence. The pain, frustration, and anger that is generated as a consequence of social rejection and victimization is prevalent on virtually every school campus. We have come to the point in our social history when we can no longer write this off as simply part of the experience of growing up. Planning for children who have serious problems relating to their peers must now become an integral part of our thinking about children's education. This volume by Karen Bierman on peer rejection can and should be a major resource for those who will undertake this kind of planning.

For those who have followed Karen Bierman's research career, this book is the natural culmination of her work to this point. As such, it is essential reading for those who want a serious understanding of the phenomenon of childhood peer rejection. For those who want the best available wisdom on the enterprise of intervening with rejected children, it is an absolute treasure. Bierman's research activity for the past two decades is reflected in the two central themes of the volume: the causes and consequences of peer rejection and effective interventions to remediate the experience of rejection among school-age children. She has been a core contributor to the basic science of the problem and is as expert as anyone in the area, but she is without equal when it comes to understanding the dynamics and complexity of intervening with children who have peer relations problems. From her graduate-student days right up to the present time, she has been involved in the creation and testing of programs for helping children improve their relationships with peers.

In the mid-1980s, Bierman and her colleagues published the results of intervention studies that were designed to examine the role of both skills training and social reinforcement procedures in improving chidren's social behavior and their social status among peers. The use of videotaping made it possible to distinguish between simply having received social skills training and actually acquiring the requisite skills. This careful differentiation among the multiple dimensions of effecting and measuring change has been the hallmark of her intervention work and served to raise the standard for intervention research that followed.

Active interest in the study of children's social relations with peers began in the 1970s, stimulated by a few longitudinal studies that included measures of peer liking and dislike among the battery of measures designed to assess developmental adjustment across the school years. To the surprise of many, the measure of peer dislike seemed to have strong predictive power in forecasting future adjustment in later childhood and adolescence. As measures of social adjustment were evaluated more closely in peer relations research, distinctions began to be made between children who were withdrawn and isolated from peers versus those who were aggressive with peers.

This volume begins with a history of the research and covers the rich expansion of developmental research on peer rejection that marked the next 20 years, providing the reader with a comprehensive understanding of critical factors in the causes of rejection, the more immediate consequences for the child, and the long-term implications for the child's adjustment. Earlier publications have covered significant portions of this tale, but Bierman brings the story up to the minute and does so in a way that personalizes the phenomenon, describing prototypical children as a way of illustrating the issues raised.

In keeping with the most current focus of the peer relations literature, Bierman has given greater evidence to developmental processes involved in becoming rejected or maintaining that status. In particular, she gives extended coverage to peer influences on both rejection and problem behaviors such as aggression, concluding that there is now considerable evidence that peer interactions across the school years shape children's behaviors in ways that go well beyond the behavioral tendencies they bring with them to school. This, perhaps, is the major influence on developmental theory brought about by the past 25 years of peer relations research, namely, that the popular tendency to ascribe the causes of child behavior to the influence of the family must now be revised to recognize the significant role played by peers.

Sometimes an emphasis on skills training or social cognition as ways of altering peer status can give the impression that rejected children are viewed as simply missing critical techniques or knowledge, as though their "software" needs to be upgraded. What distinguishes Part I is its emphasis on the integration of behavioral, emotional, and self-system patterns in rejection. This section closes with a discussion of the developing self-system that interprets the impact of habitual social patterns in terms of the child's orientation toward the social world. In doing so, Bierman has integrated disparate research on social information processing, relational schemas, competency drives, emotional reactivity, self-schemas, control beliefs, and perceived competence to provide a complex model of self-system development that helps explain such phenomena as the persistence of maladaptive social behavior in the face of repeated demands for change. The richness of this model is then translated into a framework for assessment and intervention planning that is described in the latter two parts of the book.

Parts II and III give the book its uniqueness, and it is worth a historical and personal digression to put this material in context. The chapters are organized the way a well-trained child clinician would frame them—a clinician who possessed a full grasp of what research and clinical practice had to offer on the subject. This, in fact, is Bierman's background. She is a trained clinical psychologist and has directed a clinical training program. Nonetheless, her research on peer rejection, like that of some of the rest of us who share her background, is indistinguishable from that of other peer relations researchers whose backgrounds might be in developmental psychology or education. The fact is that although peer rejection has turned out to have major significance for understanding the development of psychopathology, the study of this phenomenon did not begin with clinically oriented researchers, but with those interested in the development and education of children. For many of the early years in which interest in peer rejection simply exploded among developmental researchers, interest in the topic among clinicians was limited to the handful of researchers who happened to have clinical training but saw themselves as developmental researchers. Social skills training, for example, was seen largely within an educational framework, and this, in fact, was the background of the authors of the two or three initial and highly influential intervention studies. The use of the reinforcement paradigm in Bierman's early study did come from existing clinical research and practice, however, and reflected the possibility of merging the accumulated knowledge of these two fields of research. It was only as evidence began to accumulate that peer rejection was an important contributing factor to the development of conduct disorder and depression that most child clinicians began to take some interest in this phenomenon.

At present, it is reasonable to claim that research on peer rejection has major implications for the practice of child clinical psychology. It should pull clinicians out of the clinic and into the real-life settings of the child, particularly the school, because this is where much of a child's peer relations occur. This, then, is where the intervention, and the assessment activities that logically precede it, should take place and be evaluated. It is also the case, however, that the clinical tradition and orientation can have real value for nonclinicians who are interested in doing something about peer rejection. In the latter two parts of the book, Bierman uses the basic science findings on peer rejection in Part I as a foundation for taking the clinical approach of assessment guiding intervention that is provided in Part II, and this is played out in a careful and knowledgeable synthesis of research from both clinical and nonclinical fields.

Part II deals with the assessment of social competence and peer relations. It is not limited to coverage of peer rejection alone, but deals with the general issue of social competence and its converse. It alone is worth the purchase price of the book. In writing this section, Bierman seems to have been thinking of both the practitioner and the research scholar. She has organized this material around four major content areas: assessing peer relations (friendships, social networks, liking and disliking status in the group, and victimization), assessing the context of peer relations, the nature of children's social behaviors, and various aspects of the child's self-system relating to peer issues. These domains are properly treated as interrelated in her assessment model. Hers is as comprehensive an analysis of peer relations assessment as can be found currently. (As a side note, the book will save experienced peer relations researchers numerous hours of extended e-mail conversations each year because it can be recommended as the definitive manual for someone starting out in research in this field. It will also become the self-help manual for practitioners who want to take seriously the social context and adjustment of their child clients.) Covering the full range of research-based measurement of peer relations, discussed in the historical content of their development, Part II is important reading for graduate students in this field. For those not familiar with many of the measures, it also provides illustrative material to give a feeling for the content of measures, in some cases providing actual items.

Likewise, Part III is an essential reference for anyone considering intervention work with children who have problems relating to their peers. The existing clinical and research literatures are covered fully

and in historical context. Bierman notes the mixed patterns of effectiveness obtained across social competence training studies, despite
meta-analytic studies suggesting moderate levels of success. The para-
dox is that the number of such studies steadily decreased across the
late 1980s and the 1990s, even though it is clear that there are many
unresolved questions relating to intervention with rejected children.
Although we now understand something of the complexity of social–
emotional, cognitive, and behavioral differences among this group of
children, the combinations of intervention components necessary to
come to terms with this complexity have yet to be tested. Additionally,
more needs to be known about effective treatment processes, as well as
a technology for involving peers effectively in the treatment process. It
is as though efforts at developing more sophisticated approaches to intervention have decreased just as the field has begun to understand
what is going to be required to move in this direction. It is hoped that
this volume will serve to regenerate interest in intervention research in
this area.

    The book's final part describes virtually all of what is currently
known about intervening to improve social competence in childhood,
including specific techniques and ways of handling situations that
could only have been written by someone intimately acquainted with
the wide range of possible circumstances of competence training with
children. Admittedly, this last statement is a biased comment because I
have been a co-collaborator with Bierman on the Fast Track project, a
preventive intervention trial with children at very high risk for chronic
conduct problems. Social competence training is a core element in this
program, in that peer rejection contributes to further antisocial behavior of children already exhibiting early behavior problems. Bierman
has taken the lead role in developing the Fast Track social competence
curricula across the school years and in training staff to implement this
developmentally organized program. It would be hard to find someone
with more hands-on experience with this kind of activity, but what may
distinguish her from others with similar backgrounds is her extensive
knowledge of program evaluation underlying many of the curriculum
design issues. This knowledge is reflected, for example, in the discussion of how to select people to conduct social competence training as
well as how to compose groups to optimize intervention effectiveness.
Bierman discusses the advantages and disadvantages of using different
behavior management systems during the actual conduct of group
training sessions, getting into issues that might not be considered by
someone without prior experience.

    The goal of effective social competence training is not simply to
provide children with superficial skills in managing relationships with

others. Some critics have speculated that such programs might merely enhance the manipulative potential of children who already have sociopathic tendencies. Rather, social competence training is intended (1) to help children internalize positive social values and concern for others because these values will make it much easier to get along with other people, and (2) to foster greater self-control over destructive or self-defeating impulses. Experienced clinicians will recognize many of these dynamics as elements of good child therapy work and may become more comfortable with what might, on the surface, strike them as treatment approaches that "do not really get at the underlying problem." This is what makes *Peer Rejection* so valuable to a broad range of adults who wish to improve the social adjustment of children, whether they are trained clinicians, research-oriented preventionists, educators, social workers, counselors, or laypersons who are looking for ways to help children in a volunteer capacity.

JOHN D. COIE, PhD
Duke University

Preface

I don't know why they don't like me. I've tried everything I know how to do, but they won't leave me alone and they won't be my friend. They call me "stinky" and I tell them to stop it, but they won't. Yesterday, they chased me down the street and I had to run into my house and slam the door. Everyone else has a friend to stick up for them, but no one will stick up for me.

−JP, age 10, clinic intake interview

You want to be part of their group, but you're an outsider. They don't ask you to eat at their table; they don't want you there. You don't really have a place where you belong. You feel like nothing, like you've been tossed away.

−SS, age 11, study participant

Few childhood problems involve the level of stress and long-term damage that is caused by chronic peer rejection. Friendships are of central importance to grade school children. On a regular basis, children think about and talk about whom they like and whom they don't like. They worry about how friendships will go for them and how they will be treated by others. For some children, such as those described above, peer acceptance is elusive—a brass ring that remains out of their reach. Children who are rejected by peers, like these children, often grow up lonely and alienated, suffering through their school days, struggling with feelings of anxiety and inadequacy. As they grow into adolescents and adults, many experience continuing insecurities and difficulties in interpersonal relationships, and suffer depression and other psychiatric difficulties (Parker & Asher, 1987). The letter below illustrates the significant impact negative peer experiences in childhood can have on adult well-being.

To this day at the age of 37, I still suffer from the sting of
criticisms and rejections I received in school and elsewhere as a
child. I remember being scared of people at a very early age. As I
grew, I was not comfortable with other children. I did try but
people confused me and still do. The more the rejection and
name calling, the worse I felt. I put on a smiley face, as I do
today, but I knew in my heart that people just don't like me and
never will.

–JW, written communication

Not surprisingly, children who experience serious disturbances in
their peer relations are at risk for negative outcomes. In retrospective
(follow-back) studies, a disproportionate number of adults with serious
psychiatric disturbances (particularly antisocial personality disorder,
schizoid personality disorder or schizophrenia, and social anxiety) remember painful social experiences and describe childhood histories of
problematic social behavior and poor peer relations. Conversely, in
prospective (follow-forward) studies, a disproportionate number of
rejected children grow up to experience mental health problems and
antisocial behavior (Parker, Rubin, Price, & DeRosier, 1995).

Why do peers reject some children? For many children their social
behavior plays a critical role—they annoy and disturb others and fail to
engage in a friendly and fun way (Bierman, Smoot, & Aumiller, 1993;
Dodge, 1989). At the same time, it is important to remember that rejection is a group process, not an individual characteristic. Rejection and
victimization reflect attitudes and behaviors that peers direct toward
children, so peer group contexts and dynamics contribute to the process in critical ways. Because a child's past interpersonal experiences
and history affect his/her perceptions, goals, and expectations in new
interactions with peers, it is important to consider the transactional influences among the child's behavioral and cognitive skills, emotional
and motivational orientation, and peer group context and contingencies when assessing peer problems and designing interventions.

This book takes a developmental perspective and focuses on understanding and treating peer rejection in middle childhood during the
critical grade school years when core social skills and attitudes develop,
although some of the material is also relevant to younger children and
to adolescents. The roots of social competence begin to develop during
early childhood. However, it is in elementary school that children must
learn to adapt, conform, and negotiate a variety of complex peer group
contexts. Correspondingly, during grade school, children's concerns
about peer acceptance rise sharply (Eder, 1985); gossip and bullying increase (Eder, 1985; Olweus, 1993); and peer difficulties become more
predictive of problematic social, emotional, and academic adjustment
(see Parker et al., 1995).

The book is divided into three general parts, focusing on understanding problematic peer relations (Chapters 1–4), assessment strategies (Chapters 5–9), and intervention methods (Chapters 10–14).

Part I provides a brief summary of an extensive body of research
that has explored the causes, correlates, and consequences of peer rejection. Interview excerpts and case examples illustrate some of the various forms that peer rejection processes can take during the grade
school years, and the impact of those experiences on social–emotional
development. The four chapters in this section describe (1) research
documenting the developmental significance of peer relationships and
definitions of the key concepts of rejection and social competence; (2)
the characteristics of rejected children, along with case examples that illustrate the patterns of behavior that get children into trouble with
their peers; (3) peer group dynamics involved in rejection processes;
and (4) the interplay between peer relations and the development of
the self.

Part II describes assessment strategies, with an emphasis on assessments for intervention design and evaluation. Chapter 5 provides an
overview of assessment goals and strategies, considers the operational
definition of social competence, and describes the value of multimethod assessments. The remaining chapters in Part II consider specific strategies to assess problematic peer relations (Chapter 6), social
behavior (Chapter 7), peer interactions (Chapter 8), and self-system
processes (Chapter 9).

Part III focuses on intervention strategies, and highlights developmental and clinical research that provides guidance to the design of effective social competence coaching programs. Following a historical
overview describing the evolution of the social competence coaching
method (Chapter 10), the content and organization of coaching programs are detailed in Chapter 11, and intervention processes associated with the promotion of self-system change are described in Chapter
12. In Chapter 13, additional strategies to support the development of
social competence in school and home contexts are reviewed, including universal school-based programs and multicomponent intervention
programs. Chapter 14 identifies key issues and future directions for social competence intervention research and practice.

A major goal of this book is to highlight the importance of integrating developmental research on peer rejection processes with the
design and evaluation of interventions for rejected children—an interface that will support further advances in both theoretical and applied
domains. On the one hand, familiarity with developmental research
can inform intervention design, contributing to more sophisticated and
effective intervention strategies. On the other hand, significant re-

search is usually produced by persons who have acquired insights as a function of close familiarity with a phenomenon. Intervention efforts provide this familiarity, as they involve sustained personal contact with rejected children and offer opportunities to observe, and test empirically, processes of change. This book is designed to provide a comprehensive and critical appraisal of the empirical literature on peer-rejected children and peer rejection processes, and of its implications for intervention design and evaluation. I hope that it will serve both to clarify the current state of knowledge in this area, and also to stimulate further inquiry and progress in this field.

Acknowledgments

I would like to thank series editor Steve Asher for his insightful comments and invaluable suggestions. I would also like to thank John Coie and Janet Welsh for their wonderful reviews of my first draft and their extremely useful advice, along with the suggestions provided by two anonymous reviewers. My thoughts about at-risk children, their social–emotional development, and corresponding intervention strategies have been enriched enormously through collaboration with my colleagues (and friends) in the Conduct Problems Prevention Research Group (John Coie, Ken Dodge, Michael Foster, Mark Greenberg, John Lochman, Bob McMahon, and Ellen Pinderhughes), and I am very grateful to have had the opportunity to work with them. In addition, I have benefited greatly from the superb colleagues and rich intellectual working environment at the Child Study Center and the Prevention Research Center of the Pennsylvania State University. Much of the work described in this book relied on funding provided by the W. T. Grant Foundation, the National Institute of Mental Health, and the National Institute on Drug Abuse. Finally, I would like to thank my husband, Rick, and my children, Erin, Cale, and Lily, for the support and joy they give me every day.

Contents

PART I

UNDERSTANDING PROBLEMATIC PEER RELATIONS

Chapter 1

The Developmental Significance of Peer Relations

[handwritten: 1902 - Cooley - c's peer rel'ps as critical context]

[handwritten annotation: p's peers; support, guidance, dis'c'ne; exp'ce intim, control aggr'n, practice + master social skills, nego'n + compromise c̄='s, fantasy play, rule-based seqs + soc conv'ns]

Interest in the developmental significance of children's peer relations dates from the turn of the 20th century (see Parker, Rubin, Price, & DeRosier, 1995, and Renshaw, 1981, for historical overviews). In 1902, Cooley anticipated in theory what contemporary research has confirmed—that peer relations provide a critical context for social–emotional development and adjustment, influencing child socialization in the areas of behavior, personality, and adaptation.

Referring to "two worlds of childhood," researchers have documented that peers influence development in a manner that is different from, and complementary to, the contribution of parents (Bronfenbrenner, 1970; Hartup, 1979). With their parents, children are young dependents, receiving support, guidance, and discipline. In contrast, peers interact more often as equals, providing each other with play opportunities, entertainment, and companionship. In these interactions, the "golden rule" of reciprocity and cooperation prevails, and children must learn to negotiate and compromise to maintain their friendships successfully (Rubin, Bukowski, & Parker, 1998). With peers, children can engage in fantasy play that allows them to experiment with different ideas and roles, and they are exposed to rule-based sequences and social conventions. Thus it is in the context of peer relations that children practice and master critical social skills, including an understanding and respect for fair play, perspective taking, and negotiation and conflict management skills (Parker et al., 1995). Peer experiences also shape children's growing capacities to interact comfortably with others, to control aggression, and to experience intimacy (Hartup, 1989).

The idea that children with poor peer relations could (and should)

3

[handwritten margin notes: "early 40's — let's ID + TX kids to poor peer relns" · "'42 Chittenden — dolls as + role models" · "50's slow" · "60's on again — beh mgmt → + soc beh" · "good @ discrete beh in defined contexts but → naturalistic setting needed" · "unu → develp info'd strategies" · "preschool 1st friendships — coop'v + shared fan'y play" · "grade school larger + satisfac interaxns" · "gp interaxns benficial" · "negot'n competn conformity ach" · "longer interaxns → stable friendships"]

be identified and treated emerged in the research literature in the late 1930s and early 1940s (Renshaw, 1981). For example, in 1942, Chittenden designed a set of lessons for preschool children who had frequent conflicts with peers. She used dolls to illustrate positive strategies for getting along with others, and documented positive changes in children's behaviors (see Renshaw, 1981).

Following a hiatus in peer research during the 1950s, interest in peer-focused interventions was rekindled in the 1960s, when emerging behavioral management techniques were applied to the promotion of positive social behavior. At that time, researchers believed that child behavior was the primary determinant of positive peer relations, and that by increasing rates of positive social behaviors (e.g., smiling, greeting, eye contact) and decreasing problematic social behaviors (e.g., hitting), interventions would enable isolated or aggressive children to achieve social success (Dodge & Murphy, 1984).

Although behavioral management techniques proved effective in shaping discrete social behaviors in defined contexts, it soon became apparent that promoting positive peer relations in naturalistic settings would require a broader understanding of the developmental domain and, correspondingly, more complex and developmentally informed therapeutic strategies. Central to making progress in the design of social interventions was the recognition that peer relations and peer problems need to be understood within a developmental framework.

DEVELOPMENTAL PROGRESSIONS

Developmental research has revealed progressions in the characteristics and complexity of children's peer relations, indicating important developmental differences in the skills associated with social competence at different ages, with corresponding implications for the design of interventions for rejected children.

Whereas parents are the primary source of social and emotional support for children during the first years of life, peers become increasingly important as children age, providing companionship, entertainment, and support (Hartup, 1983). First friendships are typically established during the preschool years, when children begin to delight in cooperative and shared fantasy play (Gottman, 1983). In grade school, children benefit from larger and more structured positive peer group interactions, where their friendship skills continue to develop as they learn to negotiate issues involving competition, conformity, and achievement. Peer interactions are sustained for longer periods, and more stable friendships emerge. By preadolescence, children often experience a

pre ado - need special friend'ps c̄ >intim + support
- same-sex "chums" to model sustained close emo relps
ado - recog diff social styles + norms in "cliques" + "crowds"
- try on roles, explore self + values.
- stepping stones to repar'n fr. p's

need for special friendships that offer greater intimacy and support; many form special "chumships" with same-sex peers that provide models for the rewards and demands involved in sustaining close emotional relationships (Sullivan, 1953). During adolescence, youth begin to recognize different social styles and norms, as reflected in "cliques" and "crowds" (Brown, 1990). As youth move in and out of these groups, they have opportunities to explore different facets of themselves, and are challenged to define their personal values and sense of self. Youth may "try on" different social roles and experience a range of relationships, helping them to define the kinds of persons they are and the kinds of persons they want (or don't want) to be. Peers also provide emotional support, serving as "steppingstones" as adolescents move away from their emotional dependence upon their parents and toward autonomous functioning as adults (Steinberg & Silverberg, 1986). Thus, in many ways, childhood peer relations serve as "training grounds" for future interpersonal relations, facilitating the development of skills and feelings that will be associated with interpersonal relations in adult life, including relations with coworkers and with romantic partners.

In addition to documenting progressions in peer relations, developmental research has made important contributions to the assessment and treatment of problematic peer relations by identifying the multifaceted nature of peer relations, and clarifying the different implications for child development of peer "rejection" versus peer "neglect" (Coie, Dodge, & Coppotelli, 1982).

peers ignore, not noticed +
also few friend nomin'ns but   rarely named as friends
actively disliked + often chosen   but not actively disliked
as "least liked"

PEER REJECTION VERSUS PEER NEGLECT

- beh probs usually
ltd to social iso
+ wdrawal

hi rates of   >l. beh probs, >l. distress,
disrupt've   adjmt probs (stable + cx sit'ns)
+ agg

- inattn
- self-imposed
hostile   less stable
iso'n   over time

- feel loneliness   >l. grow out
+ social   of it or
distress'n   find new gp

more stable
over time

Neglected children are ignored by peers. They receive little notice and are rarely named as friends by their classmates, but at the same time they are not actively disliked. In contrast, rejected children, who also receive few friendship nominations by classmates are actively disliked by classmates, and frequently chosen as "least liked" (Coie et al., 1982). Across studies, rejected children are more likely than neglected children to have behavioral problems, to experience psychological distress, and to have cross-situational and stable adjustment difficulties (Coie, Dodge, & Kupersmidt, 1990). For example, whereas the behavior problems exhibited by neglected children are typically limited to social isolation and withdrawal, many rejected children show high rates of disruptive and aggressive behaviors. Both neglected and rejected children tend to struggle with academic problems and elevated anxiety. In addition, however, rejected children often show high rates of classroom behavior problems, inattentiveness, and self-imposed hostile isolation

- both - aca probs + >anx

(Bierman, 1987). Rejected children are also more likely than neglected children to express loneliness and social dissatisfaction (Asher, Hymel, & Renshaw, 1984). Developmental studies have revealed that neglected status is less stable over time than rejected status, and that neglected children are more likely to grow out of their problems or show improved peer relations when they move into new peer groups.

A particularly important study illustrating the differences in the developmental trajectories of neglected and rejected children was conducted by Coie and Kupersmidt (1983). In that study, rejected and neglected children were assigned to summer playgroups. In half of the cases, these playgroups included familiar children from the same home school and classroom. For the other groups, children were unfamiliar at the start of the summer, coming from different home schools. When Coie and Kupersmidt reassessed sociometric status in the summer playgroups, they found that the social outcomes of the neglected children depended upon the familiarity of the group. When placed with familiar peers, neglected children tended to remain neglected. However, when placed with new peers, neglected children often improved their social status, attaining average status. In contrast, rejected children reestablished their rejected status quickly (within one or two play sessions), whether placed with familiar or unfamiliar peers. Coie and Kupersmidt concluded that neglected children who are shy in the classroom and ignored by classmates are not necessarily deficient in social competence. Instead, the low levels of social involvement they display may be a reflection of their reaction to a particular peer group. Developmentally, peer neglect may be a relatively unstable classification, as the peer problems of neglected children are often situationally based; they frequently decline as children develop more confidence and move into classrooms with more familiar or more compatible peers. These findings also suggest that short-term interventions—particularly those that focus on increasing social niche and positive peer opportunities—may be more effective for neglected than for rejected children, whose peer problems tend to be more complex.

In contrast to neglected children, Coie and Kupersmidt (1983) suggested that rejected children, who garnered peer dislike quickly in new groups, had social skill deficits and behavioral control problems that made it difficult for them to initiate or maintain positive relations with peers, regardless of the peer context. Indeed, other studies have confirmed that many rejected children exhibit aggressive or disruptive problems; others are highly anxious and awkward socially (Parker et al., 1995). Even when these children move into new peer groups, their behavior quickly alienates peers. Rejected children often become ostracized or victimized by peers, contributing to feelings of resentment,

[handwritten margin notes: interv'ns for rejecteds must address underlying deficits in beh'l control + socials skills + enc. + peer response; ↑ liking ± ↓ disliking; ↑ +behs ↓ probs behs; liked ≠ not disliked]

frustration, and social anxiety over time (Coie, 1990; Rubin & Stewart, 1996). To be effective with rejected children, interventions must therefore address the behavior problems that are contributing to peer dislike, as well as promoting positive social skills and encouraging positive peer responding (Bierman, Miller, & Stabb, 1987).

[handwritten margin: avoiding rejexn ≠ gaining acceptance]

Differences between neglected and rejected children also indicate that being liked by peers is not simply the opposite of being disliked, and that different skills are needed to gain acceptance than to avoid rejection (Asher, Parkhurst, Hymel, & Williams, 1990). The primary determinants of peer liking are positive social behaviors, including congeniality, conversation skills, and cooperative behaviors (Coie et al., 1990). Peers describe well-liked classmates as helpful, friendly, nice, understanding, and good at games. In contrast, the factors that engender peer dislike typically involve behavior problems, either the acting-out kind (hostile or disruptive behaviors) or the anxious/avoidant kind (awkward and/or insensitive behaviors). Correspondingly, interventions aimed at reducing rejection need to focus on both promoting positive social behaviors to enhance peer liking and reducing problem behaviors that are contributing to peer disliking.

[handwritten margin: peer liking) comes from +soc beh (congenial, convers'n, cooper'n) -helpful, friendly, nice, understandn good @ games; dislike fr: beh probs (hostile, disruptive, awk, insens've, anx, avoidn)]

In addition to clarifying the different implications of being rejected versus neglected by peers, developmental research has illuminated differences in the developmental significance of peer group acceptance versus friendships.

[handwritten: >l. have friends v. rejecteds]

PEER ACCEPTANCE VERSUS FRIENDSHIP

[handwritten: like - dislike ≠ voluntary dyadic rel'ps reciprocal affirm'n + mutual affexn]

The quality and quantity of a child's reciprocated friendships represent a dimension of peer relations that is related to, but distinct from, peer group status. Peer "acceptance" and "rejection" refer to the degree to which members of a particular peer group (in middle childhood, usually child's classroom) like or dislike a child. In contrast, "friendships" are voluntary dyadic relationships, characterized by reciprocal affirmation and mutual affection (Furman & Robbins, 1985; Rubin et al., 1998). Although children who are well accepted by peers are more likely to have friends than are rejected children, some popular children do not have close friends, whereas some rejected children do (Parker & Asher, 1993a). In addition, although the social skills that promote peer liking (such as congeniality and cooperativeness) also foster friendships, friendships require common ground, mutual attraction, and a commitment to reciprocity as well (Hartup, 1989). Typically, friendships emerge during shared activities, when a mutual affective bond develops in that context (Asher, Parker, & Walker, 1996).

[handwritten margin: some popular kids have no close friends; some rejecteds do]

[handwritten bottom notes: social skills (eg congen'ty + cooper'n) help → liking but friends also need common ground, mutual attraxn + commitmt to recip'ty - typically emerge during shared acts]

late c'hd + early ado f'ps > imp 't tho' evident as early as preschool + imp't @ start of elem.

- satisfying + proto types for later rom'c rel'ps

Although close friendships with distinctive characteristics can be observed as early as the preschool years (Gottman, 1983), and can serve important support functions at the entry into elementary school (Ladd, 1990), theorists believe that they play a particularly important role in social–emotional development during late childhood and early adolescence (Furman & Robbins, 1985; Sullivan, 1953). In unique ways, close friendships satisfy innate needs for affection, intimacy, and reliable companionship; they foster feelings of self-worth, the development of empathy, and perspective-taking skills; and they serve as prototypes for intimate and romantic relationships later in life (Berndt, 1982).

rejexn < damaging if 1 close friend for companion'p + support

but no guarantee

Several investigators have suggested that peer rejection may be less damaging to a child if that child has a best friend who provides companionship and support (Furman & Robbins, 1985; Parker & Asher, 1993b). However, close friendships do not always exert a positive influence (Hoza, Molina, Bukowski, & Sippola, 1995). The close friendships of rejected children are often qualitatively inferior to the friendships of nonrejected children, involving more conflict and less stability (Hartup, 1989; Parker & Asher, 1993a). Conflictual friendships or friendships in which antisocial behaviors are modeled and reinforced can increase a rejected child's risk for conduct problems and for continued rejection (Dishion, Andrews, & Crosby, 1995; Kupersmidt, Burchinal, & Patterson, 1995). The implication of this research for intervention is that friendships, as well as general peer status, deserve attention in assessment and intervention design.

rejected's close f'ps often inferior to nonrejecteds (>conflict, <stable)

-antisocial modelling => >conduct probs + cont'd rejexn

so incl. f'p + peer status in Ax + Tx design

UNDERSTANDING SOCIAL COMPETENCE

beh'l Tx of 60's + 70's + substantial ↑ in c social fxn b/c missing devel'l research

Developmental research examining the multifaceted nature of children's peer relations helps explain why behavioral interventions of the 1960s and 1970s did not substantially improve children's social functioning (Dodge & Murphy, 1984). The idea that effective social interaction can be reduced to a set of discrete behaviors shaped by environmental contingencies is inconsistent with developmental research, which suggests instead that being socially competent involves the capacity to participate effectively in dynamic interpersonal processes across a range of social contexts. In this conceptualization, the appropriateness of particular behaviors depends upon a host of factors, including development, context, and culture (Parker et al., 1995; Rubin et al., 1998; Sroufe, 1996). Some behaviors become increasingly inappropriate with age (e.g., instrumental aggression), whereas others emerge in importance with age (e.g., conversation skills) (Bierman & Montminy, 1993). Some behaviors, such as withdrawal, may be viewed by others as more

social competence involves: dynamic pros a: X many social contexts

some ↑ by age inapprop

others ↑'ly > crucial as age

some > OK for f than ♂ (eg. ⌐drawal) so damage report'n >orL

[handwritten margin notes: context eg. class v. play — convers'n — fantasy]

[handwritten margin notes: so can't define social competence as discrete behs — need broader understanding]

appropriate for girls than for boys (Caspi, Elder, & Bem, 1988), and hence may have differential impacts on social reputation.

In addition, the appropriateness of a behavior often depends upon the context in which it is displayed (Foster, Inderbitzen, & Nangle, 1993). For example, different kinds of social behavior are expected in classroom settings than in play settings. Even within the context of play, different social behaviors are expected when children are playing games with rules than when they are engaging in fantasy play or focused conversations (Bierman & Welsh, 2000). Hence the extent to which a particular behavior is socially skillful depends upon the context in which it is used.

[handwritten margin notes: abil to org'za soc beh to elicit + + avoid — responses across contexts in line ā social conv'n + morals]

As an understanding of these complexities grew, it became clear that social competence could not be defined or assessed in terms of discrete social behaviors, but rather had to be understood more broadly—in terms of children's ability to organize their social behavior in a way that elicits positive responses (and avoids negative responses) from others in a variety of different social contexts and in a manner consistent with prevailing social conventions and morals (Dodge & Murphy, 1984). In this conceptualization, a repertoire of socially appropriate behaviors is necessary but not sufficient, for beyond the capacity to produce these behaviors, social competence also requires the more complicated process of using them flexibly in response to ongoing social feedback and stimuli. This process involves multiple skills, including social-cognitive capabilities and affect regulation skills that allow children to select and enact social behaviors in a way that is sensitive and responsive to the situation (Bierman & Welsh, 2000; Sroufe, 1996).

[handwritten margin notes: flexible use in response to social stim + fdbk]

[handwritten margin notes: mult skills -affect regu'n -soc-cog capabilities so can uns'ly select + respond]

The implication of this definition for intervention is that improving a child's peer relations requires more than an emphasis on specific social behaviors; it must focus more broadly on fostering the child's ability to organize and regulate social behavior in the context of dynamic, and often complex, social contexts. In addition, developmental research has made it clear that rejection is not a child characteristic but a social process, in which peer behaviors and responses play a critical role.

[handwritten margin notes: - peers control niches of social op'ty]

PEER CONTRIBUTIONS TO REJECTION PROCESSES

[handwritten margin notes: ↓ ops → some c's shut out + so miss op to devel prosocial skills]

Peers control the niches of social opportunity available to rejected children. When they decide they don't like particular children, peers become less positively responsive and less available to those children (Hymel, Wagner, & Butler, 1990). By limiting the availability of opportunities for positive bonding, peers can shut some children out of the kinds of peer interactions that could support the development of prosocial skills, contributing to increasing delays and deficits in interactional skills (Ladd & Asher, 1985). In addition, negative reputational biases reduce child opportunities for change and contribute to "self-fulfilling prophecies." Rejected children who find themselves ostracized from the mainstream network of classmates may forge alliances with other children who are socially unskilled, like themselves. Low-quality interactions fail to promote social growth; affiliations with deviant peers place youth at risk for antisocial activities and substance use (Coie, 1990).

Even more problematically, some rejected children are victimized by their peers. Victimized children are bullied, harrassed, and intimidated by their peers (Graham & Juvonen, 1998). The harassment accompanying victimization is often direct, involving physical or verbal confrontation, but it can also be more subtle, involving malicious gossip or organized social exclusion (Crick & Grotpeter, 1995; Egan & Perry, 1998). Not all rejected children are victimized, and not all victimized children are rejected, although there is substantial overlap between these two groups of children. On average, 10% of school children suffer chronic victimization, and an even greater number report occasional maltreatment by peers (Kochenderfer & Ladd, 1996; Olweus, 1993).

Certain child characteristics increase vulnerability to victimization. For example, children who are victimized tend to have low self-esteem and high levels of social insecurity and anxiety (Hodges & Perry, 1996). Victimization is also associated with behavioral characteristics, including passive submissiveness, poor social skills, and emotional reactivity (Schwartz, Dodge, & Coie, 1993). Children who display anxious, insensitive, and self-focused behaviors often elicit hostile peer responding (Eisenberg & Fabes, 1992; Rubin & Stewart, 1996). Creating a negative spiral, experiences of victimization undermine the social confidence of socially insecure children, contributing to decreased self-worth and increasing loneliness over time (Boivin, Hymel, & Bukowski, 1995; Egan & Perry, 1998). The consequences are often significant, including school avoidance, social alienation, and depression (Olweus, 1993).

The problem of victimization is not limited to the interaction between a bully and a victim; it typically occurs in the context of peer bystanders. Low levels of peer empathy or concern, beliefs that victimized children are responsible for their own problems, and a general reluctance to get involved contribute to a peer context in which victimization can escalate (Perry, Williard, & Perry, 1990; Salmivalli, Lagerspetz, Bjorkqvist, Ostermann, & Kaukianen, 1996). Thus victimization is a distinct aspect of problematic peer relations that requires attention in assessment and intervention planning.

[handwritten margin notes at top: b/c socializing devel'l, most kids do have some peer probs — short-lived + inform've neg fdbk → useful skills — little benefit to chronic, tho' — risks in later life: truancy, emo (anx, dep), anti-soc]

Child vulnerabilities and negative peer reactions can contribute to a negative cycle, in which a child's social difficulties increase over time, creating a chronic situation with a negative impact on the child's developing sense of self and mental health.

[handwritten: partly: vuln → peer probs → later maladj'mt]

CHRONIC PEER REJECTION: A NEGATIVE DEVELOPMENTAL SPIRAL

[handwritten: also active force & direct link to anx, dep, anger, etc]

Because learning to get along with others is a developmental process, most children experience some peer difficulties at some point during their youth. Sometimes these relationship problems are short-lived and represent important learning experiences. Negative feedback from peers can improve social understanding; successful experiences of working through conflicts with peers can foster the development of skills for emotion regulation and conflict resolution. However, children rarely learn useful skills from chronic peer problems.

Children who experience serious disturbances in their peer relations are at heightened risk for a number of problems in later life, ranging from truancy to emotional difficulties (anxiety, depression) to antisocial behaviors (substance use, delinquent activities) (Parker et al., 1995). To some extent, these negative outcomes may reflect the influence of child vulnerabilities that contribute both to concurrent peer problems and to longer-term maladjustment (Parker & Asher, 1987). For example, children who have significant behavioral problems or learning difficulties—including attention-deficit/hyperactivity disorder, oppositional defiant disorder, conduct disorder, developmental delays, learning disabilities, or depression—often have trouble getting along with peers and are likely to experience peer rejection, as well as other negative outcomes (Dodge, 1989). However, developmental research suggests that peer rejection is not just a "side effect" of child behavioral or emotional problems, but is also an active socializing force; it contributes directly to anxiety, depression, and anger, sometimes fueling increased counteraggression and escape behaviors on the part of the rejected child, including truancy and substance use (Parker & Asher, 1987).

In fact, children who have aggressive or hyperactive behavior problems and are also rejected by their peers show greater problems in the areas of attention deficits, emotional dysregulation, and internalizing problems than do aggressive or hyperactive children who are better accepted by peers (Bierman, Smoot, & Aumiller, 1993; Miller-Johnson, Coie, Maumary-Gremaud, Bierman, & Conduct Problems Prevention Research Group, 2002). Peer rejection can exacerbate behavioral and emotional adjustment difficulties (Parker et al., 1995). For example,

[handwritten margin notes at bottom: agg've + hyper kids who also rejected → > attn'l deficits, emo dysreg'n + int'z'ng probs — worse beh'l + emo adjmt probs eg. stable aggr'n]

peer rejection increases the likelihood that aggressive behaviors will be stable and contribute to negative outcomes (Bierman & Wargo, 1995; Cillessen, van IJzendoorn, van Lieshout, & Hartup, 1992; Miller-Johnson et al., 2002).

Coie (1990) has described the transactions among social skill deficits, behavior problems, and peer rejection as a negative developmental spiral. The spiral begins when children with poor social skills fail to gain entry into the play interactions of their peers, due to anxious/withdrawn or aggressive behaviors. As the behaviors of these poorly skilled children drive others away or make it difficult for peers to engage successfully with them, they are left playing alone or interacting in limited ways with younger and less skillful social companions (Ladd, 1983), depriving them of opportunities to learn social skills (Coie, 1990). Exposure to hostile overtures and victimization by peers fosters feelings of loneliness, resentment, anxiety, depression, and alienation (Boivin, Hymel, & Bukowski, 1995; Perry, Kusel, & Perry, 1988). The consequence of this developmental interplay is that, without intervention, peer problems can become chronic and complex, complicated by negative behavioral coping strategies and by feelings of helplessness, social anxiety, or alienation (Coie, 1990; Rubin et al., 1998).

In addition to the impact they have on children's social behavior, children's peer experiences (and their interpretation of those experiences) affect their developing sense of self and their beliefs about the social world. The internal representations that children construct to help them understand their social world appear to play a key role in shaping their social behavior, as well as in determining the extent to which negative peer experiences contribute to psychological distress, including social anxiety and depression. Based upon their negative interpersonal experiences, rejected children often find it difficult to feel secure and connected to peers, reducing their capability to approach social environments with confidence and adaptive coping.

Understanding the developmental processes associated with peer rejection, and the child characteristics and peer group dynamics that may be involved, provides an important foundation for the design of effective interventions. Developmental research indicates that the social adjustment difficulties of peer-rejected children are often complex, including behavioral, affective, and cognitive features. In addition, a child's social success is not determined by these features alone, but also by the characteristics of the social partners (peers, teachers, and parents) with whom the child interacts. Correspondingly, social skill training assessments and interventions need to address behavioral, social-cognitive, and affective/motivational aspects of children's social adjustment, as well as including a focus on the social context.

last 40yrs extensive devel + refinemt of interv'n
>'ly multifaceted + broader
- school + clinics
> consider'n for role of social partners so "nested"

IMPACT OF DEVELOPMENTAL RESEARCH
ON INTERVENTIONS FOR REJECTED CHILDREN

eg. universal school promotion to ↓ victz'n + ↑ + interaxns

The past four decades have witnessed the extensive development and refinement of interventions to promote positive peer relations and social adjustment. Fueled by developmental research elucidating the behavioral, cognitive, and affective characteristics associated with problematic peer relations and the dynamics of rejection processes, social competence interventions have become increasingly multifaceted. Such interventions have become broader in focus, with adaptations designed to enhance their effectiveness in school contexts as well as with clinic-referred children. In addition, interventions focused on building the social skills of target rejected children are increasingly considering the role of social partners. Such focused interventions are thus being "nested" within universal school-based social competence promotion efforts designed to decrease victimization and increase positive interaction in the broader peer community (see reviews in Chapters 10 and 13). Despite these advances, additional research, program development, and evaluations are needed. Gaps exist in the current research base in some particularly important areas—including gender and cultural differences, which may affect the assessment of peer difficulties as well as social competence intervention goals and methods.

still need > research, devel + eval'n
gaps.esp. re. gender + culture
may Δ Ax, goals + methods

GENDER AND CULTURAL DIFFERENCES

most research here: N. amer'n boys (>aggr'n + rejexn)

Most of the research that provides the basis for this book was conducted with North American school children. The research base includes more boys than girls, due to the higher prevalence of both aggression and peer rejection among boys. In addition, although studies incorporated a wide representation of school children, including ethnic/racial minority children who were attending those schools, the research base is limited in terms of its utility in predicting the degree to which various assessment or intervention strategies might be differentially effective with children from different cultural groups.

c's usually play in same-sex gps

The research base does indicate significant gender differences in several aspects of peer relations and social behavior. For example, across ages, children tend to play in same-sex groups (Hartup, 1983). Boys more often choose to interact with peers in large groups that emphasize competition, whereas girls more often play in dyadic or triadic groups, although both kinds of play are observed among children of either gender (Eder & Hallinan, 1978). Girls tend to report higher levels of intimacy, validation, support, help, and companionship in their

boys >
- large gps
- emph compet'n
- > agg've + hyper
- > rejexn

girls > (§ aggr'n > rel'l hostil threat'n)
- 2-3 (eg. gossip, exclude)
- > intim, validn, support, help, companion'p
- > t'r ratings of competence + prosocial beh

gender diffs Δ devel'l +'ce of some soc behs
- p's + t's > l. say P's "shy"
- ⊖drawal in boys = risk for low social + cog competence, moodiness, low s-e

bio v. cult'l?
who knows
need > research
on FX on val of Ax + Tx, too

same-sex friendships than do boys, and teachers typically give girls higher ratings in areas of prosocial behavior and social competence (Bukowski, Hoza, & Boivin, 1994; Parker & Asher, 1993b). Boys, in contrast, are more likely than girls to exhibit elevated levels of aggressive and hyperactive behaviors, and to experience peer rejection (Coie et al., 1990). Girls who are aggressive are more likely to use relational means (e.g., threatening exclusion or spreading gossip) than physical means (e.g., hitting) to express their hostility (Crick & Grotpeter, 1995).

These gender differences can affect the developmental significance of certain social behaviors. For example, parents and teachers are more likely to describes girls as "shy." Correspondingly, social withdrawal serves as an indicator of risk primarily for boys, for whom it is associated with low social and cognitive competence, moodiness, and low self-esteem (Caspi et al., 1988; Morrison & Masten, 1991). The extent to which these gender-related patterns reflect biological differences versus the influence of different cultural and socialization pressures remains a topic for debate (Ruble & Stewart, 1996). The degree to which they influence the validity or effectiveness of different peer relation assessment or intervention strategies is a matter requiring further study.

culture (local or >)
FX accept'ty of social beh

if aggr'n is normative
+> dislike

some behs >
"absolute" value

prosocial always good
disruptive/hyper always bad

Certainly there is evidence suggesting that the acceptability of social behaviors can vary as a function of cultural context (Osterweil & Nagano-Nakamura, 1992). Even the "local" culture of a particular peer group can influence peer expectations and evaluations. For example, several studies have demonstrated that in peer groups containing many aggressive children, where aggressive behavior is normative in the group context, aggressive behavior does not lead to peer disliking, as it does in typical nonaggressive peer settings (Boivin, Dodge, & Coie, 1995; Stormshak et al., 1999; Wright, Giammarino, & Parad, 1986). Some social behaviors appear to have more "absolute" value. For example, prosocial behavior contributes to peer liking across a variety of different peer groups (Stormshak et al., 1999; Wright et al., 1986). Likewise, disruptive/hyperactive behaviors elicit peer dislike, even in peer groups in which such behaviors are common (Stormshak et al., 1999).

ethnicity
FX peer ratings

-minority < + + > nomin'ns vs. majority kids

Normative biases regarding ethnicity can also affect peer ratings. For example, children who represent a minority ethnic/racial group within a particular peer group context typically receive fewer positive nominations and more negative nominations than children of majority status (Coie et al., 1982; Kistner, Metzler, Gatlin, & Risi, 1993). To the extent that racial bias inflates the rejection scores for children who have minority status within a particular peer group, peer nominations may provide a less valid indicator of child social competence, and

to that extent, peer nomin'ns < valid for minority kids so < pred've

hence may have less predictive validity (Kupersmidt & Coie, 1990). For further discussion of cultural variations in social values and their impact on the assessment of social dysfunction among children, the reader is referred to Rubin and colleagues (1998), Chen, Rubin, and Sun (1992), and Osterweil and Nagano-Nakamura (1992). More research is needed for a better understanding of how gender and cultural differences may affect the assessment and treatment of peer relation difficulties, and it is important to recognize the limitations of the current research literature in this regard.

theme: social competence
fr. complex devel'l progr'n
so Tx must be broader than
preventing rejexn +
promoting friendships

SUMMARY

This chapter has provided a review of research demonstrating the importance of positive peer relations in fostering adaptive social–emotional development. The overarching theme that emerges from this research is that social competence is the result of a complex developmental progression; hence interventions must move beyond a focus on children's behavior to encompass a broader spectrum of the factors and systems that influence children's rejection and friendships. Rejected children, who are actively disliked by peers, often have social skill deficits and behavior problems that make it difficult for them to make friends and gain acceptance from classroom peers. They can become entrapped in a negative developmental spiral in which these behaviors lead to ostracism and/or victimization by peers, which deprives them of opportunities to learn positive social skills and contributes to feelings of loneliness, resentment, anxiety, depression, and alienation.

rejected
disliked
incompetent
beh'l/y disorders
kids stuck
in neg
devel'l spiral
→ ostracism,
vic'z'n
+ even fewer
ops to lrn
+ skills
→ lonely,
resentful,
anx, dep,
alien'n

As described in later chapters, there are things that counselors, teachers, and parents can do to support the development of positive peer relations among children. In addition, they need to be ready to take action to remediate and repair peer relation problems that involve chronic rejection, hostile behavior, and victimization. The developmental research reviewed in this chapter has several implications for the design of assessment and intervention, which are discussed further in later chapters. First, this research suggests that interventions need to focus on building aspects of social competence, as well as on reducing problem behaviors; the role of behavioral, cognitive, and affective components in fostering the regulatory and organizational capacities associated with social competence must be recognized. Second, interventions must account for the role of the peer group, recognizing and treating peer rejection as a dynamic interpersonal process rather than a child characteristic. Third, interventions should address the niches of social opportunity available to children, and should focus on building friend-

coun'lrs, t'rs
+ p's:
remediate +
repair
probs of
chronic
rejexn,
hostility +
vic'z'n

Tx: ↑ social competence + ↓ probs behs
ack. beh, cog + affective → regu'n + org'z'l skills
ack role of peer gp as dynamic interpers'l process
not just inherent to rejected c.
address niches of ops for c's   — devel'ly + cult'ly
build f'ps + ↑ acceptance)   sens've

ship skills as well as improving peer acceptance. Finally, interventions should be developmentally and culturally sensitive.

In the next chapter, the characteristics of rejected children are described in more detail, and case examples are provided to illustrate the patterns of behavior that get children into trouble with their peers.

❧ Chapter 2

Characteristics of Rejected Children

*C*hildren are often rejected because their behaviors irritate and annoy others (Coie, Dodge, & Kupersmidt, 1990; Parker, Rubin, Price, & DeRosier, 1995). Children do not like behavior that is bossy, self-centered, or disruptive. It is simply not fun to play with people who won't share, who don't follow the rules, or who lose their temper when things don't go their way. There is no single "prototypic" profile of a rejected child. However, there are certain types of behaviors that act like social toxins, increasing the likelihood of rejection. This chapter describes four patterns of behavior problems linked with peer rejection in developmental research: (1) low rates of prosocial behavior, (2) high rates of aggressive/disruptive behavior, (3) high rates of inattentive/immature behavior, and (4) high rates of socially anxious/avoidant behavior. Most rejected children show at least one of these types of behaviors; children with the most severe and stable friendship problems often show two or more (Bierman, Smoot, & Aumiller, 1993; Ledingham, 1981). To provide illustrations of how these various problems present themselves in children, I include some case examples, based upon observational and interview studies my colleagues and I have conducted in past years (Bierman et al., 1993; Bierman & Wargo, 1995).

PROSOCIAL AND AGGRESSIVE BEHAVIORS

Across a large number of longitudinal studies (including cross-national comparisons), prosocial behaviors have emerged as a stable predictor of peer acceptance, whereas aggressive/disruptive behaviors elicit peer

17

rejection. A brief summary of this research is provided in the next section; for more extensive discussions of the behavioral correlates of peer
acceptance and rejection, the reader is referred to Rubin, Bukowski,
and Parker (1998), Newcomb, Bukowski, and Pattee (1993), and Coie
and colleagues (1990).

Low Rates of Prosocial and Cooperative Behavior

Children who are prosocial and cooperative are typically well liked by
peers, and elicit more support, more invitations, and more positive responding from peers than children who show low rates of prosocial
behavior (Bierman, 1987). Several factors contribute to children's
prosociality, including their display of positive behaviors, communication skills, emotion regulation skills, and social awareness and sensitivity.

Positive Behaviors and Communication Skills

Children who cooperate, share materials, invite others to play, and
take turns are attractive playmates. Classmates view these children as
friendly, nice, kind, and considerate (Coie et al., 1990). Children who
are good communicators also find it relatively easy to establish and
maintain friendships (Gottman, 1983). There is a real art to effective interpersonal communication, even at the preschool and early grade
school level. For example, skillful child communicators know how to
start off conversations with appropriate self-disclosures, sharing information about themselves and their feelings and opinions. They recognize the turn-taking sequences involved in conversation, and they ask
questions to elicit information from others. They attempt to communicate clearly, avoiding monologues. They listen to the other person and
stay on the same topic, establishing common ground. In contrast, children who communicate with peers infrequently or unskillfully have
more difficulty establishing and maintaining friendships (Gottman,
1983; Ladd, 1981).

Emotion Regulation

A child's ability to regulate emotions (particularly negative emotions)
also affects his/her social desirability as a playmate. Children who are
easygoing and affable, who laugh and smile a lot, and who have a good
sense of humor find it easier to gain peer acceptance than do children
who are moody, sulky, or glum (Coie et al., 1990). Peer play often in-

[handwritten margin notes top: - mild frus'ns in peer play common + conflict / " fixated on own ideas/desires / can't accommo others' wishes / " stay calm / nego reasonably / generate many alt sol'ns / ack + comply c others' ideas]

volves mild frustrations (e.g., losing a game) and conflicts (e.g., disagreements about which game to play or about whether a particular ball was "in" or "out"). Well-liked children remain calm under these conditions of duress, and they are able to negotiate reasonably and generate a number of alternative solutions to solve the problem (Eisenberg & Fabes, 1992). Agreeable children, who are willing to acknowledge the ideas and comply with the suggestions of others, are typically more well liked than children who become fixated on their own ideas or desires and cannot accommodate the wishes of others (Elliott & Gresham, 1993).

[handwritten: iii. social awareness + sens'ty / " social savvy - aware of + comply c / implicit expec'ns of play / - good "play etiquette" / enter grps diplomatically]

Social Awareness and Sensitivity

Well-liked children also show social savvy; they are aware of and able to comply with the implicit expectations that characterize play interactions. That is, they are sensitive to the nuances of "play etiquette." They enter a group using diplomatic strategies. For example, first they "hover" at the play site, taking stock of the state of the game and perhaps commenting upon the ongoing activity. They look for a natural break in the game sequence (such as the end of a turn or the end of a game round), and then ask permission to join in. Less skillful children may barge into the game more intrusively, or remain at the outskirts of the game, unable to find a strategy for entry (Putallaz, 1983). Well-liked children are sensitive to the feelings of others and able to assess social situations with accuracy (Dodge, Pettit, McClaskey, & Brown, 1986).

[handwritten margin notes: "hovers" - take stock - comment + maybe / find natural break in play seq (e.g. b/t turns or end round) / ask perm'n. / " barge in / stay on / outskirts / accurately fix sit'ns / assess others' flgs]

In summary, children with prosocial skills—including the ability to cooperate and communicate effectively, regulate emotion, and interact in an interpersonally sensitive and responsive way—are good companions and fun play partners, as they uphold standards of equity and show good sportsmanship. In contrast, less skillful children often show self-centered play and fail to recognize the impact of their behaviors on others.

[handwritten margin notes: " equity + good sportsman'p / " self- centred / - obliv of impact of their beh on others]

High Rates of Aggressive and Disruptive Behaviors

Aggressive behaviors can be quite destructive to peer relations, and frequently contribute to peer disliking. It is easy to understand why children dislike aggressive and disruptive peers, as no one wants to be hurt or annoyed. Interestingly, however, not all aggressive and disruptive behaviors have the same impact on peers—some are more damaging to peer relations than others (Bierman, 1986b).

Effective versus Ineffective Aggression

Broadly defined, "aggressive" behaviors include intentional acts designed to cause harm or injury to another (Coie & Dodge, 1998). Aggressive behaviors may take different forms, such as physical aggression, intended to cause bodily harm (e.g., hitting, kicking); verbal aggression, designed to derogate or coercively control another person (e.g., yelling, insulting, threatening); or indirect or social aggression, designed to cause another embarrassment, inconvenience, or loss of support (e.g., cheating in a game, tattling on someone so that he or she will get into trouble with the teacher, spreading negative gossip about someone) (Crick et al., 1999; Underwood, 2003). In general, aggressive behavior is destructive to relationships, and most aggressive behaviors elicit censure from peers. However, some aggressive behaviors are generally considered "justified" and are tolerated or even encouraged by peers, such as fighting back when provoked or defending oneself and one's honor (Perry, Perry, & Kennedy, 1992).

Some children can control their aggressive behavior and use force or verbal intimidation effectively to lead others, gain dominance, and get their own way. These "effectual aggressors" (Perry et al., 1992) often have the social skills needed to establish friendships, and rarely experience rejection or victimization. They often create problems for others in their classroom and therefore require attention in interventions, but they do not necessarily have problems making friends or gaining peer acceptance themselves.

In contrast to strategic and effective aggression, aggressive behavior can also be reactive and poorly controlled—as when a child explodes in reaction to an assault or threat made by someone else, or when a child has an outburst of emotion (a tantrum) following some frustrating or negative event (Coie & Dodge, 1998; Miller-Johnson, Coie, Maumary-Gremaud, Bierman, & the Conduct Problems Prevention Research Group, 2002). Children labeled "ineffectual aggressors" by Perry and colleagues (1992) show a pattern of disruptive, verbal, indirect, and emotionally reactive behavior, in addition to physical aggression, and are at high risk for peer rejection. These children often become targets of victimization, and often show distress and social anxiety. Effectual and ineffectual aggressors can be differentiated by the quality of their aggressive behaviors, by the additional skills or problems they have, and by peer responses to them (Coie & Dodge, 1998). Effectual aggressors typically use aggression in a proactive way to manage, direct, and control the behaviors of others. In contrast, ineffectual aggressors often show a broad pattern of multiple aggressive behaviors, which are displayed in emotionally reactive and poorly con-

- agg'n rarely sole cause of rejexn
→ controlling agg've display won't fix other skill deficits of rejected agg've kids
(→ by implic'n, not all agg've kids rejected)

trolled ways. The distinction between effectual and ineffectual aggressors has important implications for intervention design: It suggests that aggressive behavior is rarely the sole cause of peer rejection, and, correspondingly, that simply controlling the display of aggression will not remediate the additional skill deficits of rejected aggressive children (Bierman, Miller, & Stabb, 1987).

rej'd ineffectually agg've + poor emoregu'n + rel'ps → disruptive + opp'l beh - irrit, unhappy, overly sens've, easily annoyed, angry + resentful, blame others

Disruptive and Oppositional Behaviors

In addition to aggressive acts, rejected children often display disruptive and oppositional behaviors that reflect difficulties in regulating emotions effectively and maintaining positive interpersonal relationships (Coie & Dodge, 1998; Rubin et al., 1998). For example, consider the emotional and interpersonal difficulties of children who exhibit oppositional defiant disorder (American Psychiatric Association, 1994), characterized by high rates of argumentativeness, defiance, and refusal to comply with requests or rules. Emotionally, these children are often irritable and unhappy; overly sensitive and easily annoyed by others; and angry and resentful, quick to blame others for their own mistakes. Interpersonally, children with this behavior pattern appear insecure and suspicious. Often they show an intense power orientation in their play with others; they desire control (and hence are competitive and argumentative); and they are highly reactive in the face of frustration or perceived threat, escalating quickly to a "fight" response if they feel thwarted in any way (Hinshaw & Anderson, 1996). This pattern of oppositional and defiant behaviors is typically destructive to peer relations, as well as to adult–child relations. With their hostile behavior, these children elicit negative treatment from both peers and adults, thus confirming their suspicions and negative attitudes toward others, and (in their minds) justifying their hostile behaviors (Coie & Dodge, 1998).

seem insecure + suspic's
∈ intense power orien'n in play
- reactive to frus'n
- quick escal'n to fight + if feel thwarted
ruins rel'ps ∈ peers + adults
hostil elicits neg TX confirming suspic'ns, justifying hostility

Gender and Developmental Influences

girls much ↓ l. agg've phys or verbal but hostile thru gossip or exclusion (rel'l aggr'n) → rejexn

It is important to note that both gender and developmental level can affect the acceptability of aggressive behaviors. For example, girls are considerably less likely than boys to exhibit physical or verbal aggression. However, girls who are aggressive are more likely than aggressive boys to express interpersonal hostility by threatening exclusion or starting gossip, and girls who show high levels of this type of "relational aggression" may experience peer rejection (Crick & Grotpeter, 1995; Underwood, 2003). Development also affects the frequency and type of aggressive behavior that is normative. For example, instrumental physical aggres-

preschoolers commonly show instrum'l phys agg + doesn't predict rejexn this young
- atypical by middle c'hd tho'

sion is common in preschoolers, and is not predictive of peer rejection at this age (Hartup, 1983). By middle childhood, however, most children become more adept at controlling their aggressive impulses, and those who continue to exhibit high rates of physical and verbal aggression become "atypical" and face a high risk for peer rejection.

AGGRESSIVE–ACCEPTED VERSUS AGGRESSIVE–REJECTED PROBLEM PROFILES

To illustrate how aggressive behavior and prosocial skills manifest themselves in ways that do or do not lead to peer rejection, I provide two case examples from studies we have conducted in past years (Bierman et al., 1993; Bierman & Wargo, 1995). The first one is an example of an aggressive child who was well accepted by his peers. The behavior problems of this child are then contrasted with a case study of an aggressive child who was rejected by peers. Quotations are drawn from actual interviews, although the names and some of the details have been changed to protect the confidentiality of the children involved. Both examples involved boys, as they were the focus of the study from which interview excerpts were drawn.

The Aggressive–Accepted Child

The following excerpts are from interviews with the fourth-grade classmates of JP. On the basis of both teacher and peer reports, JP scored in the top 15% of the class on a scale of aggressive behaviors, being nominated frequently as one who "starts fights," "is mean to others," and "gets into trouble." He was also viewed by teachers and peers as highly sociable and well liked. As the following quotes show, JP was a powerful figure in the classroom, with strong athletic skills and a good sense of humor. At the same time, JP liked to win and expected to have a position of leadership in the group; he defended this position with aggressive behavior if necessary. He also frequently bullied less well-liked children in the classroom.

On JP's strengths, classmates commented:

"He's one of the best people in kickball and football. He pitches, kicks, he runs, receives, catches, hikes. He practices a lot."
"He has bike races, and he plays in a lot of sports."
"He usually makes home runs. He's real strong."
"He's good in math. He's smart."

At the same time, JP's classmates recognized his preference for rough play, his desire for dominance, and his tendency to tease and bully certain classmates:

"He's rowdy. He can be very rough."
"He swears sometimes."
"He bosses everyone around, and he yells at them."
"He always wants to get his own way."
"If you do something he doesn't like and he gets mad, he'll have his friends come over, and they can be pretty nasty."
"Certain people don't like him 'cause he yells at them and makes fun of them."

In fourth grade, JP's positive social skills, along with his athletic and academic skills, allowed him to establish friendships despite his domineering and competitive attitude. As his classmates summed it up,

"He's famous and most everybody knows him."
"He yells and bosses, but he's a nice person besides that."
"Inside of him, he can be really nice. I like him, no matter what."

Two years after these interviews were conducted, JP moved into middle school. By sixth grade, he had gained some control over his aggressive outbursts; he scored lower on teacher- and peer-rated aggression scales than he had in fourth grade, although he was still ranked in the high average range (top 35th percentile relative to his classmates). JP continued to perform well in sports, and he showed above-average academic attainment. He continued to be very sociable and well liked by his classmates.

JP is a good example of a boy with a focal social problem (aggressive behavior) in the context of social and academic competence. Children such as JP are more likely than less competent children to learn from their own social experiences, showing improvements in their social behaviors over time even without planned interventions. At the same time, children like JP can inflict harm on others in the classroom, particularly if they choose to exclude, tease, or bully specific children. They can be "ringleaders" in campaigns of rejection aimed at less skillful children. Because of their competence, children like JP are often responsive to interventions focused on conflict management and fair-play skills (as described in later chapters of this book), particularly if the interventions are organized in a way that takes advantage of their natural desires to be leaders. In contrast to

agg've
competent kids > l lrn fr own exp'ce w'out
planned interv'ns
-> resp've to conflict mgmt + fair-play esp. if
cap'ze on natural desire to lead

JP, who was an "effectual aggressor," other aggressive children are "ineffectual" and are soundly rejected by their peers, as in the following example.

The Aggressive–Rejected Child

GD was a first-grade boy at the time of our initial interviews. Teachers and peers both viewed him as highly aggressive, noting that he frequently "started fights," was "mean to others," "got into trouble," and "gave others dirty looks." Overall, his aggression ratings put him in the top 10% of the class in terms of problem behaviors. In addition, only one child in the class named him as a friend, whereas 60% of his classmates singled him out as one of their three least liked peers.

Classmates described GD similarly to JP as aggressive and mean:

> "He hits people and calls them names. He pushes people down. He says bad words."
> "He shoves people down on cement. He tripped me and made me smash my knee."
> "He punches and jumps on people with his boots. You can hear their bones crack."

However, when describing GD's aggressive behavior, classmates also often pointed out that it appeared unjustified and improper:

> "He fights when nobody did something to him."
> "He kicks somebody on purpose, and he just goes boom right on somebody's leg."
> "He tells on people to get them in trouble when they didn't even do it."

Unlike JP, who had prosocial skills to balance his aggressive behaviors, GD behaved in a self-focused and self-protective manner. Peers viewed him as deficient in prosocial skills:

> "He doesn't share. He doesn't let people on the swings."
> "He doesn't let anyone touch his stuff. He never helps anybody or anything."
> "He never says he's sorry."

Relative to JP, GD also showed a broader range of disruptive behaviors and rule-violating behaviors:

[handwritten marginalia: — broader range of disrup'n & rule vio — imitating + insens've on top of agg've → stable probs — become morose + edrawn]

"He cuts in line. He gets into trouble. He does bad stuff in gym class."

"He looks at other people's papers, and he copies off people."

"He steps on people's toes. He takes their things. He lies."

In addition to his aggressive and disruptive behaviors, GD exhibited a number of other behaviors that annoyed and angered his classmates. Although these behaviors were not aggressive per se, they were irritating and insensitive, and hence noxious to his peers.

"When he stands behind you in line, he grabs your back pocket and pulls on it."

"He reads our book when we are reading, and he makes us get mixed up."

"He looks in other people's desks and scribbles on their desks with crayons."

"He puts an eraser in his mouth until it's soggy, and then he throws it at someone."

"He takes people's coats down off hooks and throws them right on the floor."

"He likes to trick people, and no kids like that."

Overall, the combination of high rates of aggressive/disruptive behaviors coupled with low rates of prosocial behaviors proved to be a very damaging profile for GD socially. In their general comments about him, it was clear that peers rejected him soundly and fully condemned him:

"We always have to tell on him, because he is very, very, very bad. He is the baddest boy in this school."

"He only has one more friend left. Soon he's gonna have no friends."

"He wants to be rotten. He's nasty and he hates people. We don't want him here."

GD's problems also turned out to be more stable than JP's. When we revisited GD 2 years later, he was in third grade, and his social adjustment difficulties had worsened. GD continued to be very aggressive; he had moved into the top 2% of his class in both teacher and peer ratings of aggression. In addition, teachers described serious attentional and behavioral control problems in the classroom, as well as significant academic difficulties. Perhaps in part as a consequence of 3 years of chronic rejection by peers, GD had also become withdrawn and morose, and as a third grader was viewed by his teacher and his peers as isolated and unhappy.

some kids not hostile but inattitve, disorg'd + immature)

INATTENTIVE/IMMATURE AND SOCIALLY ANXIOUS/AVOIDANT BEHAVIORS

Behaviors do not have to be interpersonally hostile to disturb peer relations. In addition to aggressive and disruptive behaviors, behaviors that are inattentive, disorganized, and immature elicit rebuke from adults and peers alike.

"strange"
"babyish"
- whiny, dep't,
goofy

Inattentive and Immature Behaviors

Inattentive behaviors include distractibility; difficulty staying on task and concentrating on schoolwork (and peer games); difficulties following directions (and game rules); and poor listening skills. Inattention is often accompanied by socially insensitive and immature behaviors, such as dependence on adults, whining and pouting, low frustration tolerance, and attention-getting "goofy" behaviors. Peers complain that these children are "strange" and "act like a baby" (Pope & Bierman, 1999).

not dirly harmful like aggrn but
socially aversive - it acts become difficult + unpleasant
- unpred'ble, nonreciprocal + rarely rewarding)

Poor Social Regulation

Although they are not directly harmful to others in the way that aggressive behaviors are, inattentive/immature behaviors are socially aversive because they make joint activities difficult and unpleasant. The lack of sensitivity, intrusiveness, disruptiveness, and self-centered nature of these behaviors interfere with organized peer play. The failure to follow social protocol results in social interactions that are unpredictable, nonreciprocal, and rarely rewarding for the social partners (Barkley, 1996; Pope & Bierman, 1999). Whereas positive peer interactions are characterized by social regulation, in which social partners synchronize and coordinate their play behaviors, children who disregard (or are unaware of) the cues, routines, and expectations of others, and who organize their behavior around their own wants and needs, are typically avoided and disliked by their peers.

dysynchrony b/t social partners

Inattention and Hyperactivity

Inattentive and immature behaviors are often (although not exclusively) associated with attention-deficit/hyperactivity disorder (ADHD;

- impulsive, inatt've + sometimes also hyper

American Psychiatric Association, 1994). Key behavioral characteristics of this disorder include high rates of motor activity (fidgeting, squirming, difficulty remaining seated); disorganization (often losing things needed for tasks or activities, poor listening skills); impulse control problems (difficulty awaiting turn in games, talking excessively and talking out of turn); and inattention (distractibility, difficulty carrying out assignments, frequently shifting from one uncompleted activity to another). Some children show high rates of inattention and disorganization without the high rates of motor activity.

Low Levels of Self-Control

- deficits in "rule-governed" beh → inatt'n + immaturity

- preschoolers rely on adults for limits, direct'n, beh'l control then internalize

Functionally, inattentive/immature behaviors often indicate deficits in "rule-governed" behavior (Barkley, 1996). During the toddler and early preschool years, most children behave impulsively and rely on adults to set limits, provide direction, and exert control over their behavior. With development, however, children begin to internalize rules, and thus become able to control and direct their own behavior according to socially prescribed conventions. Children with ADHD show delays in this area, remaining highly dependent upon external cues and constraints for behavioral control. Not only do these deficits cause them trouble in areas of academic functioning; they make it difficult for the children to inhibit reactive behavior, delay gratification, and respect the "implicit" social rules and conventions that most grade school children take for granted. Hence these children often have trouble understanding or applying principles of fairness and reciprocity in complex peer interactions. Their impulsive, reactive, and self-serving behaviors (e.g., poor sportsmanship, cheating) lead to social censure, as do their unconventional and emotional displays. Peers perceive them as strange and inappropriate, and react with frustration, avoidance, and sometimes victimization (Saunders & Chambers, 1996).

ADHD kids remain dep't on external cues + control

- can't inhib reactivity, delay gratif'n + respect rules so don't grasp fairns or reciprocity

punished for transgress'ns + emo'l oddns

Socially Anxious and Avoidant Behaviors

Parents and teachers sometimes worry about shy children, who frequently play alone and seem "neglected" by peers. The extent to which shy behavior should be a source of worry to parents and teachers depends very much on the nature of the shyness (Rubin & Stewart, 1996). Low levels of social interaction can occur for a number of reasons, and depending upon the reason, they may or may not indicate significant risk for social maladjustment. Children who are quiet and passive in their social style, and who enjoy productive solitary play (e.g., reading, building with blocks, or other types of constructive/manipulative play),

does shyns matter?
- depends on kind
- still liked if quiet/passive social style + not vic'z'd like prod've solitary play

are not likely to be disliked by peers or to suffer victimization (Rubin &
Stewart, 1996).

Social Anxiety and Discomfort

In contrast, children who are fearful and anxious around others, who
appear uncomfortable and awkward in their social initiations; and who
spend a considerable amount of time unoccupied, or "hovering"
around the play of others because they are unable to successfully enter
the play, do warrant adult concern (Asendorpf, 1993). Sometimes these
children are ignored or teased by classmates, because of their social in-
eptitude and aspects of their social presence that appear "different"
and set them apart from other children (Rubin & Stewart, 1996). Evidence that peers are rejecting or victimizing a withdrawn child is an important "red flag" indicating that the child's withdrawal signals a risk
for maladaptive social–emotional development. The child's degree of
discomfort and distress about his/her lack of friendships and difficulty
getting along with others is another signal that the withdrawal is not a
chosen social style, but may represent a significant social handicap for
the child (Asher, Parker, & Walker, 1996).

Social Ostracism

For socially anxious and awkward withdrawn children, their inability to
interact with others creates a situation of deprivation, wherein they are
isolated or ostracized from the positive peer interactions that would allow them to develop social confidence and social skills. Hence they are
often caught in a negative socialization cycle, which contributes over
time to feelings of loneliness, depression, and worthlessness (Boivin,
Poulin, & Vitaro, 1994; Rubin & Stewart, 1996). Withdrawal is generally more normative for girls, and hence often causes girls less difficulty
in social relationships than it does boys, for whom it is more atypical
(Caspi, Elder, & Bem, 1988).

Atypical Characteristics

Children are also sometimes rejected because they have atypical or unusual characteristics (e.g., physical handicap, minority status, obesity,
or unattractiveness) (Parker et al., 1995; see also Chapter 3). The peer
group dynamics in such cases require particular attention, since negative peer reputations and negative peer treatment (exclusion, victimization) can precipitate child social behavior problems, as well as result
from such problems (Hymel, Wagner, & Butler, 1990). In some cases,

children have social behavior that is functional in some settings, but is not well adapted to peer interactions. For example, some children interact well with adults but appear aloof, bossy, or snobby to children, who prefer more egalitarian and entertaining interactions.

INATTENTIVE SOCIAL PROFILES, WITH CONCURRENT AGGRESSION OR ANXIETY

The next two case examples were chosen to illustrate the impact that inattentive behaviors have on peer perceptions and attitudes. Both of these children were rejected by their peers, and both struggled with inattentive, socially awkward, and inept behaviors. The first (ED) also displayed concurrent aggression; the second (SB) was not aggressive, but displayed anxiety.

The Rejected Inattentive Child with Aggression

ED was in third grade at the time of our initial interviews. ED scored high on teacher and peer measures of aggressive/disruptive behavior, but the quality of his problem behavior was considerably more inattentive and disruptive than GD, the aggressive–rejected boy described earlier in this chapter. Notably, peer descriptions of ED focused on the way in which his impetuous and disorganized behavior led to conflicts:

> "He pushes on the way to math. He wants to be the first to get there. He doesn't care who's in his way."
> "He pushes people in the coat closet when we're getting ready to go, because he doesn't want anyone getting in his way."
> "He runs around after and during lunch. He mouths back to the lunch ladies."
> "Mostly he gets his name on the board and gets sent back to his seat for talking. He gets everyone around him into trouble."
> "He cheats. If you get him out in kickball, he says he's not out or it didn't count."

In addition, peers noticed that ED had considerable difficulties controlling his emotions in social situations, and that he frequently responded to frustrations with aggressive outbursts:

> "If he gets out in kickball, he gets real mad. He'll start yelling and hitting everyone." "He's got a mad temper. If somebody calls

him a name, he starts getting mad. His temper goes higher and
higher, and he'll start yelling and kicking people."

"If he doesn't win a game, he starts pushing people around."

"He's always arguing with everyone, saying, 'This is better than
that,' or 'I'm better than you are,' or 'I know more than you.' "

Peers were also disturbed by ED's moody and unpredictable behaviors:

"Sometimes he likes you, and the next day he doesn't. You never
know."

"One day he lets you in his game, and the next day he won't let
you."

"He acts hot, but he cries easily. When people tease him, he cries."

ED was also viewed by peers as strange, immature, socially insensitive,
and annoying:

"He is a weird kind of person. He makes funny faces. He walks
funny."

"He'll hide in the bushes, and when you come by, he'll jump you
and throw you down."

"He says jokes that make no sense. He thinks they're funny, but
they're dumb."

"He calls kids in the class and disguises his voice."

"He brags and shows off all the time. He says, 'I bet I got more
than you do.' "

"He acts like an idiot. He totally baffles us."

Like the difficulties of many aggressive–rejected children, ED's social problems did not improve over time. In fifth grade, ED was still rejected by his peers, who continued to complain about his lack of social
skill, his unfriendly and moody nature, his inattentive and intrusive
behavior, and his emotional outbursts.

Children who show aggressive/disruptive behaviors and are rejected by their peers, like GD and ED, are at high risk for stable and
long-term adjustment problems. However, children can face chronic rejection even when they are not aggressive, particularly if they possess
other characteristics that are off-putting to peers, as in the next example.

The Rejected Inattentive Child with Anxiety

SB was a third-grade boy at the time of our initial interviews. Unlike JP,
GD, or ED, SB was not aggressive and did not fight, yell, or lash out at

others. His social problems were of a different type. SB was viewed by teachers and peers as highly inept and withdrawn, scoring in the top 5% of the class on items such as "never seems to be having a good time," "doesn't like to play," "seems sad, unhappy," and "has few friends." Teacher ratings also reflected high levels of inattentive and hyperactive behaviors. For example, teachers described him as "restless, overactive," "excitable, impulsive," "inattentive, easily distracted," and "easily frustrated."

As shown in the following excerpts, classmates were aware that SB had difficulties following classroom routines and completing his academic work. They were also aware of the teacher's displeasure with and apparent dislike of SB:

> "The teacher gets angry at him, because he doesn't get his work done."
> "The teacher is always yelling at him."
> "When we're supposed to be doing something, he doesn't listen and gets into trouble."
> "He doesn't hand in his work on time, and he doesn't listen to directions."
> "He doesn't raise his hand when he talks. He talks when the teacher's talking."

SB's difficulties in organizing himself around rules, routines, and social conventions also affected his peer play, as noted by his classmates:

> "He's bad at kickball. Kids always yell at him because he kicks it all over the place."
> "He doesn't listen to other people about the rules."
> "He doesn't let us look at his sticker book when we let him look at ours."
> "He's always copying off us."

In addition, SB showed a number of impulsive and immature behaviors that were insensitive, intrusive, and annoying to his classmates:

> "He makes noises. He burps loud."
> "He says stupid things, and he talks real loud."
> "He brags and shows off."
> "Sometimes he acts like he's a really little kid and talks in this funny voice."
> "He likes to go around and sneak up behind people and scare 'em."
> "He makes a big fuss about something nobody did."

SB's social problems were serious, but different in important ways from the aggressive behavior problems shown by the other students profiled thus far. SB showed a pattern of social problems common among children who are inattentive (including those who have ADHD) and among many children who have learning disabilities. Although SB engaged in social behaviors that annoyed others, his social difficulties would not have been solved simply by reducing these behavior problems. At a more fundamental level, SB's social problems stemmed from his lack of social understanding and social savvy, and his inability to organize his social behavior in ways that were sensitive to the (often implicit) social expectations of others.

In describing SB, one child said, "He makes people mad, and so people don't really like him, and because of that he doesn't like school." This third grader's sage observation captures the negative transactional process often experienced by children like SB. Awkward and "out of touch" socially, SB made frequent social errors, annoying and disturbing other children. When classmates withdrew from or rebuked SB, he was confused and upset. Often his solution was to engage in more "in your face" behavior to get his classmates' attention. His intensified efforts to get attention elicited increased efforts by peers to shut him down or avoid him. Bewildered, SB was left feeling increasingly frustrated, angry, anxious, and unhappy in the school environment.

Two years after our initial interviews, SB's social profile remained relatively unchanged. As a fifth grader, SB continued to show significant academic and attentional problems; teachers complained about his apathy and apparent lack of motivation for schoolwork, as well as his failure to complete tasks. With peers, SB was more moody and resentful than he had been in third grade, showing more sarcasm toward others and harboring an attitude of derogation toward his classmates and their activities. Peers continued to reject SB, describing him as socially withdrawn, "weird," and "a show-off." SB expressed an intense dislike of his school, his peers, and his teacher, and reported high levels of loneliness, depressed mood, and social anxiety.

SUMMARY

Children like GD, ED, and SB can be difficult to help, because teachers and other adults often find them as annoying as their peers. Whereas a shy, quiet child elicits nurturance, guidance, and support from adults, a similarly socially anxious and socially bereft, but intrusive and obnoxious-acting, child like SB rarely does. Aggressive children like GD and

ED elicit even less sympathy, and there is often a gut-level feeling that these children are "getting what they deserve" when peers counter-aggress and reject them. It is important that we, as adults, look beyond the obnoxious and sometimes cruel behaviors of these rejected children and examine the skill deficits and anxieties that coexist and fuel the problem behaviors. Recognizing the social incompetence that accompanies peer rejection is a critical step toward designing effective intervention plans.

In a comparison of JP with GD and ED, for example, several factors are notable. Whereas all three of these boys displayed aggression, GD and ED displayed a broader range of disruptive, inattentive, and re-active aggressive behaviors. The unpredictability and volatility of their behavior made it considerably more aversive to peers than was JP's domineering aggression. Developmentally, the pattern of aggressive/disruptive behaviors displayed by rejected boys like GD and ED (e.g., disruptiveness, negative affect, and angry reactivity) reflects deficiencies in the capability to regulate negative affect in the context of interpersonal interactions.

The socially anxious and inattentive/immature behaviors displayed by many rejected children (whether accompanied by aggression or not) are also aversive to peers. Typically it is not shy behaviors that alienate peers, but high rates of socially awkward or strange behavior that are intrusive and that reflect an insensitivity to peer expectations, a lack of understanding of social conventions, deficiencies in the ability to read social cues, and (often) high levels of social anxiety.

A consideration of the skill deficits that accompany problem behavior has implications for intervention design. To the extent that skill deficits are fueling problem behaviors, the intervention cannot focus simply on reducing problem behaviors, but must also address the skill deficits. Previous research has demonstrated that intervention programs focused solely on reducing aggressive/disruptive behaviors can lead to behavioral improvements, but do   a rule, enhance the children's social status and peer relatio   have long-lasting effects. Instead, effective interventi   ltiple goals, including promoting prosocial b   ills, emotion regulation skills, interperso   self-control, as well as reducing aggressi   osequent chapters describe intervention   kills. However, first it is necessary to consid   ther key factor that affects the process of peer r   critical role played by peers.

Chapter 3

Rejection Processes
The Role of Peers

*I*n the majority of cases, one can identify characteristics and behaviors that explain why certain children are rejected by their peers. However, it would be a mistake to conclude that these children are fully responsible for the treatment they receive from others. It should always be kept in mind that peer rejection is an interactional process—it reflects not only deficits in child skills that elicit negative reactions from peers, but also those peer reactions themselves and the reciprocal effect they have on child skills, behaviors, and feelings. Peer responses and peer group dynamics often assume a life of their own, directly affecting the developmental course of the rejected child. It is critical to recognize the role played by peers in the rejection process, as effective intervention requires attending both to the rejected child and to the rejecting peer group. There are three key ways in which peers influence the development of rejected children:

1. Peers engage in behaviors that affect the responses of rejected children, through processes of modeling, selective reinforcement, and provocation.
2. Peers develop reputational biases that affect the way they perceive, evaluate, and feel about rejected children, thus coloring their responses to those children in negative ways.
3. Peers control the niches of social opportunity available to rejected children, thereby influencing the kinds of social learning experiences rejected children can have.

Each of these types of peer influence is described in this chapter, along with a summary of the ways in which peer influence must be considered when planning interventions.

PEER INFLUENCES:
MODELING, REINFORCEMENT, AND PROVOCATION

It is often very perplexing to teachers and parents when they see children engaging in behavior that is clearly destructive to their peer relations. Almost all children want to be liked by others; yet some tease, fight, or behave so obnoxiously that they quickly alienate their peers. Adults who observe this behavior wonder what it means and why it continues when it elicits such clear reprimands from adults and rebukes from peers. Although many factors can foster misbehavior in children, one type of factor often overlooked by adults is the "functional" value of the misbehavior for the children. That is, although aggressive and disruptive behaviors are typically destructive to relationships, they also serve to manage and control relationships. To the extent that these behaviors serve a function for children, they are likely to continue, despite reprimands and punishments.

Developmental models describing how children learn aggressive behaviors typically include three components (Patterson, 1986). One component involves exposure to models who demonstrate that aggressive and defiant behaviors may be effective in controlling relationships and attaining goals. Peers can serve as models, as can contentious siblings, television characters, or parents who frequently complain or yell. In some cases (e.g., in media portrayals), aggressive tactics may even be glorified—presented as strong, masculine, and effective means of "dealing with" individuals who present frustrations or obstacles to goals (Eron & Huesmann, 1986).

A second component in the learning model involves reinforcement. Although reinforcement can involve a positive consequence or reward, aggressive behaviors are often motivated by negative reinforcement, which occurs when children are able to "turn off" or "escape" from some noxious situation by exhibiting aggression (Patterson, 1986). For example, if a child can use aggressive behavior to make a peer or sibling stop teasing, that aggressive behavior will be reinforced, because it serves as a protective self-defense mechanism for the child. Even if a teacher or parent later punishes the child for the aggressive behavior, the immediate gain (stopping the teasing) functions as a powerful immediate reinforcer.

Finally, a third component that characterizes the development of

aggressive behaviors involves the escalations and deteriorations that occur in relationships when they are characterized by frequent aggressive
interactions. Labeled "coercive processes" by Patterson (1982), these
damaging interaction patterns have been documented in the family interactions of highly aggressive children (Dodge, Bates, & Pettit, 1990;
McMahon & Wells, 1989). Literally, "to coerce" means "to restrain or
dominate by force." Coercive processes in relationships are escalating
sequences of individuals' aggressive attempts to dominate each other,
resulting in extended aversive exchanges and high levels of anger and
frustration. The positive features of the relationship are gradually un-
dermined by frequent conflict, resulting in increasing avoidance and
often depressed mood (Patterson, 1982). Documenting that coercive
processes also operate in peer interactions, Asarnow (1983) found that
aggressive boys were more likely than their nonaggressive classmates to
react negatively to conflict during cooperative peer activities, and to escalate (in an attempt to dominate) rather than resolve conflicts when
they occurred.

     Teachers often express the feeling that the child behavior prob-
lems they see at school reflect family dysfunction. Although this is often true to some degree, family influences account for only a relatively
small part of a child's school behavior and peer relations (Bierman &
Smoot, 1991; Dodge, Bates, & Pettit, 1990). For example, on average,
the correlation between parent and teacher ratings of aggressive behavior (at home and school, respectively) is only $r = .27$ (Achenbach,
McConaughy, & Howell, 1987). Similarly, Dishion, Duncan, Eddy,
Fagot, and Fetrow (1994) found the correlation between the display of
coercive interpersonal behaviors and negative attitudes in parent–child
interactions and the display of similar behaviors and attitudes in peer
playground interactions to be $r = .19$ for grade school children. These
correlations do not mean that family influences are unimportant in
shaping children's school behavior, as families certainly make contributions in a variety of ways to children's social competence and readiness
for peer socialization (see Chapter 13). However, these studies do indicate that peer relations take on a life of their own outside the family
context. With or without previous "training" at home, children can
learn to use aggressive tactics to gain supremacy in peer contexts.

     For example, in an intriguing study, Patterson, Littman, and
Bricker (1967) observed a group of children over the course of the
year, to see how their peer relations developed during their first year of
preschool. At the end of the year, they found that there were two
groups of children who showed high rates of aggressive behavior in
their peer interactions. One group consisted of children who might be
labeled "bullies." These children entered the preschool with relatively

high rates of aggressive behavior, and they were able to use their aggression successfully to dominate peers, to control play materials, and to direct play. The second group consisted of children who were "victims" early in the year, and who were the subject of other children's teasing and demands. Some of these victims turned things around for themselves by copying the aggressive behaviors of their attackers, fighting back, and then moving on to offensive strategies, using aggressive behaviors to control their peer interactions. The critical "take-home" point of this study is that although children did bring characteristics and behavioral tendencies to school with them (including behaviors learned at home), the peer interactions they experienced during the course of the year played a key role in shaping their social behaviors. Although peer influences are usually positive, this study illustrates the ways in which peers can unwittingly influence each other negatively, by providing the reinforcement that allows certain children to use aggressive behavior to gain interpersonal control and to avoid victimization. These findings have important implications for interventions designed to influence the problematic social behaviors of rejected children and to improve their peer relations, because they suggest that successful interventions cannot focus on rejected children in isolation, but must take into account the nature of the peer responses and influences that may be affecting and maintaining the children's problem behaviors.

Despite their professional training and experience, teachers are not immune to entrapment in coercive cycles of interaction with problem students that can fuel both the continuation of problem behaviors and the escalation of negative peer interactions. The classroom tends to be a particularly challenging context for children who have deficits in attentional and behavioral control skills. Disruptive and off-task behaviors occur when children do not have the control skills to focus and sustain their attention. These behaviors are often reinforced in two ways. First, off-task behaviors allow a child to "escape" from the demands of the classroom tasks, which may seem overwhelming and unpleasant for the child. Second, disruptive behaviors often elicit a response from peers, including attention, laughter, or other comments. In fact, Klein and Young (1979) conducted an observational study in elementary classrooms where they tracked peer reactions to disruptive behaviors. Rates of responding varied across classrooms, with 20%–70% of disruptive behaviors receiving attention and reinforcement by peers. Exerting effective control over peer responses to problem behaviors can be a daunting task in some classrooms, particularly in classrooms that contain a high proportion of children with aggressive or disruptive propensities (Kellam et al., 1991). Unfortunately, high-risk children often attend schools in which there is a high density of other high-risk children (Rutter, Maughan, Mortimore, & Ousten, 1979), creating a difficult teaching environment and an increased exposure to peer modeling and reinforcement of problem behavior.

Over time, teachers can be "worn down" by the problem behaviors of certain children in a manner similar to the process that operates for the parents of these children. It becomes hard for teachers to maintain a positive attitude toward children who constantly disrupt their classrooms, and they often begin to resort to more frequent and more intense criticism and punishment as a method of gaining control over the children's behavior. Although effective limit setting is certainly a critical skill in classroom management, the escalations in punishments that sometimes occur for rejected disruptive children do not function as effective limits to control their behavior. For example, I have consulted with teachers in cases in which students have lost recess privileges for weeks in advance or have been permanently isolated from others in the classroom. These sorts of escalations in punishments usually reflect the desperation of teachers who have become entrapped in coercive power struggles with children, fueled by mutual frustration, resentment, and anger. As such teachers become less positive, and as their responses to such students become less contingent and less grounded by the immediate behavior of the students, they become less able to influence the students' behavior (Strain, Lambert, Kerr, Stagg, & Lenkner, 1983). In addition, as discussed further in the next section, teachers' attitudes and behavior toward disruptive children can have a profound impact on the way in which peers think about and treat those students. If peers feel that teachers have "sanctioned" negative attitudes and behavior toward certain problem children, they often increase their negative treatment of those children. Peer teasing and ostracism can, in turn, increase the discomfort problem children feel in the classroom setting, contributing to higher rates of disruptive behavior as they seek to escape from an unhappy situation or as they seek to stop the torment they feel they are receiving from peers.

The discussion thus far has focused on the ways in which peers (and parents and teachers) can unwittingly reinforce aggressive and disruptive behaviors, and the function these behaviors may serve in controlling social interactions. When faced with high rates of aversive and aggressive behavior, peers typically develop their own self-protective strategies, in the form of self-defensive attitudes and counteraggressive behaviors, to keep themselves from being hurt or discomfitted. The response of peers is easy to understand; yet it is often a response that serves to escalate conflict and dissension in the peer group, particularly when peer defensiveness leads to negative reputational biases, ostracism, and victimization of rejected children.

REPUTATIONAL BIASES, OSTRACISM, AND VICTIMIZATION

In order to make sense out of our social world, we all develop cognitive sets to represent people with whom we have regular contacts. These "person perceptions" are built upon past interactional experiences and help us to anticipate and predict how others will treat us and respond to us (Russell & van den Broek, 1988). These expectations also serve as guides and influence the behaviors we direct toward others. At all developmental levels, social perceptions are often affectively polarized, so that interactions with some individuals are anticipated with pleasure and sought after, whereas interactions with others are anticipated with apprehension and avoided. The perceptions of young children tend to be particularly polarized, reflecting the concrete nature of their thinking. Children under the age of 7 tend to view individuals categorically as either "good" or "bad," and tend to perceive or distort information selectively so that it is consistent with their expectations (Bierman, 1988). For example, told that a boy who is a good baseball player (he catches well and hits many home runs) is a liar, most young children will deny that this boy could still be a good baseball player or that he could still catch well or hit home runs (Saltz & Medow, 1971). In the later grade school years, children become more able to recognize and understand how individuals can have both positive and negative traits. However, their person perceptions still tend to be affectively polarized, contributing to rigid reputational biases (Bierman, 1988).

Studies examining the ways that peers perceive and describe rejected children reveal the prevalence of negative stereotypes and biased or distorted perceptions (Hymel, Wagner, & Butler, 1990). For example, in an intriguing set of studies conducted at a summer camp, Koslin, Haarlow, Karlins, and Pargament (1968) examined the impact of peer popularity on children's social perceptions. After establishing the relative popularity of children in a group, by asking children who they liked best, Koslin and colleagues set up a series of events and asked children to "guess" the outcomes. For example, children were asked to guess who would win different kinds of contests. Consistently, these guesses were influenced by popularity; popular children were expected to perform in superior ways in all events, whereas unpopular children were expected to perform below par. The bias in peer perceptions was evident even on judgment tasks that did not reflect areas of child competence. For example, popularity influenced child judgments of height, with the height of popular children being overestimated and the height of unpopular children being underestimated.

Negative reputational biases affect the ways in which children perceive and interpret the social behaviors of rejected children. For example, in a study by Dodge (1980), children were told stories that included a negative event and were asked for their interpretation of that event (e.g., "Jim and Mike were building a tower of blocks. The tower got knocked down. Why do you think that happened?"). In half of the stories, Dodge (1980) used the names of boys who behaved aggressively in class; in the other half of the stories, the story characters were nonaggressive, well-liked classmates. When boys with aggressive reputations were the perpetrators of the hypothetical negative act, peers were likely to assume that the act was intentionally harmful—that the perpetrator knocked down the tower of blocks on purpose, just to be mean. When well-liked, nonaggressive classmates were named in the story, peers were likely to assume that the act was accidental, and that no harm was intended—maybe someone bumped the table by accident, or the block tower just got too high and fell down by itself. On the one hand, it is easy to see how these different expectations develop, as classmates appear to be using past experiences to make predictions about the future behavior of certain peers. However, consider the impact of these negative expectancies on the rejected children. They create a situation in which these children are never "given the benefit of the doubt" in ambiguous circumstances, but are readily blamed for unexplained events.

In another study of social perceptions, Hymel (1986) told children a series of stories about positive and negative behaviors exhibited by liked and disliked peers, and asked peers to explain why they thought the behaviors occurred. When children heard stories about well-liked peers who displayed positive behaviors, they tended to explain these behaviors in terms of the positive traits of the children ("She's kind," "He's friendly"). When they heard stories about well-liked peers who displayed negative behaviors, children tended to explain these behaviors as unusual events due to mitigating circumstances ("Maybe she was sick that day," "It was an accident; he didn't mean to do it"). In contrast, the explanations children gave for the positive and negative behaviors shown by disliked peers showed the opposite pattern. That is, children interpreted negative behaviors as evidence of the disliked peers' undesirable personality traits and intentions ("He's mean"), whereas positive behaviors were often dismissed as circumstantial or temporary ("Maybe the teacher was watching," "She can be nice sometimes if she wants to"). Similarly, Waas and Honer (1990) also found that unpopular peers were ascribed more intent in conflictual interactions, were rated as less justified in such interactions, and were described generally in a more negative light than popular peers. The important thing about such perceptual biases is that they affect the behaviors peers direct toward rejected children and severely limit the

opportunities rejected children have to change their image or their social station.

Negatively biased expectations and attributions lead classmates to
treat rejected children differently (and more aversively) than they treat
their well-accepted peers. That is, when peers expect inappropriate social behavior from a particular child, they become selectively attentive
to such behavior and unresponsive to that child's prosocial behavior
(Hymel et al., 1990). Indeed, observations suggest that peers respond
more negatively to rejected than to accepted children, even when the
two groups show no apparent differences in the quality of their social
initiations. For example, Foster and Ritchey (1985) observed children
interacting in a classroom setting. There were no differences in the
rates of positive or negative initiations made by peer-rejected children
and their peer-accepted classmates. However, rejected children were
far less likely than accepted children to receive positive peer responses.
Similarly, Solomon and Wahler (1973) observed classroom interactions
and noted that peers ignored the prosocial behaviors of identified
problem children and attended almost exclusively to the deviant actions of these children.

Negative reputations can justify ostracism and can fuel victimization. For example, consider the following case examples, drawn from
our interview study of grade school children (Bierman, Smoot, &
Aumiller, 1993). In each case, the negative treatment that rejected children received from peers extended beyond self-protective or defensive
behavior on the part of peers. In these cases, peers went on the offensive, attacking and belittling the disliked children.

One case involved a third-grade boy who was a slow learner and
had difficulty reading. This child was somewhat overweight and had a
slight facial disfigurement—physical characteristics that added to his
sense of insecurity and social vulnerability. He was not aggressive, but
was awkward and anxious socially. Peers excluded him from their play
and teased him about his deficiencies. They were unrelenting and intol-
erant of his skill deficits, which they felt provided a good reason for his
social exclusion:

"He's slow at his work. Sometimes he hardly knows anything."
"He's practically retarded!"
"He's clumsy."
"People tease him. They call him a dummy."

From an observer's point of view, it seemed that peers did not give this
child a chance. However, his classmates managed to perceive events in
a manner that allowed them to justify the exclusion of this boy and the
part they played in it:

"If we're playing baseball or football, he'll come down and go, 'Can I play?' when the teams are already fair. So somebody will push him out of the way 'cause they don't want him there, and he'll go out and push another person. He can't keep his hands to himself."

In addition, peers were aware of the low social status of this boy and the potential risk involved in befriending him:

"Other people don't like him, because all of the other kids will make fun of them if they like him."

A second case example involved a fourth-grade child who moved into a new school in the middle of a school year. He was from Australia and was unfortunate enough to move into a classroom in a rural school, where children had little exposure to or tolerance for diversity. This boy was staunchly rejected by his classmates, who gave reasons such as the following to justify their dislike:

"He packs his own lunch, and he eats things that others don't like. When he eats, he takes big bites."
"He's from Australia, and we don't like the way he talks."
"He doesn't even know how to play kickball. He plays a different kind of ball."
"We don't like his jacket. He wears the same jacket every day, and he puts his hands in the pockets all the time."

In this case, peers took offense at seemingly innocuous factors—eating unusual foods, playing different games, wearing an unusual jacket. They managed to reach a sort of consensual judgment that these differences would not be tolerated and that this boy would not be accepted into their enclave. In this case, being different (and being somewhat shy and awkward) was sufficient to elicit peer censure. This sort of exclusion can affect children who are unusual due to their appearance or abilities, and it can affect children who represent ethnic/racial minority groups in classrooms. As noted in Chapter 1, children who have minority status in the classroom typically receive fewer positive nominations and more negative nominations than children of majority status (Coie, Dodge, & Coppotelli, 1982; Kistner, Metzler, Gatlin, & Risi, 1993).

When peers engage in this type of active exclusion, it is not possible to intervene effectively by focusing intervention solely on the rejected child; instead, attending to the peer group dynamics and to the negative impact of reputational biases and victimization is critical. The negative impact of peer victimization is substantial and should not be underestimated. Rejected children may be teased, taunted, and physically roughed up or hurt by hostile peers (Perry, Kusel, & Perry, 1988). The experience is frightening and disheartening.

Victimized children often develop psychological distress, including anxiety and depressed mood (Boivin, Hymel, & Bukowski, 1995). Victimization can also affect the behavior of rejected children in negative ways. For example, Hodges, Malone, and Perry (1995) observed children over the period of two school years. They found that children who were victimized by peers in the first year showed increases in problem social behaviors the subsequent year, including higher levels of social withdrawal, pushy and intrusive social behavior, and social immaturity. Victimized children often suffer intense feelings of loneliness and social alienation (Boivin, Hymel, & Bukowski, 1995). They may become truant because they are uncomfortable in the school setting, and are at risk for school dropout. They are also at risk for substance abuse, which may emerge as a mechanism to express or escape from feelings of alienation and despair.

Children who are inhibited, anxious, awkward, and passive in their interactions are at particularly high risk for peer victimization (Olweus, 1993). Paradoxically, the experience of victimization may increase their social anxiety and withdrawal, which then elicits further victimization, creating a cycle of persistent victimization and psychological damage (Boivin, Hymel, & Bukowski, 1995). In addition, children who are reactively aggressive and who exhibit emotionally dysregulated externalizing behaviors (hyperactive/disruptive and inattentive behaviors, emotional outbursts) may also be victimized by peers (Dodge & Coie, 1987). These children, termed "provocative victims" by Olweus (1993), may aggravate peers with their intrusive and aggressive social behavior. Perhaps because of their emotional dysregulation or lack of social competence, they are unsuccessful at using their aggression to defend themselves and may become caught in escalating cycles of victimization by peers, suffering negative consequences that are similar to those experienced by "passive victims" (Olweus, 1993).

It is critical for adults to guard against their own negatively biased expectations. In work with aggressive–rejected children, it is easy to fall into the trap of expecting and responding selectively to deviant behavior. When certain children routinely engage in inappropriate behavior, adults come to expect such behavior of them. The expectations of both peers and adults can lead them to focus primarily (and sometimes unfairly) on the negative behaviors of rejected children in ways that create self-fulfilling prophecies and reduce opportunities for positive change.

Indeed, teacher opinions can influence peer preferences, reinforcing the negative reputations of disliked children. Teachers find it hard to like rejected children (Taylor & Trickett, 1989), and they may increase the risk of these children by unwittingly cuing peers about their feelings, and/or by allowing teacher–child relationships to become conflictual and nonsupportive (Pianta, 1999). Negative peer treatment is painful to children in the short run, and can stifle positive social development by seriously constricting child opportunities for positive peer contact and support.

NICHES OF OPPORTUNITY AND RISK

Positive peer interactions provide an important context for social–emotional development. In naturalistic interactions, peers act as companions, models, and sources of reinforcement and emotional support, helping children to develop aspects of social competence (such as cooperation and negotiation skills, communication skills, and perspective-taking abilities). Children who are shut out of opportunities for positive peer interactions may miss out on these learning opportunities, leading to greater deficits in interactional skills (Ladd & Asher, 1985).

Research suggests that rejected children often have few social options, and it can be difficult for them to find willing play partners. Often rejected children end up playing with fewer children than their peer-accepted counterparts, and often their playmates are younger and unpopular like themselves (Ladd, 1983). The friendships rejected children form are often of low quality, involving high levels of conflict and low levels of positive exchanges. Although these relationships provide companionship, when rejected and unskilled children band together as friends or playmates, they may hurt each other as much as they help. That is, often children in poor-quality partnerships are not able to provide each other with the social models or support that could enhance their social skill development. When these relationships involve high levels of conflict, they are also demoralizing emotionally, contributing to feelings of depression and insecurity for the children involved (Connelly, Geller, Marton, & Kutcher, 1992).

In addition, some aggressive–rejected children who feel pushed out of conventional classroom peer groups may forge affiliations with other aggressive children, forming networks of peers who share aggressive orientations (Cairns, Neckerman, & Cairns, 1989). Particularly during early adolescence, as peer influence increases, affiliations with youth who advocate aggressive/antisocial attitudes and behaviors represents a critical risk factor.

Although, in general, one might expect friendships to buffer and protect children against the negative impact of peer rejection, Kupersmidt, Burchinal, and Patterson (1995) found the opposite effect for some children: Rejected children who had a reciprocated best friend were *more* likely than friendless rejected children to develop antisocial problems. The explanation for this paradoxical finding may be in the characteristics of the friends that rejected children often associate with, given that negative peer influence and involvement with deviant peers often foster the initiation of delinquent activity, drug and alcohol use, risky sexual behaviors, and school dropout (Dishion, Andrews, & Crosby, 1995; Tremblay, Masse, Vitaro, & Dobkin, 1995).

Trying to understand better how best friendships could escalate risk, Dishion and his colleagues (Dishion et al., 1995; Dishion, Spracklen, Andrews, & Patterson, 1996) developed an observational strategy designed to examine negative support processes operating in adolescent friendships. They observed adolescent boys and their friends for a 25-minute session, as the boys planned a joint activity and discussed a problem that each boy had with his parents and with his peers. Dyads were of three types: (1) delinquent pairs (both of the participants had a previous history of arrest), (2) nondelinquent pairs (neither partner had a history of arrest), and (3) mixed pairs (in which one partner had a history of arrest and the other did not). Delinquent dyads engaged in high rates of rule-breaking talk (e.g., talk about antisocial or inappropriate activities)—rates that were double that of the mixed group and four times the rate of the nondelinquent group. In addition, sequential analyses revealed that in the delinquent dyads, youth tended to reinforce rule-breaking talk with laughter (in contrast to nondelinquent boys, who tended to reward normative topics with laughter). A longitudinal follow-up study documented predictive links between positive friend reactions to rule-breaking talk in this lab-based task and escalations in delinquent behavior over the ensuing 2 years. These findings suggest that a consideration of rejected children's opportunities for peer interaction may be important in assessment and intervention planning. Attention should be paid to the availability and promotion of opportunities for positive bonding with normative peers, as well as to reducing the opportunity and inclination rejected children may have for risky affiliations with deviant peers.

SUMMARY

The studies described in this chapter illustrate the important influence that peers have on children's social behavior and social development—

influence that operates in three kinds of ways. First, peers influence child social behavior by the ways in which they initiate and respond to that behavior. In a coercive cycle that has no winners, peers can behave in ways that provoke and reinforce aggressive, intrusive, and disruptive social behaviors. When intrusive behavior is rewarded with attention, or when aggressive behavior provides a respite from antagonism or demand, those peer responses give inappropriate social behavior "functional" value, allowing children to use those behaviors to achieve short-term gains. Second, peers influence children's behavior by the expectations they develop, which affect and bias their initiations and responses. Negative reputational biases reduce rejected children's opportunities for change and contribute to self-fulfilling prophecies. Finally, peers influence child social behavior by controlling the niches of opportunity children have for social interaction. By limiting the availability of opportunities for positive bonding, peers can shut some children out of the kinds of peer interactions that would model and support the development of prosocial skills, contributing to increasing delays and deficits in interactional skills (Ladd & Asher, 1985). Rejected children who find themselves ostracized from the mainstream network of classmates may forge alliances with other children who are socially unskilled, like themselves. Low-quality interactions fail to promote social growth; affiliations with deviant peers place youth at risk for antisocial activities and substance use.

In addition to the impact they have on children's social behavior, the experiences children have with peers and their interpretation of those experiences affect their developing sense of self and their beliefs about the social world. Theorists have speculated that the internal representations children construct to understand their social world play a key role in shaping the children's social behavior, and in determining the extent to which negative experiences with peers contribute to psychological distress, including social anxiety and depression. The next chapter describes the role that peer experiences may play in the development of the self, and the complementary role that developing self-system processes may play in influencing child social behavior and experience.

Chapter 4

Peer Relations and the Developing Self

*T*he behavior a child directs toward others is a major determinant of the social responses he/she receives, and most cases of chronic peer rejection can be traced to problematic, off-putting behaviors (Bierman, Smoot, & Aumiller, 1993). At the same time, the responses of others (peers, teachers, siblings, parents) have a marked impact on the behaviors rejected children show, often provoking and reinforcing asocial, inappropriate, or hostile reactions from these children (Hymel, Wagner, & Butler, 1990). One of the factors that can make problematic peer relations difficult to change is that patterns of social interaction develop over time and become embedded in the dynamics of social networks; they constrain behavioral flexibility and lead some children to "fall into a rut," repeating the same disharmonious relationship cycles over time, in new settings, and with new partners (Cairns & Cairns, 1991).

Sometimes teachers and parents remark with dismay that a child seems unwilling to change his/her problematic social behavior, even after repeated instructions, encouragement, or reprimands, as if that child is not interested in having friends (e.g., "I've told him again and again not to do that because children don't like it, but he does it anyway"). In most cases, the resistance to change is not a reflection simply of poor motivation (e.g., the child does not want friends); rather, it reflects the power of habitual patterns of social responding that become part of the child's affective, cognitive, and behavioral orientation toward his/her social world. Indeed, the way a child perceives and thinks about his/her social world (and his/her corresponding sense of self) develops in order to enhance the predictability and controllability of

47

the social world, but can also contribute to continuity of the "status quo" in relationships—in some cases, fueling the maintenance and repetition of problematic styles of social interaction.

The idea that children's mental representations of their social relationships might contribute to the maintenance of problematic social behaviors and corresponding peer relationship difficulties was documented in developmental research and influenced intervention models as early as the 1970s. The central focus was the influence of children's social cognitions (e.g., social knowledge, social goals, problem-solving skills, and reasoning about relationships) on their social behavior, and thereby on their social acceptance. Theoretical models and research linking broader conceptualizations of self-system development with the quality of children's social adjustment have since emerged, but have been slow to influence intervention strategies to improve peer relations.

In this chapter, I first review briefly the research literature linking social information-processing skills with problematic social behaviors and peer rejection, and the impact of this research on intervention design. Then I describe broader theoretical models of self-system process development, examining recent research and discussing the potential importance of these broader conceptual models for understanding peer problems and designing effective interventions.

SOCIAL INFORMATION-PROCESSING MODELS OF THE 1980s

By the mid-1980s, substantial research had accumulated documenting links between children's social information-processing skills and their social behavior and peer acceptance. On the basis of this research, these skills were being incorporated into social competence interventions.

Comparisons of Popular and Unpopular Children

For example, based upon documented differences between popular and unpopular children, Ladd and Asher (1985) suggested that three social-cognitive factors warranted attention in social competence interventions: (1) limited knowledge about effective social interaction strategies, (2) asocial goals, and (3) low levels of perceived efficacy in social interactions. Their recommendation to focus on social knowledge was based on studies demonstrating that, compared with popular children, unpopular children were less able to articulate normative social strategies for a variety of peer situations, including making friendships

(Gottman, Gonso, & Rasmussen, 1975), helping others (Ladd & Oden, 1979), initiating interactions, and resolving conflicts (Asher & Renshaw, 1981). Unpopular children described goals that interfered with positive social interaction (e.g., winning games rather than having fun with friends), leading to competitive and self-serving play behavior (Renshaw & Asher, 1983). In addition, unpopular children expressed less confidence than popular children about their ability to handle peer interactions effectively (Wheeler & Ladd, 1982), suggesting possible benefits from interventions that increased their feelings of perceived efficacy for prosocial interaction strategies. Ladd and Asher labeled these social cognitions "underlying processes," recognizing that their influence on social behavior was covert and not readily observable by others, and that these factors often operated outside the conscious awareness of the children themselves.

Comparisons of Aggressive and Nonaggressive Children

Concurrent with research on the social cognitions of popular and unpopular children, research was conducted comparing the social cognitions of aggressive and nonaggressive children. By the mid-1980s, Dodge (1986) had integrated this research and articulated a five-step model of social information processing that proved to be highly influential in both research and intervention contexts. The five steps were as follows:

1. *Encoding*—perceiving and appraising the social situation (processes influenced by the child's social goals, attention, cue utilization, and memory skills).
2. *Representation*—interpreting, evaluating, and making attributions about the meaning of others' behavior.
3. *Response search*—generating alternative responses.
4. *Response decision*—selecting a response based upon the child's self-perceived capacity to enact the various response options successfully, and upon anticipation of the potential outcomes.
5. *Enactment*.

This model presumed that these steps of social information processing occur at a rapid rate, often automatically at an unconscious level, becoming conscious primarily when individuals are faced with unusual or difficult social situations requiring more careful problem-solving efforts. Dodge suggested that biases or deficits at any one of those steps could increase the likelihood of a child's aggression and thereby impair the child's social competence.

Indeed, a series of studies comparing aggressive with nonaggressive children has demonstrated differences at each of these information-processing steps. For example, aggressive children more often endorsed goals that focused on instrumental gains or retribution rather than the maintenance of positive peer relations (Dodge, Asher, & Parkhurst, 1989). Aggressive children were more impulsive and less comprehensive in their cue utilization, gathering less information about a social situation than nonaggressive children did before making interpretations and attributions (Dodge & Newman, 1981; Milich & Dodge, 1984). When encoding social information, they were more likely to focus on aggressive cues in the environment than were their less aggressive peers, and they had more trouble shifting their attention away from such aggressive cues (Gouze, 1987). The social interpretations made by aggressive children were also subject to bias. Particularly when faced with negative events and ambiguous interpersonal intentions, aggressive children were more likely than nonaggressive children to attribute hostile intentions to peers (Dodge, Murphy, & Buchsbaum, 1984; Dodge, Pettit, McClaskey, & Brown, 1986). Aggressive children also generated fewer prosocial or assertive and more aggressive responses to social situations (Asarnow & Callan, 1985; Dodge, 1986). They expressed more confidence in their ability to use aggression effectively than nonaggressive children did, and they expected aggression to be more effective in obtaining rewards, decreasing aversive treatment from others, and bringing about more positive self-evaluation (Crick & Ladd, 1990; Perry, Perry, & Rasmussen, 1986). Each of these tendencies in social information processing made it more likely that aggressive children would select hostile or power/domination strategies for solving social problems than collaborative or prosocial strategies.

Incorporation in Intervention Designs

Based upon evidence that deficits or distortions in social information-processing skills were associated both with problematic social behavior (especially elevated aggression) and with low peer acceptance, it made sense to include these skills as targets in interventions designed to improve social behavior and promote positive peer relations. Attempts to incorporate a social-cognitive focus in interventions primarily involved the use of explicit instructional strategies and practice opportunities (for a comprehensive review of social competence interventions, see Chapter 10).

For example, based on research indicating that unpopular and aggressive children exhibited deficits in their social knowledge, coaching programs included instructions, discussions, modeling, and examples to enhance children's cognitive understanding of and knowledge about socially appropriate behaviors and strategies (Ladd & Mize, 1983). Positive social goals were introduced, and performance feedback provided reinforcement to children for selecting prosocial response options. It was anticipated that explicit instruction, modeling, and reinforcement would increase children's social knowledge, reinforce social goals, and increase their perceived efficacy for prosocial behavior, thus promoting cognitive as well as behavioral change to support improved peer relations (Ladd & Asher, 1985).

Also targeting social-cognitive skills related to social competence, social problem-solving interventions were designed to enhance the thinking skills involved in effective social information processing. The premise of these interventions was that children's cognitive capacities to recognize and accurately assess social problems, to generate and evaluate multiple potential responses, to set goals, and to self-monitor their behavioral performance in light of those goals would provide the critical building blocks for flexible, socially responsive, and adaptive behaviors (Weissberg & Allen, 1986).

Although built upon solid theoretical premises, interventions that focused primarily on the cognitive skills of social problem solving tended to have a stronger impact on what children were able to say about their social goals and social problem-solving strategies than on their generalized social behavior and peer relations (Allen, Chinsky, Larcen, Lochman, & Selinger, 1976). Even coaching programs, which embedded social-cognitive instruction with behavioral rehearsal and feedback, had difficulty promoting the generalization of intervention gains to real-life peer interactions (see reviews by Gresham, 1994, and La Greca, 1993).

Although many factors may account for these limited intervention effects, two possibilities warrant consideration here. First, it is possible that the domain of social-cognitive skills being targeted in intervention (or, correspondingly, the model of social information processing guiding these interventions) was incomplete, and failed to include key aspects of self-system development that were contributing to children's problematic social behavior and low peer acceptance. Second, it is possible that the model for promoting change was insufficiently developed. Social belief systems may be more difficult to change than originally thought, and adult instruction, exhortation, and reinforcement may not be sufficient to influence social thinking or social behaviors outside the settings that adults control.

Recent years have witnessed the expansion of conceptual models linking emotional and motivational aspects of self-system development with social behavior problems and problematic peer relations. Correspondingly, social information-processing models themselves have developed and expanded (see Crick & Dodge, 1994, for a reformulated model). However, the translation of this research to interventions has remained limited; social competence interventions continue to rely heavily on the provision of information and encouragement to enhance children's social knowledge and change their social beliefs. Coaching programs for disliked children still operate from the premise that when children are introduced to and reinforced for new ways of thinking and behaving during intervention sessions, these changes will in turn promote changes in the children's broader self-system development, including emotional, motivational, and self-evaluative features. Yet theoretical models of self-system development suggest that social belief systems may not be so easily changed, as they are anchored in children's social experiences, both past and present.

In the remainder of this chapter, I consider characteristics and models of the developing self-system that interface with but extend beyond social information processing to influence social competence and peer relations. First, research and theory describing self-system processes as developmental, adaptive, and functional are reviewed. Next, research and theory emphasizing the emotional and motivational bases of self-system development are discussed. Whereas social competence interventions have focused on changing cognitions and behaviors, this research suggests that emotions, motivations, and control beliefs may require more attention in interventions (Izard, 2002). Finally, the interface between perceptions about others and oneself is considered. The development, function, and adaptive significance of these multiple dimensions of the self-system suggest potential new directions for intervention design.

THE FUNCTIONAL SIGNIFICANCE AND ADAPTIVE VALUE OF SELF-SYSTEM PROCESSES

The social knowledge and social problem-solving skills that have been targeted in social competence interventions represent features of a broader set of self-system processes. Conceptually, these processes reflect the human ability to develop perceptual and interpretive systems that are informed on the basis of past experience, and allow a child to navigate a complex social world with efficiency, familiarity, and comfort (Crick & Dodge, 1994; Dodge & Murphy, 1984; Harter, 1998; Lochman & Dodge, 1994). That is, in order to manage the dynamic array of social stimuli surrounding them, children develop mental representations that help them organize and make sense out of their social world and understand its relation to them. These mental representations act as heuristics, allowing them to "figure out" how the social world is organized in order to move effectively within it. Conceptions

of the outside world and others are intertwined with a child's conceptions of the self and of his/her perceived ability to influence or act on
the social world in effective ways (Baldwin, 1992; Skinner, 1995). Central to these heuristics are "relational schemas," which, as described by
Baldwin (1992), include information about the other, the self as experienced in the context of that relationship, and the pattern of interaction
characterizing the relationship. With development, relational schemas
grow in complexity to include a broad range of social knowledge, beliefs, and theories. As organized representations of past behaviors and
experience, these schemas include both declarative social knowledge
(e.g., information about specific others and the self) and procedural
knowledge (e.g., rules for social exchange, social roles, scripts, and prototypes) (Abelson, 1981; Baldwin, 1992). All of these schemas and
scripts include knowledge about events, as well as associated expectations, thoughts, feelings, goals, and motivations (Fiske & Taylor, 1984).

Relational schemas and associated mental representations of the
social world allow a child to move away from a dependence on the immediately available social stimuli, and instead to guide behavior in a
more organized and strategic way. Theorists have emphasized three important functions served by the schemas children construct about their
social world and their relation to it. When they are functioning well,
these representations (1) provide a basis for the prediction and control
of the outside world; (2) preserve a system of internal synchrony or
consistency in a child's sense of self; and (3) promote self-protection,
maintaining a favorable sense of self to motivate action and adaptive
problem solving (Cairns, 1991; Epstein, 1991; Harter, 1998). Interestingly, it may be that the functional value of self-system processes, which
allow children to develop strategic and habitual patterns of social responding, can also contribute to social dysfunction and resistance to
change by limiting the malleability of relationship patterns.

From a functional perspective, the social information-processing
patterns shown by aggressive children do not represent distortions or
deficits. Rather, as Cairns (1991) has argued, aggressive children may
be attuned to aggressive cues because aggressive exchanges are well
represented in their relational schemas and have historical meaning.
That is, their hostile biases do not reflect a distorted paranoia, but a
reasonable appraisal based on their past experiences that others are
threatening them. Given the typical behavior of an aggressive child,
and his/her prior experiences of coercive and conflictual interactions
with others, the child may be correct and prudent to anticipate hostility
from peers and take a self-protective stance; consider, for example, the
research documenting the negative reputational biases faced by disliked children (reviewed in Chapter 3). Given their situation, it may be
self-protective for aggressive–rejected children to assume that they are

in danger (e.g., to assume hostile intentions in ambiguous circumstances), rather than to assume a benign situation and risk being caught "off guard."

Regardless of the source of their social-cognitive beliefs, the bottom line for aggressive youth is that an orientation toward the social world as threatening, and the mounting of counteraggressive behaviors, contribute to self-fulfilling prophecies that increase the long-term stability of both hostile peer treatment and continued aggressive orientations. Yet one might approach intervention differently, depending upon one's conceptualization of social cognitions as distortions or adaptive predictions. Whereas distortions may be remedied with an instructional approach, one would not anticipate that adaptive predictions about a hostile peer environment would be likely to change unless substantive changes occur concurrently in the nature of that peer environment.

In addition to considering the functional value of children's self-system processes, Izard (2002) has argued compellingly that the role and function of emotion in children's relational schemas and social behavior deserves greater consideration, particularly in terms of the implications for intervention design.

AFFECT AND SELF-SYSTEM DEVELOPMENT

Emotion plays a central role in motivating and regulating social interaction, and emotional well-being depends upon social connection and support (Sroufe, 1990). This section considers the motivational drives that may activate and organize the construction of relational schemas and related self-system processes, as well as the regulatory role of emotion in social interaction.

Motivational Drives

In 1991, Connell and Wellborn integrated available theory and research to suggest that self-system development is driven by three basic human needs—the needs for relatedness and secure connections with others; the need for autonomy and self-direction; and the need for competence and the capability to predict and control outcomes.

Relatedness

Theorists have suggested that infants come into the world biologically prepared to develop affectively charged informational schemas that allow them to navigate safely within the social surround (Ainsworth, Blehar, Waters, & Wall, 1978). Attachment theorists describe a process that begins during the first year of life as the development of "internal working models," which enable infants to predict the behavior of primary caregivers in relation to themselves (Bowlby, 1969; Bretherton, 1995; Sroufe, 1990). The adaptational significance of this capability is evident, as it motivates the identification of dependable caregivers (providers of warmth, food, and comfort), and it reduces anxiety and promotes feelings of well-being (Bowlby, 1969).

The desire to form secure attachments continues to motivate social behavior throughout the life span, and plays a central role in the organization of relational schemas (Connell & Wellborn, 1991). Relational schemas are affectively charged to maximize their salience, with some interpersonal experiences associated with pleasure and comfort, and others associated with anxiety and distress (Epstein, 1991). In a broad sense, these schemas promote children's ability to distinguish between friends and enemies—persons they should trust and persons they should fear—allowing them to maximize their opportunities for social support and to reduce social exclusion or rejection (Baldwin, 1992; Cairns, 1991).

When they are functioning well, relational schemas and corresponding self-conceptions foster a child's ability to develop secure friendships and to feel comfortable in social situations. However, children with problematic peer relationships often show evidence of relational schemas that contribute to their interpersonal difficulties, making it hard for them to experience security or intimacy in their friendships. For example, in a longitudinal study, Sroufe and Egeland (1989) found that children who demonstrated insecure attachment with their caregivers in infancy showed lower levels of teacher-rated peer competence in third grade than their securely attached peers did. They postulated that early experiences in insensitive or unresponsive caregiving situations increased children's vulnerability to feelings of insecurity and anxiety in their later relations with peers. Studying elementary school children, Rudolph, Hammond, and Burge (1997) found that representations and expectations children had for support and hostility in their concurrent relationships with their mothers and peers showed similar features, providing additional support for the hypothesis that children's mental constructions of relationships may foster continuity in positive (or negative) interpersonal expectations across contexts.

Researchers have also documented associations between indices of insecure attachment and aggressive behavior problems. For example, Speltz, Greenberg, and DeKlyen (1990) found that preschool-age children with aggressive and oppositional behavior problems were more likely to show evidence of insecure attachments in a maternal separation and reunion task than were peers without such problems (84% vs. 28%, respectively). Their hypothesis was that these children who were faced with inconsistent or insensitive caregiving situations and associated feelings of insecurity were reacting to (or coping with) these feelings by engaging in high-demand acting-out behaviors, which forced maternal responding and thus helped them to control their mothers' attention and proximity (Greenberg & Speltz, 1988). These studies suggest that children who develop insecure models of relationships, anticipating that others are not supportive and trustworthy (and, correspondingly, that they themselves are not likable), may be vulnerable to social adjustment problems, including low levels of prosocial behavior and elevated acting-out behaviors.

Autonomy

Whereas relational schemas that develop during the first year of life primarily serve the motivation to connect securely with others, the focus and purpose of these schemas begin to broaden in later years, as the cognitive capabilities of young children develop and their social world expands. Usually emerging during the second year of life, children show a desire to experience autonomy—to make choices about the behaviors they will and will not do (Connell & Wellborn, 1991). A child's need to direct his/her own behavior toward chosen goals exerts a powerful influence on interpersonal processes during the second and third years of life (Deci & Ryan, 1985). In parent–child relations, autonomy striving is reflected in "the terrible twos"; in peer relations, autonomy striving emerges in attempts to choose one's play, control resources, and direct one's destiny in everyday activities, such as going first and getting to play with a desired toy.

The social information-processing biases demonstrated by aggressive children are consistent with the hypothesis that many of them are particularly sensitive to perceived threats to their autonomy. That is, one could argue that due to their experiences in coercive environments, the relational schemas of aggressive children are oriented around power and control issues; they therefore show particular vigilance toward the protection of their autonomy, and reactively defend themselves against interpersonal threats that involve perceived domination or autonomy constraint. Their focus on instrumental gains (Lochman & Dodge, 1994), vigilance to aggressive cues in the environment (Gouze, 1987), and tendency to interpret the ambiguous behavior of peers as hostile (Dodge et al., 1984, 1986) are all consistent with this affect-based representational explanation.

Competence

A third drive that shapes the development of self-system representations involves the desire to experience competence (Connell & Wellborn, 1991; Skinner, 1995). Theoretically, a child's sense of competence reflects his/her perceived capability to produce desired events and prevent undesired events in particular action domains (Patrick, Skinner, & Connell, 1993). Perceived competence motivates engagement and problem solving; a lack of perceived competence is associated with disengagement and helplessness (Skinner, 1995). Perceived competence may affect developing peer relations in direct ways, in terms of children's beliefs that they can (or cannot) control interpersonal outcomes, such as peer liking or peer treatment (Crick & Ladd, 1990). It can also have an impact in indirect ways, by motivating (or inhibiting) engagement in activities that provide a foundation for positive peer interactions (Skinner, 1995).

A number of theoreticians have identified links between individuals' perceptions regarding the causes of particular negative events and their corresponding affective reactions to those events, feelings of self-worth, and coping attempts (Skinner, 1995). The models of such links have focused on locus of control (Dweck & Elliott, 1983), causal attributions (Weiner, 1985), self-efficacy (Bandura, 1977), and learned helplessness (Seligman, 1975). Feelings of competence reflect generalized beliefs that the self can produce desired and prevent undesired outcomes, which in turn depend on beliefs concerning the means that will produce the outcomes (knowledge about strategies) and beliefs concerning the capability of the self to utilize those strategies (beliefs about capacity) (Skinner, 1995). When individuals believe that they are unable to control outcomes (particularly negative events), feelings of depression and anxiety ensue, along with the cessation of coping attempts. In the reformulated model of learned helplessness, for example, Abramson, Seligman, and Teasdale (1978) contend that when individuals explain negative events in terms of internal, stable, and global causes (e.g., such events are their fault because of the kinds of persons they are), they believe they cannot prevent similar negative outcomes in the future, resulting in depression and passive withdrawal or avoidance. In this way, the exposure to negative social outcomes, coupled with the interpretations children make about the causes and controllability of those outcomes, affects their feelings about themselves (e.g., depression, anxiety, shame) and their motivation to act in ways that might prevent or change those social outcomes (Nolen-Hoeksema, Girgus, & Seligman, 1986; Skinner, 1995).

Incorporating Emotion and Motivation into Models of Social Information Processing

Social information-processing models have been expanded to incorporate the growing literature regarding the role of emotional and motivational processes in social competence. In Crick and Dodge's (1994) reformulated model of social information processing, attachment-related experiences and mental representations of relationships are stored in the form of an affect-laden informational database that influences social information processing at the levels of social perception and appraisal, causal interpretations, and decision making about social responding. This influence works at an unconscious level, creating an affective bias that influences child sensitivity and reactivity to certain social cues.

For example, children who have experienced rejection in the past may become particularly vigilant to signs of potential rejection in the future, and therefore focus selectively on cues consistent with this expectation in their social perceptions. This affective bias may also influence their social goals and decision making. That is, in order to protect themselves from harm, they may more often select self-protective over other-oriented social goals, attribute hostile intentions, and respond with aggression or avoidant withdrawal (Crick & Dodge, 1994). These types of responses further decrease the likelihood of positive responses from others. In this way, stored memories of negative interpersonal experiences may contribute to biases in social information processes that promote a self-fulfilling prophecy, in which children who fear rejection or hostile interpersonal treatment behave in ways that increase the likelihood of rejection and victimization (Crick & Dodge, 1994).

Although Crick and Dodge (1994) have focused primarily on the impact of attachment-related experiences on social information processing, one could anticipate that experiences related to autonomy and competence also fuel the construction of the self-system and influence children's social information processing (Connell & Wellborn, 1991). Poorly met needs in any one (or more) of these areas could conceivably contribute to a hypervigilance or hypersensitivity in that aspect (or aspects) of social relationships, increasing emotional and behavioral reactivity to certain interpersonal events or experiences (Baldwin, 1992).

For example, low levels of perceived security (relatedness) may increase emotional reactivity to signs of perceived rejection or lack of support. Corresponding behavioral reactions in social situations may include withdrawal and avoidance—or, alternatively, intrusive and demanding behavior, which forces others to respond by creating demand characteristics that cannot be easily ignored (Greenberg & Speltz, 1988;

Jacobvitz & Sroufe, 1987). Children with elevated sensitivity around issues of interpersonal power and control (autonomy) may be particularly vigilant and reactive to perceived goal blocking, disagreement, or
behavioral constraints, because these threaten their capacity for self-
determination. Perhaps fueled by a history of coercive exchanges, these
children may show high levels of oppositional, defiant, and bossy
behavior (wanting to do things their way) and high levels of reactivity in
situations involving goal frustration (e.g., when they can't go first, when
they lose a game). Alternatively, children may also avoid asserting their
desires, showing passive submissiveness. Children who feel uncertain
about the implicit rules and routines that characterize social situations
or who question their capacity to elicit fair treatment from peers (competence) may show poor coping skills, withdrawal, or disengagement in
the face of social challenge. In a new or difficult social situation involving an initial failure or rebuff, they may give up easily, showing reduced
capacity for frustration tolerance and sustained coping. They may
blame themselves for their failures (contributing to feelings of depression and low self-worth), or they may blame others (contributing to reactive anger).

   To a large extent, these models suggest that emotion and motivation have their impact on social behavior by the way in which they influence social information processing (including social perception, appraisal, response generation, and response selection) (Crick & Dodge,
1994). Although, as noted earlier, social competence interventions
have included an explicit focus on social cognitions (notably social
knowledge, social goals, and social problem solving), the roles of emotions and motivations (and corresponding implications for intervention
design) are rarely discussed. The change model assumes, implicitly,
that changing social cognitions will in turn affect the emotions and motivations that contribute to those cognitions. Izard (2002) calls for more
explicit attention to emotions in social competence intervention models.

Emotion Reactivity and Dysregulation

Although Izard (2002) agrees that emotions have a profound influence
on perception, cognition, and action, he emphasizes the reciprocal nature of the relationship between thinking and feeling. He notes the
contribution of noncognitive processes (as well as cognitive processes)
to emotional experiences, suggesting that intervention models that
confine themselves to a child's thinking processes as a way to address
emotional issues are incomplete.

   Certainly the role that emotional reactions play in disrupting effective social interaction has been documented—primarily by behavioral observations or teacher ratings, which have indicated links among "reactive" aggression, emotionally dysregulated behavior, and peer rejection (as described in Chapter 2). Social information-processing models recognize that emotional arousal may derail strategic planning with "fight-or-flight" responding, fostering preemptive action in which a child responds quickly with reactive patterns of self-protection, typically aggression or withdrawal (Dodge et al., 1986; Izard & Youngstrom, 1996). These models suggest that such emotional reactions, sometimes termed "hot cognitions," can lead to impulsive and reactive behavioral actions. Children may be able to show the capability for thoughtful social information processing under conditions of "cold cognition" (e.g., generating a list of potential responses to conflict when discussing hypothetical situations), and yet may show preemptive action with little evidence of alternative response generation in real-life conflict settings when they are emotionally aroused and upset, under conditions of "hot cognition" (Dodge & Newman, 1981).

In some cases, patterns of emotional reactivity in interpersonal relations may become characteristic of individuals; when these patterns contribute to narrow and rigid response hierarchies that lead to social impairment, they are reflective of "emotion dysregulation" (Cole, Michel, & Teti, 1994). Dysregulated patterns of problem behavior can involve high levels of negative affectivity, emotional outbursts, inattentiveness, and low frustration tolerance—all detrimental to effective peer relations (Eisenberg & Fabes, 1992). Dysregulation is evident in the high rates of inattentive and hyperactive behaviors often exhibited by peer-rejected children, reflecting poorly developed abilities to inhibit impulsive responding, focus and sustain attention, and regulate behavior according to internalized rules (Barkley, 1996).

Although both theoretical models and empirical studies suggest that emotion plays an important role in social interaction and peer relation difficulties, our intervention models have remained focused primarily on social-cognitive and behavioral change efforts. Intervention design may need to consider both how emotions and motivations relevant to social interaction could be addressed as targets for change (e.g., expanding the focus of social competence interventions), and also what the appropriate change mechanisms might be (e.g., expanding intervention techniques and our understanding of change processes). Chapter 12 addresses this theme in more detail.

In addition, although this section has focused on how children perceive others, it is important to consider how self-system processes affect the way children view themselves in the context of their social interactions.

SELF-SYSTEM PROCESSES AND SELF-CONCEPTIONS

Within relational schemas, social cognitions regarding others are intertwined with individuals' social constructions of themselves. Relational schemas include expectations about how one will be treated by
others, the degree to which one can affect the responses of others,
and corresponding self-evaluations about how one deserves to be
treated and how lovable or worthwhile one is (Greenberg, Speltz, &
DeKlyen, 1993). Modern conceptions of social influences on developing self-systems continue to reflect basic principles articulated by
Cooley in 1902. Coining the phrase "the looking-glass self," Cooley
suggested that children develop and evaluate themselves by imagining
how they look to others and how they believe others are evaluating
them. Interpersonal responses may begin to shape self-conceptions in
infancy. Broader social comparison processes, and particularly the
use of reference groups for self-evaluation, begin to emerge around
age 8, as children become able to assess their competence in relation
to the perceived social standards of groups to which they belong or
aspire (Ruble & Frey, 1991).

The utility of a schema is that it makes information processing
more efficient, enables prediction and anticipatory planning, and
thereby fosters competence. The self-conceptions that are part of children's relational schemas represent expectations about how they are
likely to be treated by particular social partners and how they are likely
to behave, together with associated thoughts and feelings (Baldwin,
1992). Such self-conceptions represent generalizations about the self
that are based upon repeated patterns of interaction and experience
(Markus & Wurf, 1987). When a person has an established set of self-
expectations (as in a relational schema), information about the self
(similar to information about the other) is processed more efficiently
and recalled more easily when it is consistent with this established
schema (Markus & Wurf, 1987). The system is designed to develop consistency in views of self and other, and works to maintain synchrony.
Simply put, this effect reinforces past experiences, such that individuals
who have a positive sense of their social competence and self-worth
tend to construe events and process information in a way that promotes the maintenance of these positive self-perceptions, which in turn
serves to preserve feelings of self-worth (Taylor & Brown, 1988). In
contrast, individuals with more negative self-perceptions tend to encode, store, and retrieve information in a way that focuses on the
schema-consistent negative information about the self, filtering out or
deemphasizing schema-inconsistent positive information (Quiggle, Garber, Panak, & Dodge, 1992). Negative self-conceptions are associated

with psychological distress, including feelings of depression, anxiety, and loneliness (Boivin & Begin, 1989).

Peer Rejection and Negative Self-Schemas

Not surprisingly, children who have experienced peer rejection are likely to view themselves as less socially competent than higher-status children, and to express lower levels of perceived self-competence and social worth (Bukowski, Hoza, & Boivin, 1994). Rejected children also report greater loneliness and social dissatisfaction than do nonrejected children (Asher, Parkhurst, Hymel, & Williams, 1990). Interestingly, however, not all rejected children express negative self-evaluations and distress about their social problems (Boivin & Begin, 1989; Williams & Asher, 1987). To some extent, psychological distress varies as a function of the severity of a child's peer problems. For example, children appear more likely to feel incompetent and to experience loneliness and distress when their rejection is chronic as opposed to transitory (Burks, Dodge, & Price, 1995).

Researchers have also suggested that negative self-evaluations are more characteristic of nonaggressive–rejected than of aggressive–rejected children. For example, compared to children of average sociometric status, nonaggressive–rejected children report greater feelings of loneliness and lower self-esteem, whereas aggressive–rejected children do not differ from children of average status (Boivin, Poulin, & Vitaro, 1994; Parkhurst & Asher, 1992). Correspondingly, nonaggressive–rejected children are more likely than aggressive–rejected children to express a desire for help with their peer relations (Asher, Zelis, Parker, & Bruene, 1991). Investigators have found that aggressive children tend to be unaware of the degree to which they are disliked by peers (Cillessen, van IJzendoorn, van Lieshout, & Hartup, 1992), and that they overestimate the extent to which they are accepted (Hughes, Cavell, & Grossman, 1997).

In order to clarify the basis for these apparent distortions in the self-evaluations of aggressive–rejected children, Zakriski and Coie (1996) conducted a series of three studies. First, they compared the number of "like most" and "like least" ratings that children expected to get from their classmates with the number they actually got. Both nonaggressive–rejected and aggressive–rejected children expected to get more "like most" nominations than they actually received. However, whereas nonaggressive–rejected children expected (and received) more "like least" nomination than average-status children, aggressive–rejected children did not expect (but did receive) more "like least" nominations than average-status children. In the second study in this series, Zakriski and Coie demonstrated that aggressive–rejected boys were just as accurate as nonaggressive–rejected and average-status boys in judging the social status of other children; this suggested that their self-evaluations were not distorted by any general deficit in social sensitivity or lack of awareness regarding the signs of rejection. Finally, in the third study, Zakriski and Coie manipulated the interpersonal responses that children got as each child played a board game with a peer confederate. In one condition, the confederates signaled dislike by making negative comments about the activity (commenting that they did not want to be there); failing to respond to some of the questions asked by their partners; acting competitively; and noting, when asked as part of the game, that they could not think of anything they particularly liked about their partners. When aggressive–rejected children watched videotapes of other children playing the game with negative peer feedback, they accurately identified the signs of peer dislike. However, when they themselves experienced this feedback, they gave themselves and their partners higher liking ratings, estimating that they liked their partners more and their partners liked them more than the children they watched on the videotape. The nonaggressive–rejected children did not show this bias. Zakriski and Coie concluded that even when aggressive–rejected and nonaggressive–rejected children are given identical negative social feedback, aggressive–rejected children interpret this feedback in a more positive way, and correspondingly feel less distress about their social situation.

Although this research suggests that aggressive behaviors may protect rejected children from experiencing low self-evaluations and corresponding loneliness (Hughes et al., 1997; Zakriski & Coie, 1996), some aggressive children suffer from depressed affect and negative self-evaluations. For example, when Rudolph and Clark (2001) created subgroups of children based on teacher ratings of aggression and self-ratings of depressed mood, they found that 49 of the 128 identified aggressive children (38%) also showed elevated levels of depressed mood. Based upon teacher ratings of children's peer status, both subgroups of aggressive children (depressed and nondepressed) were at elevated risk for rejection by peers. The aggressive children who were depressed rated themselves as more socially incompetent, and rated peers and friends as less trustworthy and more hostile, than nonaggressive comparison children. In contrast, the other aggressive (nondepressed) subgroup showed a self-protective bias (similar to that reported by Hughes et al., 1997, and Zakriski & Coie, 1996), giving themselves social competence ratings that were equivalent to those of the nonaggressive comparison children. These results suggest that it is not aggressive behavior per se that protects children from negative self-evaluations. However, there may be ways of thinking about one's self and one's social interactions that are more common among aggressive–rejected than nonaggressive–rejected children, and that protect more of the aggressive–rejected children from negative self-views and corresponding psychological distress. Control beliefs and perceived self-efficacy may be central to this process.

The Role of Control Beliefs and Perceived Competence

The way that children interpret the causes of their social experiences, particularly negative social events, may determine the impact of experiences of rejection or victimization on children's self-conceptions and associated feelings of distress. Nondistressed rejected children are more likely to blame others for their social failures, whereas distressed rejected children are more likely to blame themselves (Vitaro, Tremblay, Gagnon, & Boivin, 1992).

Several studies have documented the importance of children's social interpretations and causal attributions in linking negative social experiences with psychological distress and perceived incompetence. For example, Graham and Juvonen (1998) found that victimized youth who blamed their characters (i.e., who believed they were teased because of the kinds of persons they were—an uncontrollable and stable attribution) were significantly more likely to experience social anxiety, loneliness, and passivity than were youth who blamed their behavior (which could be changed in the future to elicit a different outcome). Similarly, rejected children who attributed their social failures to internal and stable factors were more likely to feel lonely and anxious, and to respond with behavioral withdrawal and social avoidance, than were youth who blamed situational or external factors (Renshaw & Brown, 1993).

The impact of negative self-perceptions may be to perpetuate maladaptive approaches to social interchanges, thereby increasing vulnerability to future episodes of peer rejection or victimization. For example, Egan and Perry (1998) found that self-regard served as a moderating condition, influencing the likelihood that grade school children with behavioral vulnerabilities (e.g., physical weakness, poor social skills) would experience peer victimization. Among behaviorally at-risk children, those with higher levels of self-regard and confidence in their social competence appeared protected from future victimization, whereas those with a sense of social failure and feelings of social inadequacy were at increased risk for future victimization.

It may be that some children who are aggressive are protected from negative self-evaluations in two ways: (1) They are more likely to blame others than themselves for their problems (Dodge et al., 1986); and (2) they may feel that they are capable of using their aggression to protect themselves and control negative outcomes (Cairns, 1991; Perry et al., 1986).

RISK OR PROTECTION?

Hughes and colleagues (1997) raised critical questions about the degree to which the positive control beliefs and inflated self-perceptions of aggressive children represent a risk or a protective factor. On the one hand, aggressive youth who are unaware of the degree to which peers dislike them, and who fail to recognize their own culpability in their social difficulties, may have little motivation to change. In contrast, other investigators suggest that although aggressive children often provide an inflated estimate of their competence and skills compared to how teachers and peers evaluate them, this inflation is needed to buffer the children's sense of self from the very low regard in which others hold them and to motivate coping attempts (Cairns, 1991). Accepting the viewpoint of others might prevent these children from maintaining a sense of potential competence, which would motivate continued engagement and efforts at social relationships. When levels of perceived competence are very low, affect is depressed, and motivation for coping is compromised (Skinner, 1995). Hence change efforts may be more effective when they target the promotion of new prosocial goals and strategies to supersede old ones than when they attempt to dismantle the scaffold supporting a child's social engagement.

IMPLICATIONS FOR INTERVENTION

Habitual patterns of social responding are not easy to change, particularly when they have served adaptive functions in the past and have become an established part of a child's affective, cognitive, and behavioral orientation toward his/her social world and sense of self. Unfortunately, we know relatively little about how children reconstruct perceptual and interpretive systems, particularly those that serve self-protective functions. Given the developmental processes associated with the construction of self-system processes and their adaptive functions, it is doubtful that they will be easily changed by adult instruction, exhortation, or reinforcement alone. Rather, reworking internal models may require intervention strategies that introduce new ways of looking at and interpreting social interaction, in combination with new interpersonal experiences that validate the functional value of those alternative social attitudes, affects, and behaviors (Price & Dodge, 1989; Selman & Schultz, 1990).

To accomplish this goal, intervention designs may need to pay more attention to a child's affect and self-system orientation. That is, social competence programs for disliked children typically target social cognitions and behavior for change, with the assumption that affect and self-perceptions will improve as a function of the increased positive peer responding that accompanies improved social behavior. Yet the primacy of emotion in social interaction, and the tendency for self-system processes to maintain synchrony (Cairns, 1991), may create resistance to change if they are not addressed in intervention (Izard, 2002; Price & Dodge, 1989).

The need to address these issues may not be met simply by adding lessons to existing intervention program curricula. Although lessons on skills such as emotional understanding and anger regulation may be helpful, these kinds of lessons still rely on changes in children's "cold cognition" (their capacity to think about and talk about feelings outside a problem situation) as a mechanism for driving changes in the underlying feelings and motivations that affect their functioning in the "hot-cognition" conditions of real-life interactions. As an addition to "cold-cognition" lessons, scaffolded experiences that allow for commentary, inquiry, and support during "online," emotion-charged social interactions may provide critical learning opportunities (Selman & Schultz, 1990). This idea is explored further in Chapter 12, which suggests that unexplored features of coaching sessions may affect the impact of those sessions. Specifically, the ways that coaches choose to elicit and respond to interpersonal affect and dynamic interpersonal exchanges during sessions may affect the impact of those interpersonal experiences on children's working models of peer relations and their corresponding affect-charged orientation toward others and toward themselves (see Chapter 12 for more details).

In addition to expanding our models of social competence acquisition, consideration of developing self-system processes suggests that attention to children's real-world peer interactions is also important. Even with extensive effort during coaching sessions, it is difficult to prepare children to sustain a positive and efficacious cognitive and affective orientation toward peers if their peers' responses do not validate this orientation. Interventions have been designed to enhance the positive responsivity of peers to target children (see Chapter 13); however, these techniques have not been fully integrated with coaching strategies.

In addition, an unaddressed issue involves the degree of malleability in children's attraction to different peers. Particularly among aggressive–rejected children, attraction to other aggressive children contributes to deviant partnerships that support problematic social behaviors (Dishion, Andrews, & Crosby, 1995) and may buffer children against a need or desire to change. Cairns, Neckerman, and Cairns (1989) have suggested that many aggressive youth are attracted to (and comfortable in) a social world that fits their social cognitions and expectations. As a function of this attraction, their experiences in aggressive peer interactions accumulate, thereby reinforcing both their aggression-prone social styles and their comfort level with aggressive peer interactions. Developing intervention strategies that prepare the naturalistic peer environment to provide alternative niches of social opportunity for rejected and aggressive youth, and increasing the attraction value of those niches to the target youth, are challenges for future program designs.

SUMMARY

In summary, children who develop patterns of problematic interaction often find themselves embedded in dynamic social networks that support the maintenance of their rejected status and constrain their opportunities for change. Their developing representations, which help them organize and make sense of their social world, affect the way in which they perceive, interpret, store, and recall information about peers and about themselves in relation to their peers. Children with problematic peer relations often develop relational schemas that contribute to their social difficulties—limiting their capacity to feel securely connected to peers, interfering with their ability to balance autonomy striving with interpersonal sensitivity and reciprocity, and reducing the degree to which they approach social interactions with confidence and adaptive coping.

Given the developmental and functional significance of relational schemas and self-protective social-cognitive processes, they may be difficult to change without altering the interpersonal context in significant ways to provide a different set of interpersonal experiences for a child—a set of experiences that would support the restructuring of existing relational schemas and the construction of new relational schemas. In general, intervention efforts need to proceed with a recognition of the way in which beliefs about others and about the self are intertwined and embedded in interpersonal experience. Generalized change may require repeated exposures to new models and therapeutic peer contexts, in which behavioral improvements become systematically aligned with positive affective experiences and competence-promoting cognitive processing. To promote generalization to peer contexts, new attitudes and behaviors need to have functional value, with the capacity to accurately predict and influence peer responding in naturalistic settings. In Part II, I move on to discuss issues and methods for the assessment of social competence and peer relations, as a prelude to the discussion of intervention designs.

PART II

ASSESSING SOCIAL COMPETENCE AND PEER RELATIONS

Chapter 5

Assessment Goals and Strategies

Child characteristics, family relationships, peer interactions, and school experiences all can contribute to the development of deficits, habits, or insecurities that negatively affect social adaptation. The social adjustment difficulties of peer-rejected children are often complex, including behavioral features (e.g., excessive displays of aggressive, avoidant, or immature/inattentive behaviors, and deficient displays of prosocial and cooperative behaviors); affective features (e.g., negative expectations for interpersonal relationships, and easily aroused feelings of anxiety, anger, or ambivalence in interpersonal contexts); and cognitive features (e.g., impulsive and inaccurate perceptions, negatively biased evaluations, and inadequate or aggression-prone problem-solving skills). In addition, a child's social success is not determined by these features alone, but also by the characteristics of the social partners (peers, teachers, and parents) with whom the child interacts.

Correspondingly, social skill training assessments and interventions need to address the behavioral, social-cognitive, and affective/motivational aspects of children's social adjustment. In addition, assessments and interventions need to address the interpersonal contexts in which social behaviors and peer interactions take place. Within this general developmental framework, the particular structure and focus of selected assessment procedures will vary as a function of the purposes and goals of a particular project.

PURPOSES AND GOALS OF ASSESSMENT

Assessment techniques are utilized by researchers and by practitioners in somewhat different ways. Typically, research projects are focused on building and evaluating descriptive models that identify the nature, facets, dynamics, developmental course, and outcomes associated with children's social competence and peer relations. In contrast, for practitioners, assessments serve more practical functions; they provide a basis for the selection of participants, guide the focus of intervention efforts, and enable the evaluation of intervention effects. Whereas researchers are typically interested in group averages (and individual variations around those group averages), practitioners (particularly those working outside a research setting) are typically interested in child-specific evaluations and, whenever possible, seek standardized norms that allow them to interpret the meaning of a child's absolute score on a particular measure. In addition to these differences in orientation, assessments planned by researchers and by interventionists often vary as a function of the resources available for assessment (including data collection, scoring, and statistical analyses), which typically are greater in the research context than in the school or clinic context.

Chapters 6–9 provide an overview of measures that, for the most part, have been developed in the context of developmental, clinical, and school-based research. Their utility in intervention settings varies somewhat, depending largely on the resources required for implementation and scoring, and on the degree to which they provide norm-based or comparative guidelines for score interpretation. However, they provide an important array of empirically validated assessment strategies from which practitioners can draw for their assessment needs.

Focusing specifically on assessment processes associated with social interventions, Gresham and Elliott (1984) describe two phases and types of measurement. The first phase involves the identification and selection of children with significant peer problems, using diagnostic measures designed to determine the severity and nature of the children's social difficulties. This process typically involves the assessment of peer status and the identification of problem behaviors affecting peer relations, via standardized peer and teacher rating measures. Given the heterogeneity evident in the group of children who have peer relation problems, this phase of assessment provides information about individual differences in dimensions of problem behaviors and prosocial deficits that may influence the appropriateness of various intervention approaches (Coie & Koeppl, 1990). The second phase involves assessment to guide the planning and evaluation of intervention. These measures, termed "intervention measures" by Gresham and Elliott, enable a functional analysis of the factors contributing to a child's social problems. These measures may include more focused behavioral observations, the collection of information about child perspectives, and assessments of affective and social-cognitive factors, as well as an analysis of social dynamics and contextual reinforcement contingencies.

This conceptualization of the phases and functions of an assessment are similar to those identified by Guralnick and Weinhouse (1983): (1) to identify children who have a problem that warrants intervention; (2) to describe the nature and severity of the problem, providing a clear "operational" definition identifying the problem in a way that can be specified and measured; and (3) to develop a "functional" model of the factors contributing to the problem to guide intervention efforts. It is important for assessment to be conducted within a developmentally and culturally informed framework. In addition, for the purposes of intervention evaluation, the selected measures should be sensitive to change over time.

Although there are some differences in the goals and functions of assessments developed for research versus intervention purposes, effective assessment frameworks should be built upon the foundation of our empirical and developmental understanding of the key factors associated with peer relations. For example, based on the empirical research described in Chapters 1–4, Figure 5.1 represents the different

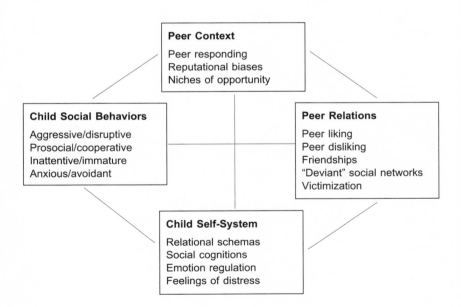

FIGURE 5.1. A model for the assessment of problematic peer relations.

dimensions appropriate to a formulation and assessment of a child's peer relations.

The first phase of assessment described by Gresham and Elliott (1984) and Guralnick and Weinhouse (1983) involves a description of the child's peer relations and social behaviors. The prior review of the empirical literature suggests that the description of a child's peer relations should include the extent to which the child is liked and disliked by the peer group, the number and quality of his/her friendships, the extent to which the child is embedded within problematic or "deviant" social networks, and the degree of victimization the child may be experiencing. The description of the child's social behavior should include aggressive/disruptive, inattentive/immature, and avoidant/withdrawn behaviors, as well as prosocial/cooperative deficits. The second phase of assessment, providing a clear "operational" definition of the problem and developing a working model of the factors contributing to the problem (Guralnick & Weinhouse, 1983), must additionally address the child's self-system and the peer context. Characteristics of the child's self-system—particularly his/her relational schemas, social cognitions, affective reactions to interpersonal experiences, and self-perceptions—may all affect the child's perceptions, interpretations, and behavioral choices in social interactions. In addition, the nature of the peer group and social interaction support available to and impinging upon that child is important, as peer responding and niches of opportunity for social interaction operate as constraints that intervention must address.

USING MULTIPLE ASSESSMENT METHODS

Whenever possible, the use of multiple evaluation methods is desirable. As reviewed by Coie and Dodge (1988) and by Pepler and Craig (1998), peer ratings, teacher ratings, direct observations, and child interviews provide complementary information. Each type of method has particular advantages and limitations. For example, gathering information directly from peers can be cumbersome; yet peers are in the best position to describe the aspects of a classmate's social behavior that they find aversive. At the same time, their perceptions can be colored by the child's social reputation (Hymel, Wagner, & Butler, 1990). Typically, teachers are the preferred adult informants, as they have multiple opportunities to observe children's interactions with peers in a normative group context across a sustained period of time. However, a teacher's ratings can be influenced heavily by a child's classroom behavior, because it is in this context that the teacher has the greatest opportunities to observe the child's peer relations (Newcomb, Bukowski, & Pattee,

1993). Teachers often underestimate the peer acceptance of effective aggressive children (who behave aggressively but are nonetheless liked by peers), and overestimate the peer acceptance of children who behave appropriately in class but lack the skills to connect or collaborate well with peers in play settings (Coie & Dodge, 1988). Direct observation can provide an objective measure of children's peer interactions, but particularly in the older elementary grades, observations become difficult to accomplish unobtrusively. In addition, some behaviors that may be "critical events" in terms of their social impact (such as fighting or stealing) may occur with low frequency, and thus may be difficult to capture in time-limited observations (Foster & Ritchey, 1985). Given the strengths and limitations of each measurement technique, the use of multiple measures provides a more comprehensive basis for interpretation than does the use of any one method alone (Coie & Dodge, 1988).

In clinical settings, parents are often the source of the referral and the most readily available source of information about a child's social problems. It is important to note that although parents are often able to describe aspects of the child's social behavior and peer contacts outside school, the information they have about a child's school-based peer group relations is typically limited and secondhand, making it important to gather direct information from the school context as well as to interview the parents (Graham & Rutter, 1968). In addition, whereas teachers are able to observe children in the context of a normative peer group, parents often lack access to this normative database, making it more difficult for them to identify atypicalities in their children's peer relations (Coie & Dodge, 1988).

It is important for an assessment to include the social settings in which a child has difficulty. The appropriateness of various social behaviors and the kinds of skills needed for behavioral performance differ across settings. For example, classroom settings call for constrained and routine social behavior. Behavioral expectations are fairly clear in the classroom setting, and there are external signals to help guide behavior (e.g., classroom rules, teacher directions). At the same time, classroom settings require high levels of behavioral inhibition and focused attention, which can strain the regulatory capabilities of some children. In contrast, free-play situations offer fewer external guides or constraints, thus presenting a more flexible but also a more ambiguous social context. They allow for more spontaneous social behavior, but also require children to orient their behavior around more subtle social cues and conventions. Games with rules represent yet a different structure and demand situation, as they reward competitive behavior but require internalized arousal regulation and rule compliance. Depending upon their social-cognitive skills, behavioral repertoires, and emotional regulatory capacities, children may have difficulty in one or more of these social settings, and their social problems may be evident in one setting but not another (Foster & Ritchey, 1985).

CONCEPTUALIZING SOCIAL COMPETENCE

In addition to the gathering of information, the manner in which this information is conceptualized or framed can have an important impact on the focus and design of remedial interventions. Many rejected children show patterns of excessive problem behaviors (e.g., aggressive/disruptive behaviors) as well as low levels or deficits in socially appropriate behaviors (e.g., cooperative behaviors, communication skills). The way that one thinks about the relationship between prosocial skill deficits and problem behaviors can influence decisions regarding intervention design (McFall, 1982). For example, if the difficulties of rejected children are conceptualized primarily in terms of their excessive levels of problematic behaviors, intervention efforts might focus primarily on prohibitions and environmental contingencies designed to reduce those inappropriate behaviors. However, if these behavioral difficulties are conceptualized as social skills deficits or faulty social-cognitive processing, and are viewed as influenced by environmental contingencies, the focus of intervention might shift to social skill promotion or social-cognitive "retraining" instead of (or in addition to) environmental control strategies (McFall, 1982). A case example serves to illustrate.

RT

RT was a second-grade boy who was rejected by the majority of his classmates, and had no reciprocated friendships in his classroom. He had a lot of trouble getting along with peers in unstructured settings, particularly the playground. Peers complained that RT would not follow rules in games, and he was frequently accused of cheating. Playground squabbles often escalated into yelling and pushing fights as RT denied the charges, and then threatened, derogated, and attacked those accusing him of wrongdoing. Teacher ratings confirmed a problem profile involving high levels of aggressive and disruptive behaviors, along with poor frustration tolerance and frequent anger outbursts.

RT's difficulties could be conceptualized as high rates of problem behaviors (e.g., cheating in games, pushing others, calling names, fighting, and breaking playground rules), with the corresponding intervention goal being the reduction of these problems. If the difficulties were framed this way, intervention efforts might emphasize the use of environmental contingencies proven to be effective at problem behavior reduction, such as time out or response cost methods. For example, RT might be placed in time out during recess if he cheated, called names, or pushed someone. He might be excluded from recess games that were problematic for him, and required to earn the privilege of playing by showing he could follow playground rules, perhaps earning a certain number of "good behavior" points. If RT did get involved in a fight, he might be required to play alone, or he might be suspended from recess altogether and required to pass the time in the classroom. Any one of these strategies might be effective in reducing RT's problem behaviors. Certainly, if RT spent recess alone in the classroom, he would not have the opportunity to fight with peers. However, it is unlikely that this approach would substantially improve RT's ability to get along with peers in the long run, as it would not address RT's capacity for skillful social interaction with peers.

An alternative conceptual frame would be to consider RT's problem behaviors in terms of social skill deficits. For example, we might hypothesize that RT had deficits in: (1) fair-play skills, (2) conflict management skills, and (3) anger regulation and coping skills. Within this framework, intervention would logically proceed with attempts to teach RT these three sets of skills, which could enable him to play recess games successfully with peers. Effective skill training should function both to reduce problem behaviors and to improve peer relations. That is, if RT became more adept at playing games fairly, the cycle of escalation (e.g., cheating to squabbles to fights) should be eliminated. In addition, if he could become a more fun play partner, RT would have a much improved chance of gaining acceptance from his peers and making friends.

This example illustrates that the decision to conceptualize the difficulties of rejected children as primarily in terms of behavior problems or social skill deficits (behavioral, emotional, or cognitive) is not simply academic, but has major implications for the design of preventive and remedial interventions. To the extent that the behavioral difficulties of these youth are conceptualized as "markers" of deficits in underlying affective, cognitive, and behavioral regulatory processes, the focus of intervention becomes the provision of supportive relationships and interpersonal learning experiences that may assist them in developing various aspects of social competence, which in turn should foster more appropriate social behavior and reduced behavior problems. At the same time, this conceptual frame raises the question regarding the definition of social skills or social competence. How are these constructs to be understood and measured?

Defining Social Competence

Researchers have struggled to develop an operational definition of "social competence" to represent a child's overall capacity to establish positive relations with peers (Dodge, 1989). Initial approaches to assessment during the 1970s attempted to isolate and measure specific behavior capabilities that might account for social success or difficulty (Dodge & Murphy, 1984). Discrete social skills were identified with observations comparing popular and unpopular children. Then simulated role-play assessments were developed to determine the frequency with which children used these specific social skills (e.g., eye contact, smiling, giving compliments, etc.). The hope was that interventions could be designed to target the specific skill deficiencies exhibited by children, and, by remediating these deficiencies, to improve children's peer relations. The Behavioral Assertiveness Test for Children (Eisler, Hersen, Miller, & Blanchard, 1975) is a good example of this type of assessment method. However, as documented in a review by Dodge and Murphy (1984), this approach to social skill assessment and intervention proved too limited. The studies that failed to validate this approach to assessment revealed that social competence involves more than a repertoire of specific behaviors, and cannot be reduced to any static set of actions. Rather, it became clear that social competence involves the capacity to participate effectively in an interpersonal process; it requires an individual to initiate, respond, and adapt behavior in a dynamic social context. In this conceptualization, the degree to which particular behaviors are socially competent in particular social settings depends upon a host of factors.

For example, the social appropriateness of many discrete behaviors varies as a function of development, context, and culture (Rubin, Bukowski, & Parker, 1998; Sroufe, 1996). As discussed in Chapter 1, the prevalence and contributions of particular social behaviors or peer attitudes to peer rejection vary, depending upon the age, gender, and developmental status of the child (Parker, Rubin, Price, & DeRosier, 1995). Some behaviors become more and more inappropriate with age, whereas others increase in importance with age (Bierman & Montminy, 1993). In addition, some behaviors may be viewed by others as more appropriate for one gender than for the other (Caspi, Elder, & Bem, 1988), and thus may differentially affect social reputation.

Moreover, a behavior's appropriateness often depends upon the context in which it occurs (Foster, Inderbitzen, & Nangle, 1993). For instance, different kinds of social behavior are expected in classroom settings than in play settings, and even within the play context, different social behaviors are expected during games with rules than during fantasy play or focused conversations (Bierman & Welsh, 2000). Thus the extent to which a particular behavior is socially skillful depends upon the context in which it is displayed.

Furthermore, the social impact of a particular behavior may depend upon subtle aspects of its performance (Dodge & Murphy, 1984). For example, timing and interpersonal sensitivity may determine whether a joke is perceived as a congenial tease or a hostile put-down, or whether a hit is perceived as boisterous roughhousing versus inappropriate aggression (Dodge, Coie, Pettit, & Price, 1990). In such cases, the social appropriateness of the behavior is not evident in its form, but only in its execution and in the response it elicits (Bierman & Welsh, 2000; Dodge & Murphy, 1984).

Finally, some researchers have suggested that social impact may be determined less by a child's typical behavior than by the way in which he/she handles social challenges, termed "critical events." For example, a child who reacts with extreme distress or hostility whenever he/she loses a game may have trouble getting others to play, even if that child behaves appropriately at other times (Foster et al., 1993).

As I have described in Chapter 1, it became clear by the mid-1980s that social competence could not be defined or assessed in terms of discrete social behaviors. Instead, it had to be viewed more broadly, in terms of a child's ability to organize social behavior in a way that attracts positive responses (and avoids negative responses) from others in various social contexts and in a manner congruent with existing social conventions and mores (Dodge & Murphy, 1984; Rubin et al., 1998). From this perspective, a repertoire of socially appropriate behaviors is necessary but not sufficient for social competence; in addition to the capacity to produce these behaviors, social competence requires the more complex process of flexibly using them in response to continuing social feedback and stimuli. This process involves many skills, including social-cognitive capabilities and emotion regulation skills that permit children to select and engage in social behaviors sensitively and appropriately in different situations (Bierman & Welsh, 2000; Dodge & Murphy, 1984). Sroufe and his colleagues (Sroufe, 1996; Waters & Sroufe, 1983) have described social competence as an "organizational construct," recognizing the central importance of the child's ability to generate and coordinate flexible adaptive responses to various interpersonal demands and interpersonal opportunities.

The implication of this definition for assessment is that evaluations of a child's social competence and peer relations must be based on information abut the child's functioning and relationships in real-life peer and social settings. Assessment must include information about the social behaviors that are representative of the child's performance in natural social settings, and also information about the responses and evaluations a child receives from peers. In addition, assessments should consider the child's capabilities for emotional regulation and social information processing, which provide a foundation for effective organization of social behavior.

The implication of this definition for intervention is that improving a child's peer relations requires more than attention to specific social behaviors. Intervention must focus more broadly on fostering the child's ability to organize and regulate social behavior in the context of changing, often complicated social contexts.

Identifying Intervention Foci

The conceptualization of social competence as an organizational construct stands to some degree in contrast with the way social skills are represented in much of the intervention literature. That is, the approach taken to intervention in the social skills training literature is based on an educational model, in which skills are isolated, defined, and targeted for instruction. For example, Cartledge and Milburn (1986) have used the prescriptive teaching model as a framework for social skills intervention. In this model, the elements of skill training involve (1) defining the skills to be taught in specific behavioral terms, (2) documenting the initial level of skill capability, (3) systematically providing instruction in the deficient behaviors, (4) reassessing the skill capability, and (5) providing opportunities for practice and generalization of skills to new situations. Skill inventories have been developed to make it easier to apply this kind of teaching model by identifying discrete social skills to target with instruction (see, e.g., Goldstein, Sprafkin, Gershaw, & Klein, 1986; Stephens, 1977). Target skills have been defined both in terms of behaviors (e.g., prosocial cooperation and conversation skills) and in terms of emotional and social-cognitive capabilities thought to underlie prosocial behavior—for example, emotional understanding or social problem-solving skills (see Chapter 11). Although a focus on target skills provides an important guide for intervention design, it is important not to lose sight of the ultimate intervention goal, which is to foster the child's ability to organize and regulate social behavior in the context of dynamic social contexts. The process is parallel to the teaching of other complex skills, such as chess. For example, although the learning process begins with the discrete task of learning how each piece moves, being a good chess player requires attention to higher levels of dynamic game strategies.

Along this line, a useful distinction is made by Trower (1980) between "skill components" and "skill processes." Skill components are single elements of behavior or specific capabilities evident in performance tasks that provide a foundation for effective social interaction, such as eye contact, greetings, or the ability to identify another's emotional state. Social processes, in contrast, involve individuals' ability to organize themselves in the context of naturalistic social interactions, in order to generate behavior that is culturally and situationally appropriate, responsive, and effective. The degree to which skill components can be used effectively to produce successful social processes depends upon nonobservable cognitive and affective elements (such as perceptions, expectations, thoughts, and decisions), as well as such factors as timing, responsivity to the immediate social context, and the receptivity of the social partners. Assessment and intervention models should not be limited to a focus on skill components, but must also tap a child's capacity to enact complex skill processes in situations that represent naturalistic levels of affective, cognitive, and social challenge.

Behavior, Emotion, and Cognition: Separate Components?

A critical issue in this regard involves the theoretical conceptualization and pragmatic ramifications of one's model regarding the separation of the behavioral, emotional, and cognitive elements of social behavior. The question is whether, when breaking complex skills down into components, one should separate skills along the lines of behavioral capabilities (e.g., sharing, helping, taking turns), emotional capabilities (e.g., emotional understanding, emotion regulation), and cognitive capabilities (e.g., social information-processing skills). Although this kind of division is commonplace in current social competence training programs and reflects the lines along which many developmental studies are focused (see Chapter 10), it is not consistent with the theoretical model that characterizes social competence as an organizational construct. Within this organizational framework, a child's capacity to perform skillfully is a function of his/her ability to *coordinate and integrate* behavioral, emotional, and cognitive regulation, rather than a reflection simply of the child's separate capabilities in behavioral, emotional, and cognitive domains.

As noted in Chapter 4, there is evidence that a child's capacity to display certain behavioral or cognitive skills in conflict-free and affectively benign contexts (i.e., under conditions of "cold cognition") is different than when that child is affectively aroused in emotionally loaded contexts (i.e., under conditions of "hot cognition") (Izard & Youngstrom, 1996; Sroufe, 1990). At the cognitive level, affective arousal can disrupt strategic planning with "fight-or-flight" responding, fostering defensive action in which the child responds quickly with reactive patterns of self-protection, usually either aggression or withdrawal (Dodge, Pettit, McClaskey, & Brown, 1986; Izard & Youngstrom, 1996). At the behavioral level, emotional arousal can contribute to behavioral dysregulation, eliciting regressive self-serving reactions or aggressive reactivity in situations in which children feel threatened socially (Cole, Michel, & Teti, 1994). One could argue that these data suggest that a child's capacity to regulate his/her emotions is a moderator of that child's cognitive and behavioral skill performance. From this perspective, the child's capacity for emotion regulation is separate and distinct from the child's cognitive and behavioral skills, although it affects the performance of those skills. Alternatively, the argument from an organizational framework—a perspective in which emotional, cognitive, and behavioral capabilities are viewed as dynamically intertwined—would be that attempts to train emotion regulation skills in isolation from the social-cognitive and behavioral skills that, in coordination, affect the child's social performance are bound to fall short in the promotion of the child's functional social competence. The implications of these two contrasting perspectives are illustrated first in the context of a case study and then in the context of intervention design, in which they lead to different ways of conceptualizing the skill training process.

JC

JC was a third-grade boy who was friendly, outgoing, and cooperative much of the time. However, in certain social situations—particularly when his wishes were thwarted or he lost in a game—he became hostile and self-centered, displaying mean-spirited and vengeful behaviors in order to "get back at" those he felt had betrayed him. As a function of this behavior, he was disliked and feared by the majority of his peers. His teacher and parents were confused and distressed about his apparent ability to behave in socially skillful ways, but his periodic unwillingness to do so. They viewed him as hot-headed, stubborn, and willful.

Conceptually, JC's teacher and parents framed his difficulties as motivational. They believed he possessed the skill components needed to behave prosocially, but simply refused to use them at times. They conceptualized JC's problem as a performance problem rather than a skill deficit problem. This conceptualization assumes that the capacity to behave prosocially represents the same skill, whether it is performed when a child is angry or calm—that is, that the "skill" is limited to its behavioral components, with performance determined by motivational and situational factors.

Alternatively, from an organizational perspective, JC's problems reflected a skill deficit. That is, although under calm conditions JC had a well-developed repertoire of cooperative and friendly prosocial behaviors, under conditions of autonomy threat—when his indignation and anger were aroused—JC was unable to access these behaviors. As such, his "organizational capacity" to display prosocial behavior when upset represented a deficient social process. In JC's case, affective and cognitive aspects of social situations elicited emotional reactions or negative expectations and thoughts that interfered with his capacity to perform certain social behaviors. In this framework, the "skill" involved in accessing prosocial behavior when JC was angry represented a different "skill" from displaying the same behaviors under calm conditions, because in the former condition the skill involved a much more complicated process of affect regulation, self- and other-analysis, and strategic decision making.

Intervention Design

There are two ways in which social skill training interventions treat behavioral, cognitive, and affective components of skillful social interaction as separate and distinct. One way is by separating lessons on behavioral skills (e.g., game-playing skills, such as joining in, taking turns, following rules), affective skills (e.g., managing anger, relaxation skills), and cognitive skills (social problem-solving skills). In some programs, each of these skills are targeted in separate lessons. It is anticipated that after receiving separate training in these different skill components, a child will be able to integrate them in practice. The second way in which social skill training interventions separate these skills is by using a calm, "cold-cognition" approach in training sessions, where children have a high level of support to practice cognitive and behavioral skills. This leaves a large gap between the training context and the naturalistic performance context, which is often affectively charged.

   In contrast, if "skills" are understood to be organizational capabilities, skill training interventions need to be designed in ways that provide children with more practice in the integration and coordination of behavior, cognitions, and affect in increasingly complex and challenging social situations. For example, anger regulation skills would be taught within the context of game playing, and intervention would provide increasingly challenging levels of exposure to affect-charged game playing situations, while providing scaffolded support for children to practice their regulatory skills in the context of socially complex and arousing situations. Initial lessons might focus on fair-play skills in "easy" games with low levels of arousal (e.g., taking turns and sharing during cooperative games), whereas later lessons would increasingly include skills needed to handle more emotionally challenging game situations (e.g., handling a loss in competitive games).

   Research comparing differences in the effectiveness of these two

approaches is lacking; however, we might hypothesize that an integrated approach (rather than a piecemeal approach) would be more likely
to foster JC's capability to employ anger regulation skills in the context
of the high-arousal games that characterized his problem situations at
school. I return to this theme in future chapters (see Chapters 11 and
12). In the context of assessing and conceptualizing children's peer difficulties, the "take-home" point is that assessments of children's peer
problems should be based on information about their social functioning-
ing in their naturalistic peer contexts. It is for this reason that my
colleagues and I emphasize assessments that incorporate peer and
teacher informants (who see children in multiple social settings), and
we focus on measures that incorporate functional skill domains rather
than assessing specific discrete behaviors.

SUMMARY

As described in previous chapters, children with significant peer
problems exhibit a wide and complex range of characteristics (Parker &
Asher, 1987). Their social effectiveness is multiply determined—
influenced by characteristics of the peer context and self-system, as
well as by their social behavior. Assessment models and strategies
should reflect this complexity, addressing the behavioral, social-cognitive,
and affective/motivational aspects of children's social adjustment and
the interpersonal contexts in which their peer interactions take place.
Assessments have multiple goals, including the identification of children who have social problems that warrant intervention, the description of the nature and severity of those problems, and the specification
of factors that may be contributing to those problems—pieces of information that may guide the design and serve to evaluate the effectiveness of intervention. The articulation and assessment of target skill
components may aid in the design and evaluation of intervention,
though the distinction between the acquisition of skill components and
the capacity for effective social process must be recognized. Ultimately,
the goals of intervention will extend beyond the promotion of target
skill components to the promotion of social competence, which involves the child's capacity to generate and coordinate adaptive responses flexibly in response to a variety of interpersonal demands and
opportunities. Assessments should include multiple methods and sources
of information, including the perspectives of key social partners and
observers (particularly peers and teachers) and the children themselves.

The following four chapters are organized to provide a descriptive overview of specific measures and strategies that have been used by developmental researchers to assess children's social competence and peer relations. Chapter 6 reviews measures designed to identify children with significant peer problems and to assess the quality of their relationships with peers. Chapter 7 focuses on assessments of children's social behavior in peer settings, including socially competent behavior as well as behaviors that may be contributing to low acceptance and peer dislike. Chapter 8 reviews the use of observational strategies to assess peer interactions, including both naturalistic observations and observations of "staged" performance tasks, which can provide information for more in-depth functional analyses of children's social strengths and social difficulties (including opportunities to observe the contingent responding of peers). Finally, Chapter 9 examines measures and strategies used to assess children's social cognitions, relational schemas, self-perceptions, and psychological distress, which also serve to expand and clarify factors that may contribute to a child's social difficulties.

Chapter 6

Assessing Problematic Peer Relations

As noted by Gresham and Elliott (1984), assessments designed to determine the need for targeted social competence interventions begin by identifying children with problematic peer relations, and evaluating the severity and nature of their social difficulties. This chapter focuses on measures of peer regard (i.e., peer liking and disliking) and interpersonal attraction (i.e., friendships, peer affiliations), which are associated with, but distinct from, the way the child behaves with peers (described in Chapter 7). Here I review strategies to assess the four dimensions of peer relations identified in Chapter 5: (1) the degree to which children are liked and disliked by their peer group; (2) the number and quality of their friendships; (3) their social networks, with a particular concern for problematic peer affiliations; and (4) the degree to which children are victimized by peers.

ASSESSING PEER LIKING AND DISLIKING

In research studies, peer nominations and/or ratings are typically used to assess the degree to which a child is liked or disliked within a defined peer group (usually the classroom peer group) and to identify a child's sociometric status.

Sociometric Nominations

In early sociometric studies, individual investigators used a variety of questions to assess peer status, and typically focused on positive choices (whom children liked) rather than negative choices (whom children disliked) (Newcomb, Bukowski, & Pattee, 1993). However, as research accumulated, it became clear that wording was important, and that different kinds of questions elicited different information about peer preferences. In particular, researchers realized that questions about whom children liked in their peer group and questions about whom they disliked in that group tapped different dimensions of peer preference, not simply opposite poles of a unidimensional continuum (Coie, Dodge, & Kupersmidt, 1990; Newcomb et al.,1993; Peery, 1979). These two dimensions have different correlates: Peer liking is associated primarily with positive social behaviors, such as conversation skills, cooperative, and supportive behaviors, whereas peer disliking is linked with problematic behaviors, including aggression, disruptiveness, and anxiety–withdrawal (Coie et al., 1990). Certainly some children are liked by few classmates and disliked by many ("rejected" children), but other children are both liked and disliked by many classmates ("controversial" children), or liked and disliked by few classmates ("neglected" children) (Coie, Dodge, & Coppotelli, 1982). These distinctions have proven important in developmental studies. For example, across studies, rejected children are more likely than neglected children to be aggressive, inattentive, and disruptive; to express loneliness and social dissatisfaction; and to have cross-situational and stable adjustment difficulties (Asher, Parkhurst, Hymel, & Williams, 1990; Bierman, 1987; Coie et al., 1990).

This research led to the widely used convention of establishing sociometric status by asking children to name both the classmates they like ("like most" nominations) and the classmates they don't like ("like least" nominations). Although nominations are sometimes limited to the top three, unlimited nominations appear to have even stronger psychometric properties (Terry & Coie, 1991). An example of a sociometric interview is provided in Table 6.1. To score these measures, nominations are summed across classmates and divided by the number of raters, in order to compute a score representing the proportion of peers who particularly like or dislike each child. Scores are standardized within class or group, to control for differences in class size. In some cases, researchers score sociometric nominations within each gender rather than across the whole classroom—a decision that depends upon the goals and purpose of the assessment (for a review of these issues, see Foster, Bell-Dolan, & Berler, 1986). In the widely used Coie and Dodge (1983) system, two additional scores are calculated to assign sociometric status classification—social preference ("like most" minus "like least" nominations) and social impact ("like most" plus "like least" negative nominations) (Coie & Dodge, 1983). Five types of

TABLE 6.1. Example of a Sociometric Interview

Introduction: "I am interested in finding out how friendships have been going this year in your classroom. There are no right or wrong answers to these questions, and I won't be telling other kids what you say. I'm just really interested in finding out what you think."

Review of class roster: "I'm going to show you a list of the kids in your class. I'll read through the names, and I'd like you to tell me if there are any you don't know or who go by a nickname or different name."

Request for "like most" nominations: "There might be a lot of kids in the class who you like. I'd like you to tell me the kids in your class who you like the most—the ones who are your best friends in the class."

Request for "like least" nominations: "Even though you like almost everyone, there might be some kids in the class that you don't like quite as well as the other kids. I'd like you to tell me the kids that you don't like as well as the others."

Request for play preference ratings: "I'm interested in how much you like to play with different kids in the class. Next to the name of each person on the list, I'd like you to circle a number. If you like to play with the person all the time, every day, circle a 5. If you like to play with them most of the time, circle a 4. If you like to play with them some of the time, circle a 3. If you like to play with them every once in a while, circle a 2, and if you usually don't like to play with them, circle a 1.

Closure: "Well, that's all of my questions. I really appreciate your help, and I enjoyed talking with you. You can feel free to talk with your teacher or parent about this interview, but please do not tell the other kids your answers. Thanks again for helping me."

---

sociometric status are identified: "popular" (many "like most" and few "like least" nominations), "controversial" (many "like most" and many "like least" nominations), "neglected" (few "like most" and few "like least" nominations), "rejected" (few "like most" and many "like least" nominations), and "average." Rejected status is a valid predictor of current and future maladjustment, particularly when combined with elevated aggressive/disruptive behaviors or anxious withdrawal (Parker & Asher, 1987; Rubin & Stewart, 1996).

In general, "like most" and "like least" nomination scores are quite stable during the grade school years, with correlations in the range of $r = .50-.70$ for a 1-year period and $r = .30-.40$ over 3–4 years (Coie & Dodge, 1983). During the grade school years, on average, 12% of children meet the criteria for rejected status based on the nomination procedure (Coie et al., 1982); however, the actual prevalence depends upon the calculation methods used and cutoffs selected, which vary somewhat across studies (Hymel, Bowker, & Woody, 1993; Newcomb et al., 1993). For example, researchers often use a fairly stringent social preference cutoff of 1 standard deviation below the class mean to identify rejected children (Coie et al., 1983); this cutoff is sometimes relaxed to a slightly less stringent level (e.g., 0.8 standard deviations below the mean in Zakriski & Coie, 1996), identifying a slightly larger group of rejected children. Gender differences sometimes emerge, with boys receiving more negative sociometric scores that girls (O'Neil, Welsh, Parke, Wang, & Strand, 1997).

Although the specific number of "like most" and "like least" nominations a child receives depends in part upon the number of children in the classroom group who are providing nominations, striking differences often exist in the numbers of nominations received by children in different status groups. To give readers a sense of these differences, Table 6.2 provides the breakdown of raw nomination scores for 7,087 third-grade children participating in sociometric interviews as part of a longitudinal prevention program (the Fast Track project; Conduct Problems Prevention Research Group, 1992, 1999b). In these interviews, children were allowed unlimited nominations; thus their selections were unconstrained, and they could list as many children as they wanted. Under these conditions, it was very rare for a child to receive no "like most" nominations at all (only 5% of the sample received none,

TABLE 6.2. Number of Unlimited "Like Most" and "Like Least" Nominations Received by Children in Different Social Status Groups

Nomination type and social status group	Number of nominations				
	0	1–3	4–6	7–9	10+
"Like most" nominations					
Popular (n = 1,119)	0	4	232 (21%)	534 (48%)	349 (31%)
Average (n = 3,471)	0	969 (28%)	1,935 (56%)	529 (15%)	38 (1%)
Controversial (n = 395)	0	10 (2%)	215 (54%)	139 (35%)	31 (8%)
Neglected (n = 976)	98 (10%)	693 (71%)	185 (19%)	0	0
Rejected (n = 1,126)	261 (23%)	774 (69%)	91 (8%)	0	0
"Like least" nominations					
Popular (n = 1,119)	632 (56%)	487 (44%)	0	0	0
Average (n = 3,471)	441 (13%)	2,366 (68%)	637 (18%)	27(1%)	0
Controversial (n = 395)	0	114 (29%)	217 (55%)	64 (16%)	0
Neglected (n = 976)	361 (37%)	599 (61%)	16 (2%)	0	0
Rejected (n = 1,126)	0	68 (6%)	493 (43%)	366 (33%)	199 (18%)

Note. Data from Conduct Problems Prevention Research Group (1992).

and these were all children of "rejected" or "neglected" sociometric status). Among children of rejected status, 23% of them received no "like most" nominations, whereas 10% of the neglected-status children shared this unfortunate situation. Most children received 4 or more "like most" nominations, with most children of popular status receiving 7 or more (see Table 6.2). When the "like least" nominations are examined, it is clear that many children received a few (1–3) "like least" nominations from their classmates when classmates could give unlimited nominations. However, whereas the majority of children received no more than 3, almost all of the rejected children received 4 or more. Indeed, half of the rejected children received 7 or more "like least" nominations. These numbers provide a striking description of the unsupportive and often hostile interpersonal context that rejected children face in their classrooms, where they have very few or no classmates who like them and a large number of classmates who actively dislike them.

Peer Preference Ratings

Peer rating procedures have also been used to assess peer liking and disliking. In this procedure, initially developed by Roistacher (1974), children are given a roster with the names of all of their classmates, and a set of numbers (1–5) next to each name. Children are asked to circle a number next to the name of each individual to indicate the extent to which they like to play with that child (e.g., from 1 = "not at all" to 5 = "very much"). In some cases, children have been asked to rate the degree to which they would like to work with each classmate, as well as the degree to which they would like to play with each classmate—questions that elicit somewhat different assessments of peer preferences (Asher & Hymel, 1981). Asher and Hymel (1981) calculated separate "play with" and "work with" preference scores for individual children by averaging the ratings they received from each classmate on the two kinds of questions (other investigators have used just the "play with" ratings).

This rating scale technique has the advantage of providing data on how each group member feels about all others. It provides a score that is correlated with "like most" nominations ($r = .55$; Gresham, 1981), capturing each child's overall acceptability to peers. The average rating score on this measure does not distinguish well between rejected and neglected children, who both receive preference ratings at the low end of the distribution (Asher & Hymel, 1981). However, as described below, the measure can be scored in a way that provides a reasonable differentiation between rejected and neglected children (Asher & Dodge, 1986).

Concerns about Negative Nominations

Despite their documented validity, parents, school personnel, and researchers have all worried about whether sociometric procedures—particularly the solicitation of "like least" nominations—might increase the problems of disliked children. Although children are routinely asked to keep their nominations confidential, one study suggests that many (nearly 50%) violate this confidentiality agreement (Bell-Dolan, Foster, & Christopher, 1992). Even though children often gossip about peers they like and dislike, the possibility exists that adult interviews sanction this kind of negative talk about others in a way that might increase or validate negative gossip. The concern then is that sociometric nomination procedures might increase the social ostracism of unpopular children, leading to increases in negative peer treatment, and in the corresponding level of the children's distress (Asher & Hymel, 1981; Bell-Dolan, Foster, & Sikora, 1989).

However, studies designed to evaluate the potential negative effects of sociometric nominations have failed to document any increases in feelings of rejection or heightened peer negativity toward rejected children as a result of sociometric assessment (Bell-Dolan, Foster, & Sikora, 1989; Hayvren & Hymel, 1984). Even in the Bell-Dolan and colleagues (1992) study, in which 25% of the sample of third- through fifth-grade girls said that they disliked giving negative nominations and almost 50% talked with peers about their choices, the vast majority of children reported enjoying the interviews overall. In addition, a wide array of measures (including reports by the children, parents, and teachers) detected no negative impact on either rejected or non-rejected children as a result of these interviews.

Although no adverse effects have been documented for negative nomination procedures, two alternatives have been explored by researchers to provide similar information without directly asking children to identify classmates whom they "like least." One alternative involves the "repeated-positive-nominations" procedure, in which each child is given a class roster (or set of pictures) and asked to identify the classmate with whom he/she most likes to play. With that name (or picture) removed, the child is asked again to identify the classmate with whom he/she most likes to play (among those left). This process is repeated until the entire class has been rank-ordered. Compared with classifications based on standard "like most" and "like least" nominations, this repeated-positive-nominations technique correctly identified 82% of the rejected children, suggesting that it can provide a reasonable alternative for assessing peer rejection (Bell-Dolan, Foster, & Tishelman, 1989).

A second alternative, developed by Asher and Dodge (1986), utilized ratings of 1 on a peer preference rating scale as a proxy for negative "like least" nominations (the correlation between these two indices of rejection was $r = .80$). When 1 ratings were combined with "like most" nominations, 91% of the rejected children were identified accurately (compared to classification based upon traditional "like most" and "like least" nominations). Lewin, Davis, and Hops (1999) used peer preference ratings alone to create social preference scores by scoring ratings of 1 as "like least" nominations and ratings of 5 as "like most" nominations; however, standard sociometric scores were not available in their study to test the degree to which this scoring strategy replicated the more conventional nomination method.

Developmental Issues

Most of the research documenting the value and validity of sociometric nomination and rating measures has involved grade school children. However, nomination and rating procedures have also proven to be reliable with preschool and kindergarten children (Asher, Singleton, Tinsley, & Hymel, 1979; Brendgen, Vitaro, Bukowski, Doyle, & Markiewicz, 2001; Ladd & Mars, 1986; O'Neil et al., 1997). Simplified measures and individual administration are required. For example, rating scales for preschool children typically use a 3-point scale rather than a 5-point scale, and use pictures of faces (happy, neutral, sad) to indicate the rating anchors. Children are shown the picture of a classmate and asked to point to a face to show how much they like to play with that peer (Asher et al., 1979). Alternatively, they are given photographs of peers and asked to sort them into three containers marked with a smiling, neutral, or frowning face (Vaughn et al., 2000). With young preschool children, paired-comparison methods tend to be the most reliable, although somewhat tedious to administer (Vaughn et al., 2000). In this procedure, children are shown all possible pairs of photographs of classmates, and for each pair are asked to choose which child they especially like. Peer acceptance scores are calculated as the total number of choices received from peers divided by the number of classmate raters.

Among 3- to 4-year-old children, correlations between play ratings and sociometric nominations are in the .30–.40 range (Vaughn et al., 2000). Peer nominations are less stable at the preschool than at the grade school level, although stability correlations are significant at the preschool level (see Hymel, 1983, for a more detailed discussion of the use of sociometric measures with preschool children).

Teacher Simulations of Peer Nominations and Ratings

Although teacher assessments are considered less valid than assessments of peer preferences derived directly from peers, teachers have sometimes been asked to simulate peer "like most"and "like least" nominations or play preference ratings, particularly when the use of peer nominations or ratings is not possible. There is no standard way of gathering simulated teacher ratings. Working with preschool children, Connelly and Doyle (1981) asked teachers to rank-order the children in the classroom, according to the frequency and extensiveness with which each child was selected as a playmate by peers. Teacher ratings of child sociometric preference gathered in this way were correlated in the $r = .35-.55$ range with nominations given by preschool children when they were asked to select three children they most wanted to play with. Teachers have also been asked to identify, for each child in the classroom, the three positive nominations and three negative nominations they believe the child would make. Among grade school teachers, these kinds of simulated nominations were significantly correlated with peer positive and negative nominations collected in the conventional manner (r's $= .50$ and $-.59$, respectively; Landau, Milich, & Whitten, 1984). In another variation of teacher-simulated nominations, Rudolph and Clark (2001) provided teachers with descriptions of the five sociometric status categories (popular, controversial, average, neglected, and rejected) and asked teachers to identify the children who fit each category. Unfortunately, in that study they did not collect conventional peer nominations, so the degree of correlation between teacher-identified and peer-nominated sociometric status categories could not be compared.

These studies suggest that when peer ratings are not available, teacher ratings represent the next best alternative for the assessment of peer acceptance and rejection (Glow & Glow, 1980). However, it is important to note that despite significant correlations between teacher and peer ratings, correlations are rarely above the $r = .50$ level, suggesting that the more well-validated peer nomination or rating method should be used when possible.

ASSESSING FRIENDSHIPS

Assessing peer regard (including the degree to which a child is liked by and disliked by the peer group at large) is important, because it is this dimension of peer relations that has shown robust validity in longitudinal studies predicting mental health outcomes. However, other aspects of peer relations also appear to play an important role in shaping social development and affecting psychological well-being, notably a child's dyadic friendships (Parker & Asher, 1993a; Price & Ladd, 1986). Although measures of peer regard and sociometric status are collected from a group of peers, they are generally interpreted as measures that provide information about a child and that child's general capacity to get along with peers. This is particularly true for rejected status, which has proven to be fairly robust across peer contexts (Coie & Kupersmidt, 1983).

In contrast, by its very nature, a dyadic friendship is the product of the personal characteristics of both participating children, along with the dynamic transactions that have characterized their relationship history and circumstances (Parker & Asher, 1993a). Hence, whereas a child's peer group status is assessed by external raters (usually peers, sometimes teachers), the existence and quality of a child's mutual friendships cannot be assessed well without including the perspectives of the partners involved—the child and his/her friend. Although researchers have not reached a consensus regarding the optimal strategies for assessing friendships, they agree that it is important to assess both the child's participation in reciprocal friendships and the quality of those friendships.

Identifying Friendships

Both nominations and rating scales have been used to identify reciprocated friendships (Furman, 1996). For example, children are asked to nominate their three best friends, or to circle the names of their best friends on a classroom roster (Asher, Parker & Walker, 1996; Parker, & Asher, 1993b). Investigators have also designated reciprocated friendships when children nominated each other as someone they "like most" (see review by Newcomb & Bagwell, 1995), although assessments that specifically ask children to identify their friends provide a more precise identification of friendships than the more generic "like most" questions (Parker & Asher, 1993a). Friendships are considered "reciprocal" when both children nominate each other, and "unilateral" when only one child nominates the other. When the "three best friends" nomination method is used, on average 6%–11% of all children in the third through sixth grades of elementary schools are friendless (Parker & Asher, 1993a); however, the prevalence varies somewhat across studies, depending upon the number of nominations children are allowed and the specific criteria used to determine reciprocity (e.g., the children have each other on their list of friends vs. they both list each other first). Although less precise, researchers have also identified reciprocal friends on the basis of play preference ratings, considering children to be friends when they give each other the highest ratings (e.g., mutual ratings of 5 on the 1–5 scale) (Schwartz, McFadyen-Ketchum, Dodge, Pettit, & Bates, 1999). In some cases, researchers have used dual criteria, in which mutual friendships are those in which at least one member nominates the other as a "best friend," and both children give each other a rating of 4 or 5 on a play preference scale (Berndt, 1982). As Parker and Asher (1993a) have articulated, in addition to assessing participation in mutual friendships, a second issue involves the assessment of the quality of those friendships.

Perceptions of Friendship Quality

A number of measures have been developed to assess qualitative aspects of children's friendships. Most of them are designed for older grade school children or adolescents, and focus on measuring the unique characteristics hypothesized to account for the role friendships play in promoting social competence and emotional well-being. Six of the most commonly used measures are described below.

The Intimate Friendship Scale (Sharabany, 1994) uses 32 items to assess eight dimensions of friendship: frankness/spontaneity, sensitivity/knowing, attachment, exclusiveness, giving/sharing, imposition, common activities, and trust/loyalty. On this instrument, children are asked to identify one particular friendship and to rate it on a 6-point scale for each item (1 = "strongly disagree," 6 = "strongly agree"). Items include "I feel close to him/her," "I know which kinds of books, games, activities he/she likes," and "I can use his/her things without asking."

The Friendship Qualities Scale (Bukowski, Hoza, & Boivin, 1994) assesses the quality of children's and early adolescents' friendships in five domains: (1) companionship (e.g., "My friend and I spend all our free time together," "Sometimes my friend and I just sit around and talk about things like school, sports, and things we like"); (2) help/support (e.g., "If I forgot my lunch or needed a little money, my friend would loan it to me," "My friend would stick up for me if another kid was causing me trouble"); (3) security (e.g., "If I have a problem at school or at home, I can talk to my friend about it," "If my friend or I do something that bothers one of us, we can make up easily"); (4) closeness (e.g., "If my friend had to move away, I would miss him," "I feel happy when I am with my friend"); and (5) conflict (e.g., "My friend and I argue a lot," "My friend can bug me or annoy me even though I ask him not to").

Children identify a best friendship and rate that relationship on a

5-point scale (1 = "not true at all about the friendship," 5 = "really true") for each item. The scales have shown high levels of internal consistency (ranging from .71 to .86), have differentiated reciprocated from non-reciprocated friendships, and have predicted the stability of friendships (Bukowski et. al., 1994).

The Friendship Qualities Questionnaire (Parker & Asher, 1993b) contains 40 items, each rated on a 5-point scale, designating how true a particular quality is of a specific friendship (0 = "not at all true" to 4 = "really true"). Similar to the Bukowski and colleagues (1994) measure, the items tap multiple scales, including companionship and recreation (e.g., "do fun things together a lot"), help and guidance (e.g., "help each other with our school work a lot"), validation and caring (e.g., "cares about my feelings"), intimate exchange (e.g., "tell each other our problems"), conflict and betrayal (e.g., "argue a lot"), and conflict resolution ("make up easily when we have a fight"). Using this scale, Parker and Asher (1993b) demonstrated that the qualities of the best friendships of children who were not well accepted by the peer group were often inferior to those of well-accepted children. In addition, friendship quality made unique contributions to children's reports of loneliness (beyond those made by group acceptance and having a best friend).

Three additional scales warrant mention here, although they are not specifically measures of friendship quality. The following measures focus more broadly on a child's network of relationships and perceived support, although they include information about friendships as well.

The Friendship Questionnaire (Bierman & McCauley, 1987) focuses on the extensiveness of the peer network rather than the quality of friendships per se. It includes information about the degree to which friends are available to provide companionship across different social settings (in school and out of school), as well as the child's perception of exposure to negative peer treatment in these contexts. Children are asked to list their friends and to rate the extent to which they regularly experience specific positive and negative peer interactions in school and home settings. Items include "Is there someone who saves you a seat at lunch? (How often?)"; "Is there someone who teases and makes fun of you? (How often?)"; and "Is there someone you have sleep overnight at your house? (How often?)"

The Network of Relationships Inventory (Furman & Buhrmester, 1992) focuses on multiple close relationships, including siblings, parents, and romantic partners, as well as same-sex friends. It was designed to evaluate the functions of and subjective importance of relationships by asking young people about the quality of their interpersonal interactions. It also assesses multiple domains of relationship quality, such as conflict, intimacy, affection, and support. Items include "How much free time do you spend with this person?" and "How much do you share your secrets and private feelings with this person?"

Similarly, My Family and Friends (Reid, Landesman, Treder, & Jaccard, 1989) was designed to assess multiple relationships, but focuses on the support functions that various individuals fill for the child. In this individualized interview, the interviewer describes a particular social situation in one of five domains (emotional support, informational support, instrumental support, companionship, and conflict), and children name an individual who helps them and indicate how successful they are at eliciting the desired aid. Items include "Who do you go to when you want to share your feelings?"; "Who do you go to when there is something that you don't know too much about or when you need more information?"; and "Who do you go to when you want to hang out or do fun things?" This measure does not focus on friendships alone, but allows the evaluator to assess the extent to which friends are listed as sources of various types of support.

A note on the use of these measures with both parties in a friendship is in order here. When given to the target child alone, these friendship quality and social network measures provide an assessment of the child's perception of support derived from friendships, which is associated with other child feelings of social satisfaction and well-being (Parker & Asher, 1993b). To provide a full assessment of the relationship quality, however, the viewpoints of both participants—child and friend—must be considered (Price & Ladd, 1986).

ASSESSING SOCIAL NETWORKS

In addition to assessing the degree to which children are liked or disliked, and the number and quality of their reciprocated friendships, it can be useful to look at the characteristics of children's friends and affiliates. Although such characteristics are rarely included as an assessment index in social competence interventions, developmental research suggests that they can contribute in positive or negative ways to the child's social behavior. For example, aggressive children often choose to affiliate with each other, and when they do, the risk for the escalation of their aggressive and antisocial behavior over time is increased (Cairns, Neckerman, & Cairns, 1989). In addition, the degree to which children are isolated from or peripheral to particular social networks in the classroom could inform the choice of strategic peer partners for intervention.

A standard method of examining social network affiliations is to gather peer reports and then to construct a "social map" of relationships in a classroom (Cairns, Neckerman, & Cairns, 1989). A simpler method involves a more limited assessment of the affiliations of target children, without mapping the broader classroom context (Vitaro, Tremblay, Kerr, Pagani, & Bukowski, 1997). In general, neither method has been used to inform the design of or assess the impact of social competence interventions, although Farmer, Pearl, and Van Acker (1996) suggest that this perspective could be useful for both intervention design and evaluation.

Constructing Social Maps

The methods used by Cairns and his colleagues provide an example of network assessment involving social map construction. To elicit information from peers to construct maps, this research group conducts individual interviews that begin with this question: "Now tell me about your [school, class]. Are there some people who hang around together a lot?" Follow-up questions are used to identify the classmates constituting each cluster (Cairns, Cairns, Neckerman, Gest, & Gariepy, 1988; Cairns, Perrin, & Cairns, 1985). Decision rules have been established to combine information across child informants and to identify peer clusters in the social network and the relations among children in each cluster (Cairns et al., 1985). A computer program is available to score social maps (SCM 4.0 program) from the Center for Developmental Science at the University of North Carolina–Chapel Hill. The scoring program denotes the centrality of social clusters in the classroom (i.e., nuclear, secondary, or peripheral) and the centrality of each student in his/her cluster (i.e., nuclear, secondary, or peripheral). It also identifies children who are "isolates" and not associated with any cluster.

Problematic Peer Partnerships

Even when resources do not allow for a social mapping of the whole classroom, it may be useful to examine the behavioral characteristics of the peers that target children choose as their friends and affiliates. In this method, standard sociometric nominations and/or ratings are used to identify those peers with whom the child associates. Then the behavioral characteristics of those children (as rated by peers and/or teachers—see Chapter 7) are examined (Vitaro et al., 1997). This information could be used in intervention design, with efforts undertaken to strengthen affiliations with peers who could provide positive social models, and conversely to weaken affiliations with peers who may be reinforcing aggressive behaviors and antisocial attitudes. The next section describes assessment strategies for one additional aspect of peer relations—the degree to which children are experiencing victimization by peers.

ASSESSING VICTIMIZATION

Although rejected children are not liked by their classmates, they may or may not be the recipients of hostile treatment (Perry, Kusel, & Perry, 1988). Both peer reports and self-reports have been used to assess victimization.

Peer Reports

Peer nominations and ratings have been used to identify the degree to which various children are visibly victimized and harassed by their peers. For example, Graham and Juvonen (1998) asked middle school students to nominate peers who fit these descriptions: "gets picked on or pushed around" and "gets put down or made fun of by others." Egan and Perry (1998) used three similar items to assess victimization among elementary school students, adding them to the Peer Nomination Inventory rating form: "kids make fun of him," "he gets hit and pushed by other kids," and "he gets picked on by other kids" (see full description of this measure in Chapter 7).

In addition, multi-item peer rating scales have been developed to assess victimization. Perry and colleagues (1988) developed a peer nomination instrument, with 7 items describing hostile treatment by peers, which demonstrated a high level of internal consistency and stability (for 3-month stability, $r = .93$). Similarly, Crick and Bigbee (1998) developed a peer report version of the Social Experience Questionnaire (SEQ-P) to assess peer perceptions of children's positive and negative treatment by peers (there is also a parallel self-report version of this scale, the SEQ-S). This scale included two victimization scales, one involving overt aggression (6 items, including "gets hit a lot," "gets beat up," and "gets picked on by bullies") and one involving relational aggression (6 items, including "a kid tells lies about them so other kids won't like them anymore," "gets left out of something if someone is mad at them or wants to get even," and "other kids tell rumors about them behind their backs"). The third scale assesses positive treatment by peers (5 items, including "other kids say nice things about them," "other kids cheer them up when they are sad," and "other kids help them when they need it"). Crick and Bigbee found that girls were more likely to be relationally victimized, whereas boys were more likely to be overtly victimized, and that both forms of victimization were associated with peer rejection and feelings of loneliness.

Self-Reported Victimization

Self-report measures have also been developed to assess children's perceptions of peer victimization (Crick & Grotpeter, 1995; Kochenderfer & Ladd, 1996). Self-reports are only moderately correlated with peer reports; the reported correlations are in the range of .14–.42 (Ladd & Kochenderfer-Ladd, 2002). Self-reports tend to yield higher estimates of victimization, with some different correlates (Graham & Juvonen, 1998). That is, whereas peer nominations of victimization correlate most highly with sociometric measures of rejection, self-ratings of victimization correlate most highly with other psychological variables, including loneliness, social anxiety, and low self-worth (Graham & Juvonen, 1998). In an interesting longitudinal study, Egan and Perry (1998) found that self-perceptions may affect future risk for victimization. Low perceived competence and a sense of social inadequacy predicted an increase in victimization over time, beyond the risk predicted by specific behavioral problems that were visible to peers. In contrast, confidence in one's standing in the peer group served to protect behaviorally at-risk children from becoming victimized. Hence perceptions of victimization and associated feelings are important both in their own right, and also because of the vulnerability they create to future victimization and distress.

The specific rating items used to assess perceptions of victimization show some variability across studies, but usually include items describing physical, verbal, and relational aggression. For example, Kochenderfer and Ladd (1996) asked children to rate the extent to which they had experienced four kinds of aggression, using a 4-point scale (from 1 = "no, never" to 3 = "a lot"). Items included physical aggression (being hit by peers), direct verbal aggression (peers saying mean things to a child), indirect verbal aggression (peers saying bad things about a child to other kids), and general (being picked on by peers). In subsequent work, Ladd and Kochenderfer-Ladd (2002) evaluated the utility of an expanded self-report scale that included 12 victimization items, but they found that the additional items did not extend the validity of the scale. Four items appeared sufficient to assess the construct.

SUMMARY

Accessing the perspectives of the peers who constitute a child's social community at school provides a critical first step in an assessment of peer relations. Peer nomination and rating methods establish the degree to which a child is liked and disliked, provide information about reciprocated friendships, and identify a child's social status. Teachers provide the next best estimate of peer liking and disliking when peer respondents are not available, although it is easier for teachers to describe student behavior than it is for them to estimate the degree to which peers are attracted to (or repelled by) those students.

In addition to assessments of the degree to which a child is liked and disliked by the peer group with peer informants (ideally) or teacher informants (next best), both the child's and peers' perspectives are needed to assess the number and quality of the child's reciprocated friendships, the degree of child attraction to and affiliation with different social clusters in the classroom, and the degree to which the child is experiencing victimization by peers. At the same time, these measures do not describe the nature of children's behavioral difficulties with peers. As Parker and Asher (1993a) note, these measures describe *whether* a child is disliked, but not *why* a child is disliked. In the next chapter, I discuss strategies and measures designed to assess child social behavior.

Chapter 7

Assessing Social Behavior

*I*n addition to evaluating peer regard, assessments need to determine the nature and severity of the social behavior problems that may be contributing to children's peer difficulties. As noted in Chapters 1 and 2, most cases of peer rejection are related to problematic social behavior, including aggressive/disruptive, inattentive/immature, and/or avoidant/withdrawn behaviors, as well as prosocial skill deficits. Intervention designs need to take into account the pattern of problematic behavior shown by various children.

By the time children reach elementary school, peer and teacher informants are the best source of information regarding the children's typical social behavior. Teachers and peers have many opportunities to observe the children's customary behavior in peer interaction contexts, such as the classroom, lunchroom, and playground, whereas parents are less likely to have the same opportunities or normative base against which to evaluate their children's behavior with peers (Coie & Dodge, 1983). Teachers and peers are particularly reliable at rating overt behavioral excesses, such as aggressive behavior. Teacher and peer ratings do have their limitations, as they are subject to negative reputational biases, and are primarily useful in identifying the behavioral manifestations of a child's social difficulties rather than elucidating the kinds of feelings or thoughts that may underlie these social difficulties. This chapter discusses peer, teacher, and parent measures of child social behavior. The following chapters describe behavioral observation methods that can support a functional analysis of a child's behavior, including the contribution of peer responses (Chapter 8), and self-ratings that provide information about a child's thoughts and feelings (Chapter 9).

PEER NOMINATIONS AND RATINGS

During the grade school years, peer nominations and ratings are often used to describe the social behavior of children, as well as to assess peer liking and disliking. Behavioral measures help identify why a child is liked or disliked (Parker & Asher, 1993a).

Descriptive Peer Nominations

Using the same technique as that used to elicit "like most" and "like least" nominations, children may be asked to nominate classmates who fit various behavioral descriptions. For example, students may be asked to name the children in their classroom who "start fights or say mean things" or who "cooperate a lot—they help others and share" (see more examples in Table 7.1). Although this nomination method relies on scale scores comprising only a few items or even a single item, the availability of multiple peer informants provides a broad base for measurement. Indeed, this peer nomination method has proven effective in producing stable and predictive descriptions of children's social behavior (Coie & Dodge, 1988).

A more elaborate peer nomination method that yields behavioral descriptions is used by the Revised Class Play (RCP; Masten, Morison, & Pellegrini, 1985). In the RCP, children pretend to be the directors of a imaginary play who "cast" their classmates in a variety of positive and negative roles. Nominations of each type are then summed, so that

---

TABLE 7.1. Examples of Behavioral Nominations

Request for behavioral nominations: "I'm going to ask you about some things that kids might do. I'm going to ask you whether any of the kids in your classroom do these things."

Aggressive: "Some kids start fights, say mean things, or hit others. Who in your classroom does that?"

Hyperactive/disruptive: "Some kids get out of their seat a lot. They make a lot of noise and bother people who are trying to work. Who in your classroom does that?"

Withdrawn/anxious: "Some kids are shy and afraid. They play alone most of the time. Who in your classroom does that?"

Prosocial: "Some kids are friendly and cooperative. They help others and share. Who in your classroom does that?"

---

each child receives a score for three behavioral dimensions: (1) Sociability–Leadership (e.g., "good leader," "plays fair"); (2) Aggressive–Disruptive (e.g., "picks on other kids"); and (3) Sensitive–Isolated (e.g., "very shy"). A validation study involving students in grades 3–6 revealed that the three scores derived from this measure were reliable and stable at intervals of 6 and 17 months, and showed concurrent relations with other measures of competence. For example, scores on the Sociability–Leadership dimension were associated with other aspects of social and intellectual competence, whereas scores on the Aggressive–Disruptive and Sensitive–Isolated dimensions were associated with school adjustment difficulties (Masten et al., 1985).

Descriptive Peer Ratings

A second approach involves the use of a multi-item questionnaire, on which peers rate the behaviors shown by each classmate. This approach has the advantage of providing some information on all children in the classroom, in contrast to the nomination methods in which children are usually asked to pick one to three classmates for each item. A widely used peer rating measure is the Pupil Evaluation Inventory (PEI; Pekarik, Prinz, Liebert, Weintraub, & Neale, 1976). The original version of the PEI presents children with 35 items describing social behaviors, listed vertically on a page, and a roster containing the names of classmates, listed horizontally across the top of the page. Students place a check mark under the name of classmates who fit each behavioral description. Each child then receives a score indicating the proportion of classmates who rated him/her on each item. These items factor into three scales (Aggression, Withdrawal, and Likability), and have demonstrated a high level of reliability and predictive validity (Ledingham, 1981; Ledingham & Schwartzman, 1984).

A very similar approach is used by the Peer Nomination Inventory (PNI), developed originally by Wiggins and Winder (1961) and modified by Egan and Perry (1998). Like the PEI, the PNI presents children with behaviors and a roster of peers, and they check off the names of classmates who manifest the behavior described in each item. The revised measure factors into three scales (Egan & Perry, 1998): (1) Externalizing Problems, which include aggressive and disruptive behaviors (e.g., "he makes fun of people," "he hits and pushes others around," "he tells lies," "he makes noise or bothers you in class"); (2) Internalizing Problems, which include withdrawn, anxious, and depressed behaviors (e.g., "on the playground he just stands around," "he doesn't talk much," "he is afraid to do things," "he seems unhappy"); and (3) Social Skills (e.g., "in a group, he shares things and gives other people a turn," "he is always friendly").

In 1991, Pope, Bierman, and Mumma developed a revised version of the PEI (the PEI-R) by condensing the existing scales and adding items describing inattentive/immature and disruptive/hyperactive behaviors. Factor analyses verified the presence of five distinct dimensions of the peer perceptions of elementary school boys: Aggressive, Inattentive–Immature, Disruptive–Hyperactive, and Withdrawn–Internalizing behaviors, plus Likability (see Pope et al., 1991, for details; items are listed in Table 7.2). The distinction among the Aggressive, Disruptive–Hyperactive, and Inattentive–Immature dimensions is important, given research suggesting that disruptive and inattentive behaviors best differentiate aggressive children who are accepted from aggressive boys who are rejected by peers, with aggressive-rejected boys being more likely to show elevations on the Disruptive–Hyperactive and Inattentive–Immature scales (Bierman, Smoot, & Aumiller, 1993; Dodge & Coie, 1987; French, 1988; Miller-Johnson, Coie, Maumary-Gremaud, Bierman, & Conduct Problems Prevention Research Group [CPPRG], 2002). Information about the specific pattern of acting-out behaviors displayed by disliked children may assist in formulating hypotheses about core deficits that may need attention in intervention. For example, the disruptive and inattentive behavior problems exhibited by many aggressive children may reflect deficiencies in developmental capabilities to regulate negative affect in the context of interpersonal interactions (Calkins, 1994), impairing the children's ability to respond flexibly and strategically in emotionally arousing situations in order to engage in goal-directed social behavior (Eisenberg & Fabes, 1992).

In addition, a number of nonaggressive–rejected children exhibit inattention and negative affect. These children would be overlooked if measures such as the PEI-R assessed only aggressive behaviors, without separate scales assessing disruptive-hyperactive and inattentive-immature behaviors (Bierman et al., 1993). For example, Martin and colleagues (1994) found inattention to make separate and distinct contributions to the prediction of substance abuse, above the prediction made by aggressive and hyperactive behaviors. Pope and Bierman (1999) replicated this finding and additionally found that high Inattentive–Immature ratings in grade school contributed significantly (beyond the prediction based on Aggressive or Withdrawn–Internalizing alone) to the stability and severity of elementary school peer relation problems and adolescent rejection, victimization, and antisocial activity. Hence obtaining peer ratings on the dimensions of Disruptive–Hyperactive, Inattentive–Immature, and Aggressive behaviors, as well as Likability and Withdrawn–Internalizing behaviors, as provided by the PEI-R, can help specify the particular profile of problematic behavior that is disturbing to peers.

TABLE 7.2. Descriptive Peer Nomination and Rating Items

Aggressive (alpha = .92)

Those who start a fight over nothing
Those who make fun of people
Those who are mean and cruel to other children
Those who say they can beat everybody up
Those who act stuck up and think they are better than everyone else
Those who tell other children what to do
Those who try to get other people into trouble
Those who give dirty looks

Disruptive–Hyperactive (alpha = .85)

Those who get out of their seat a lot
Those who do strange things
Those who talk a lot
Those who fidget or move around in their seat a lot
Those who play the clown and get others to laugh
Those who run around the room a lot
Those who make a lot of noise
Those who bother people when they are trying to work

Inattentive–Immature (alpha = .80)

Those who don't pay attention the teacher
Those who can't sit still
Those who act like a baby
Those who are upset when called on to answer questions in class
Those who exaggerate and make up stories
Those who complain, nothing makes them happy

Withdrawn–Internalizing (alpha = .75)

Those who aren't noticed much
Those who are too shy to make friends easily
Those who are unhappy and sad
Those whose feelings are too easily hurt
Those who never seem to be having a good time
Those who are upset when called on to answer questions in class
Those who often don't want to play
Those who are usually chosen last to join in group activities
Those who have very few friends

Likability (alpha = .75)

Those who are especially nice
Those who are liked by everyone
Those who help others
Those who are your best friends
Those who always seem to understand things

Note. Items are drawn from the PEI-R (Pope, Mumma, & Bierman, 1991; Pekarik, Prinz, Liebert, Weintraub, & Neale, 1976).

Gender Differences

A recent study by Lewin, Davis, and Hops (1999) suggests that the factor structure of the PEI may be different for boys and girls. For example, whereas a clear overt aggression scale emerged for the boys (including items such as "start a fight over nothing," "mean and cruel to other children," "say they can beat everybody up"), for girls the item "mean and cruel to other children" was associated with domineering and snobbish behavior (e.g., "act stuck up," "tell other children what to do"), and the item "starts a fight over nothing" was associated with gossip ("exaggerates and makes up stories").

These findings underscore the recommendations made by Crick and colleagues (Crick & Bigbee, 1998; Crick, Casas, & Mosher, 1997; Crick & Grotpeter, 1995) that careful attention be paid to the assessment of relational as well as overt aggression in social assessments. As noted in earlier chapters, overt aggression involves the use or threat of physical damage to harm or intimidate others (e.g., pushing, hitting, kicking, or threatening to beat up a peer), whereas relational aggression involves the use or threat of social exclusion or the spreading of rumors. Crick and Grotpeter (1995) developed a peer nomination measure to access ratings for relational as well as overt aggression, called the Children's Social Behavior Scale. The Overt Aggression subscale of this measure consists of five items (e.g., "Name three classmates who start fights," "Name three classmates who hit or push others"); the Relational Aggression subscale consists of five items (e.g., "Name three classmates who tell their friends they will stop liking them unless their friends do what they say," "Name three classmates who try to keep certain people from being in their group when it's time to play"); and the Prosocial Behavior subscale consists of four items (e.g., "Name three classmates who do nice things for others," "Name three classmates who try to cheer up other kids when they're sad or upset"). Crick and Grotpeter report a high level of internal consistency (e.g., subscale alphas of .83, .94, and .91, respectively for Relational Aggression, Overt Aggression, and Prosocial Behavior), and a moderate correlation between Relational and Overt Aggression ($r = .54$), indicating distinct yet related constructs. Rejected children scored higher than popular children on both aggression scales. In addition, in research completed by Crick as well as by other investigators (Rys & Bear, 1997; Tomada & Schneider, 1997), aggressive boys often obtain high scores on both Overt and Relational Aggression, whereas aggressive girls are much less likely to score high on Overt Aggression than boys, more often being rated high on Relational Aggression alone. Hence a failure to assess Relational Aggression could result in an underidentification of at-risk girls.

Crick and colleagues have also developed and validated a pre-school version of her peer nomination measure (the Preschool Social Behavior Scale; Crick et al., 1997). For these young children, Crick and colleagues (1997) adapted the items and the presentation method. To administer this measure, the interviewer displays photographs of class-mates and then asks children to point to those who engage in various behaviors (e.g., "Point to the picture of a kid who pushes and shoves other kids").

Descriptive Peer Interviews

A third method of gathering information about children's social behav-ior from their classmates involves the use of semistructured interviews. For example, we (Bierman et al., 1993) conducted individual interviews with peers, asking them five open-ended questions about target chil-dren:

1. Describe [child's name]; tell me what he/she is like.
2. What might some children like about [child's name]?
3. What might some children not like about [child's name]?
4. Why might some children not want to be friends with [child's name]?
5. Why might some children want to be friends with [child's name]?

In addition to descriptions of aggressive, disruptive, and withdrawn be-haviors, this interview elicited comments about nonbehavioral charac-teristics and about insensitive or atypical behaviors that were affecting children's peer relations but were not well assessed by standardized teacher and peer ratings or by observations (Bierman et al., 1993). For example, in the Bierman and colleagues (1993) study, in addition to physical aggression, verbal aggression, rule violations, and shy behav-iors that were contributing to children's peer difficulties, open-ended interview responses elicited information about behaviors that children felt were atypical, annoying, and insensitive to peer norms. Atypical characteristics included features that peers described as non-normative or odd, such as physical disabilities or unusual appearance, whereas in-sensitive behaviors included behaviors that were non-normative and an-noying, such as peculiar habits, poor hygiene, and egocentric or imma-ture behaviors (e.g., "shows off," "acts like a baby"). These atypical characteristics and insensitive behaviors proved to be important distin-guishing characteristics of rejected children that were not well assessed by other measurement methods (e.g., observations, standard peer or teacher ratings) (Bierman et al., 1993; Bierman & Wargo, 1995).

Developmental Considerations

It is important to consider the developmental level of the participating children when one is selecting peer rating methods. Although even preschool children can give reliable behavioral descriptions of their classmates—that is, descriptions demonstrating test–retest and inter-rater consistency (Ladd & Mars, 1986)—their behavioral perceptions tend to be polarized and not well differentiated. For example, although young children differentiate prosocial behavior from problematic so-cial behavior (the good vs. bad dimension), they are less able than older children to make finer discriminations among different kinds of prob-lematic social behaviors, such as aggression versus withdrawal (Youn-ger, Schwartzman, & Ledingham, 1986). Hence, at the preschool level, teacher ratings may provide more valid and predictive behavioral de-scriptions of rejected children than peer ratings may (Connelly & Doyle, 1981). In particular, behaviors that are more subtle indicators of potential social difficulties, such as anxious withdrawal, are difficult to assess well with peer ratings at the preschool or early grade school level (Younger et al., 1986). At older ages, however, peers are the preferred raters, as their descriptions of child behaviors are more predictive of observed child social behavior than are teacher ratings (Landau, Milich, & Whitten, 1984).

Summary of Peer Nominations and Ratings

Several different types of measures have been developed to assess peer perceptions of classmates. With adaptations, several of these measures can be used at the preschool level. They are widely used at the grade school level and have also been used with adolescents (Graham & Juvonen, 1998; Parkhurst & Asher, 1992). Typically, an assessment would include a measure to indicate peer liking and disliking (e.g., "like most" and "like least" nominations or play preference ratings) and a measure to elicit behavioral descriptions (e.g., behavioral nominations or one of the peer rating inventories). In addition to peer ratings, teacher ratings provide a well-validated source of information about children's peer relations.

TEACHER RATINGS

A number of standardized teacher rating instruments have been devel-oped to assess child behavior in the school setting. Some of these measures were designed primarily for clinical purposes, to identify problem behaviors associated with conduct disorder, attention-deficit/ hyperactivity disorder (ADHD), or other related conditions (see McMahon & Wells, 1998, for a review). In terms of their utility for assessing and evaluating interventions targeting peer relations, teacher rating scales of child behavior problems are more useful when they (1) focus on the behavior problems linked with peer liking and disliking, including aggressive, hyperactive/disruptive, inattentive, and socially awkward/anxious behaviors; (2) focus on social behaviors that are commonly observed in the school classroom and playground setting; (3) use multipoint item rating systems, to provide sufficient variance to identify individual differences and detect intervention effects (e.g., 4- to 6-point rating scales for items rather than 2- to 3-point scales); and (4) are not overly long or cumbersome for teachers. For example, two measures commonly used in school-based research examining the behavioral correlates of peer problems are the Social Behavior Questionnaire (Tremblay et al., 1991; Tremblay, Pihl, Vitaro, & Dobkin, 1994; 22 items assessing antisocial behavior, hyperactivity/inattention, and anxiety/withdrawal) and the Walker Problem Behavior Checklist (Strain, Steele, Ellis, & Tim, 1982; Walker, 1983; 50 items assessing acting-out behaviors, distractibility, disturbed peer relations, withdrawal, and immaturity) (see also McMahon & Wells, 1989). In general, however, teacher rating scales that focus exclusively on problems are not as useful for assessments of social dysfunction as scales that include ratings of prosocial behaviors and other social skills. In this section, I focus on teacher rating measures that assess both social behavior problems and social competence. It should be noted that in addition to the measures developed specifically for teachers and described here, several of the peer rating inventories described earlier have been used as teacher rating measures. For example, the PEI (Pekarik et al., 1976) has demonstrated validity as both a teacher rating instrument and a peer rating measure (Ledingham, Younger, Schwartzman, & Bergeron, 1982).

First I consider two social competence measures that, although well validated and often used, consist of many items and are time-consuming to administer, yet result in rather undifferentiated assessments of child social behavior. Then I examine social competence measures that are more useful for intervention design because they provide more differentiated assessments, including separate subscales assessing the key behavioral correlates of peer status.

Measures That Provide "Broad-Band" Ratings of Social Behavior

Initial scales developed to assess social competence involved relatively long scales with many items describing discrete social behaviors. Although these measures are still commonly used, and this approach results in social competence scores that are reliable and valid, the scales are time-consuming to administer due to their length, and result in relatively undifferentiated assessments of child social behavior problems.

For example, the Matson Evaluation of Social Skills with Youngsters (MESSY; Matson, Rotatori, & Helsel, 1983) was one of the first comprehensive teacher rating measures designed specifically to assess children's social skills. The measure was designed to assess the social skills of children with a variety of developmental, behavioral, and educational disabilities, across a wide age range. The measure has 64 items, each rated on a 5-point Likert scale, which are scored into a behavior problem scale (labeled Inappropriate Assertiveness/Impulsiveness) and a social competence scale (labeled Appropriate Social Skills). The problem scale includes 38 items describing a range of aggressive, domineering, dishonest, impulsive, and intrusive behaviors. The social competence scale includes 20 items describing prosocial behaviors and positive communication skills.

The Walker–McConnell Scale of Social Competence and School Adjustment (Walker & McConnell, 1988) includes 43 behavioral items, each rated on a 1 ("never") to 5 ("frequently") Likert scale, which are scored into three scales. A scale labeled Teacher Preferred includes 15 items that focus primarily on self-regulation (e.g., "can accept not getting his/her own way," "controls temper"). A scale labeled Peer Preferred includes 18 items describing peer interaction and communication (e.g., "invites peers to play and share activities," "plays or talks with peers for extended period of time"). The third scale, School Adjustment Behaviors, includes 10 items describing work habits and attention (e.g., "has good work habits," "listens carefully to teacher instructions.") The scales are psychometrically sound with regard to both test–retest reliability and internal consistency (Lewin et al., 1999; Walker & McConnell, 1988), and provide more differentiation than the MESSY. Nonetheless, the scale labels are somewhat misleading (as both self-regulation and prosocial behavior are valued by teachers and peers alike), and the measure uses more items to describe fewer dimensions of social behavior than alternative scales described below, making it less efficient.

Measures That Provide Differentiated Assessments of Social Behavior

Over the last two decades, considerable effort has gone into the development of teacher rating measures to assess children's social behavior. In general, the trend has been to move away from assessments of a few broad-band dimensions (such as those represented by the MESSY and the Walker–McConnell Scale) toward assessments of more differenti-ated dimensions that better reflect the domains of behavioral corre-lates of peer status: (1) high rates of aggressive/disruptive behaviors, (2) high rates of inattentive/immature behaviors, (3) low rates of prosocial behaviors, and (4) high rates of socially anxious/avoidant be-haviors (see Chapter 2).

In addition, whereas the items in earlier scales were often more narrowly defined behaviors (e.g.,"compliments others regarding per-sonal attributes," "maintains eye contact when speaking to or being spoken to"), most of the more recent scales use items that refer to more general classes of behavior (e.g., "fights," "inattentive"). In large part, these changes reflect developments in the conceptualization of so-cial competence and in the study of the correlates of peer acceptance and rejection. Conceptually, the field has moved away from a model of social competence based on a set of discrete behaviors, to a model that understands social competence in terms of a child's capacity to regu-late and organize behavior in social contexts. Correspondingly, it makes less sense to ask teachers to identify specific, discrete behavioral deficits; rather, greater utility results from using teacher ratings to assess more general classes of behavioral excesses and deficits. Four measures that reflect this "competence correlates" approach to social competence assessment are described next.

The Teacher–Child Rating Scale

The Teacher–Child Rating Scale (T-CRS; Hightower et al., 1986) is a 36-item measure designed to provide further differentiation in the as-sessment of child behavior problems and social competence by includ-ing 36 items assessing six dimensions of child adjustment (three dimen-sions of problems and three dimensions of competence). Items are rated on a 5-point scale (for problem items, 1 = "not a problem" to 5 = "very serious problem"; for competence items, 1 = "not at all" to 5 = "very well"). Each scale consists of six items. The problem scales are Acting Out (e.g., "disruptive in class," "fidgety," "overly aggressive to peers"); Shy–Anxious ("withdrawn," "anxious, worried," "unhappy, de-pressed, sad"); and Learning Problems ("underachieving," "poor work habits," "limited attention," "difficulty following directions"). The com-petence scales are Frustration Tolerance (e.g., "accepts things not going his/her way," "mood is balanced and stable," "copes well with failure"); Assertive Social Skills ("defends own views under group pres-sure," "comfortable as a leader," "questions rules that seem unfair/ unclear"); and Task Orientation (e.g., "completes work," "well orga-nized," "works well even with distractions"). In a set of validation stud-ies, more than 200 teachers rated 1,379 children in grades K–6 on the

T-CRS, in a variety of urban and suburban schools (Hightower et al., 1986; Work, Hightower, Fantuzzo, & Rohrbeck, 1987). Test–retest reliability coefficients (10-week and 20-week) ranged from .61 to .88 (median = .85) for each of the three problem subscales, and from .64 to .91 (median = .76) for each of the three competence subscales. The median internal-consistency coefficient over the six subscales was .91 (Cronbach's alpha). All scales were significantly correlated with standardized reading achievement scores, parent ratings of child behavior problems, math grades, and teacher ratings. All scales except Acting Out correlated significantly with child self-reports of anxiety and emotional distress. In addition, children referred for mental health services within the school showed more problematic scores than a normative, nonreferred matched sample on all scales except Assertive Social Skills.

The Child Behavior Scale

The Child Behavior Scale (CBS; Ladd & Profilet, 1996) was developed specifically to assess the social behavior of young children during the preschool and early school years. The goal was to assess six distinct behavioral constructs related to peer status: Aggressive behaviors, Hyperactive–Distractible behaviors, Prosocial behaviors, and three different patterns of withdrawn behavior (Asocial behaviors, Anxious–Fearful behaviors, and being Excluded by Peers). The seven-item Aggressive subscale assesses physical and verbal forms of aggression (e.g. "fights," "bullies," "argues"; alpha = .89–.92; test–retest r = .69–.71). The four-item Hyperactive–Distractible subscale includes overactive and inattentive items (e.g., "restless," "squirmy," "inattentive"; alpha = .88–.93; test–retest r = .82–.83). The seven-item Prosocial subscale assesses empathic and cooperative behaviors (e.g., "helps," "recognizes feelings," "cooperative"; alpha = .91–.92; test–retest r = .62–.65). The six-item Asocial subscale describes self-imposed solitude (e.g., "prefers to play alone," "avoids peers"; alpha = .87–.89; test–retest r = .54–.59). In contrast, the seven-item Excluded by Peers subscale describes peer ostracism (e.g., "not much liked," "excluded from peers' activities"; alpha = .93–.96; test–retest r = .67–.72)). Finally, the four-item Anxious–Fearful subscale assesses emotional distress (e.g., "is worried," "fearful or afraid," "cries easily"; alpha = .77–.79; test–retest r = .59–.68). In a study involving 412 kindergarten children, the scales all showed high levels of internal consistency and moderate to strong levels of stability over the 4-month period between the fall and spring school assessments (Ladd & Profilet, 1996). A regular pattern of significant correlations emerged between teacher ratings on this measure and observations and observer ratings of child behavior in the kindergarten classroom.

The Teacher Observation of Child Adaptation—Revised

The Teacher Observation of Child Adaptation—Revised (TOCA-R; Werthamer-Larsson, Kellam, & Wheeler, 1991) was designed to assess the behavior and adjustment of grade school children. It includes three scales, each composed of items rated on a 6-point scale (1 = "almost never" to 6 = "almost always"). The 10-item Authority Acceptance scale assesses aggressive and disruptive behaviors (e.g., "stubborn," "fights," "breaks rules," "yells at others"). The 12-item Cognitive Concentration scale assesses school performance, including distractibility and concentration (e.g., "pays attention," "works well alone," "completes assignments," "stays on task"). The four-item Social Contact scale describes sociability vs. withdrawal (e.g., "loner," "avoids social contact," "plays with others," "social contact with others"). A validation study including ratings on 1,471 children, and 1-month test–retest assessments for a subsample, revealed strong psychometric properties.

In 1998, the CPPRG added a 9-item scale (called the Social Health Profile or SHP) to the TOCA-R to provide a social competence subscale. This scale includes 9 items describing prosocial behaviors (e.g., "friendly," "helpful to others," "understands others") and emotional regulation (e.g., "controls temper," "thinks before acting"). The SHP demonstrated predictive validity for peer nominations, with teacher ratings collected at the end of kindergarten predicting peer sociometric nominations collected a year later at the end of first grade (r = .25 with "like most" nominations and r = −.28 with "like least" nominations.)

The Cassidy and Asher Scale

Cassidy and Asher (1992) developed an even shorter teacher rating scale, using three items to tap each of four subscales: Aggressive Behavior ("starts fights," "mean to others"); Disruptive Behavior ("acts up in class," "interrupts others"); Prosocial Behavior ("cooperates," "friendly and nice"); and Shy/Withdrawn ("does not play much with other children," "seems fearful of others"). To reduce potential response bias, each item was listed on the top of a page, with child names listed down the side. Each child was rated on a 5-point scale from 1 ("very uncharacteristic") to 5 ("very characteristic"). Used with a sample of 457 kindergarten and first-grade children, the scale revealed a good four-factor structure, and high levels of correlation with peer nominations (r's = .75 for Aggressive Behavior, .40 for Shy/Withdrawn, and .69 for Prosocial Behavior).

Comparing Measures

When one compares the scale and item focus of these four measures, one can see a growing consensus regarding the dimensions of social behavior that warrant evaluation in social competence assessments. Table 7.3 illustrates the items that, across these measures, tap into the four behavior pattern correlates of peer rejection identified in Chapter 2 (i.e., aggressive/disruptive behaviors, inattentive/immature behaviors, low rates of prosocial behaviors, and socially anxious/avoidant behaviors). Consistent with evidence linking aggressive behaviors to peer rejection, the teacher rating scales each contain multiple items representing this domain. Five items have nearly identical wording on two or more of the scales. Similarly, the dimension of inattentive/ immature behaviors is represented on all three measures, although its label and factor structure vary across measures. A dimension of prosocial and self-regulatory behaviors is also represented on each of the four scales, although there is relatively little content overlap in the items selected to represent this dimension across the four scales. Finally, the dimension of shy and anxious/avoidant behaviors is represented on each scale, with six items having nearly the same wording on two or more scales. The overlap in behavioral dimensions and item content represents the beginning of some consensus regarding the behavioral correlates of child social adjustment that can be accurately assessed by classroom teachers.

Despite this growing consensus, there are certainly still areas of difference among scales assessing social competence and their conceptual foundations. For example, in some scales inattentive behaviors are assessed as part of a broader dimension of school performance (the TOCA-R), whereas in other scales they are assessed with hyperactive behaviors as part of a broader dimension of ADHD symptoms (the CBS). The degree to which hyperactive/disruptive behaviors are differentiated from hostile/aggressive behaviors also varies across scales (one dimension in the TOCA-R and T-CRS; separate dimensions in the CBS and the Cassidy & Asher scale). Finally, in some scales, items describing prosocial behaviors (friendly, cooperative, kind behaviors) are considered separately from self-regulatory behaviors (capacity to cope with frustration and to control temper), whereas in other scales these dimensions are combined. Communication skills are represented in some scales of prosocial behaviors and not others. There are also teacher rating measures that have been developed to tap specific aspects of social behaviors for particular studies. For example, Crick and her colleagues developed the Children's Social Behavior Scale— Teacher Form (Crick, 1996) and the Preschool Social Behavior Scale—

TABLE 7.3. Comparison of Teacher Rating Measure Items That Address Dimensions of Social Behavior Associated with Peer Sociometric Evaluations

Dimension of behavior and item content	T-CRS	CBS	TOCA-R with SHP	Cassidy & Asher
Aggressive/disruptive behaviors				
Fights	×	×	×	×
Aggressive	×	×	×	
Fidgety, difficulty sitting still	×	×		
Stubborn	×		×	
Disruptive	×			×
Disturbs others while they are working	×			
Constantly seeks attention	×			
Teases		×	×	
Bullies		×		
Kicks, bites, hits		×		
Threatens		×		
Argues		×		
Restless		×		
Takes others' property			×	
Lies			×	
Yells at others			×	
Breaks things			×	
Trouble accepting authority		×		
Breaks rules		×		
Mean to others			×	
Hurts others			×	
Acts up in class			×	
Interrupts others			×	
Inattentive/immature behaviors				
Poor concentration	×	×	×	
Inattentive		×	×	
Difficulty following directions	×			
Poor work habits	×		×	
Completes assignments	×		×	
Distractible	×		×	
Self-reliant	×		×	
Works well without support	×		×	
Underachieving	×		×	
Poorly motivated to achieve	×		×	
Well organized	×			
Carries out requests responsibly	×			
Stays on task			×	
Mind wanders			×	
Prosocial and self-regulatory behaviors				
Helps	×		×	×
Understands others' feelings	×		×	

TABLE 7.3. (*continued*)

Dimension of behavior and item content	T-CRS	CBS	TOCA-R with SHP	Cassidy & Asher
Kind	×			
Cooperative	×		×	
Concerned about others	×			
Concern for moral issues	×			
Accepts things not going his/her way		×		
Mood is balanced and stable		×		
Copes well with failure		×		
Has a good sense of humor		×		
Generally relaxed		×		
Friendly			×	×
Suggests without bossiness			×	
Controls temper in a disagreement			×	
Resolves problems on own			×	
Appropriate expression of feelings			×	
Thinks before acting			×	
Can calm down when excited or upset			×	

Shy, anxious/avoidant behaviors

Dimension of behavior and item content	T-CRS	CBS	TOCA-R with SHP	Cassidy & Asher
Withdrawn	×	×		×
Worried	×	×		
Shy, timid	×			
Nervous, fearful, afraid	×	×		×
Does not express feelings	×			
Unhappy, depressed, sad	×			
Prefers to play alone		×	×	×
Likes to be alone/loner		×	×	
Solitary child		×	×	
Avoids peers		×	×	
Keeps peers at a distance		×		
Appears miserable, distressed		×		
Cries easily		×		

Note. Items with similar wording were placed in the same category, as were items that referred to the same behavior but with reversed scoring (e.g., "inattentive" and "good attention span"). For comparison purposes, items are grouped by conceptual category based on item content, which is not necessarily the category in the reported factor structure for the instrument.

Teacher Form (Crick et al., 1997) to assess relational aggression (e.g., "this child spreads rumors or gossips about some peers") separately from overt aggression (e.g., "this child hits, shove, or pushes peers").

Ultimately, the degree to which different dimensions of behavior should be discriminated on teacher rating measures will become clear as the research base continues to grow, indicating the reliability and relative utility of those discriminations for the prediction of social adjustment and for intervention design and evaluation. For the present, researchers and clinicians should select the empirically validated measure that best suits their goals and target participants.

Task-Focused Assessments of Social Competence

One additional approach to teacher assessments of child social competence warrants discussion. The two teacher rating measures described below were designed with the goal of providing more differentiation regarding the specific types of skill deficits various children were experiencing. Each of them focused on defining key social tasks and asking teachers to rate children's ability to cope appropriately with those social tasks. The idea was that the assessment of children's social competence should be contextualized, with an emphasis on identifying the social challenges or social contexts that were most problematic for various children. Conceptually, this kind of specific assessment of the social tasks that were problematic for children might directly inform intervention design.

For example, the Teacher Rating of Social Skills—Children (TROSS-C; Clark, Gresham, & Elliott, 1985) includes 52 items designed to assess children's social skills in regard to the social tasks of initiating interactions (15 items—e.g., "invites peers to play," "appropriately joins an activity or group"); sustaining interactions with cooperative behaviors (17 items—e.g., "waits turn when playing a game," "follows rules when playing games"); and being a reinforcing and rewarding playmate (7 items—e.g., "praises peers," "congratulates peers on accomplishments"). Teachers rate each item on a 3-point scale (ranging from 0 = "not true of the student" to 3 = "very true or often true of the student"). Scores on this measure were moderately correlated with academic achievement scores (median r = .63) and (inversely) with school behavior problems (Clark et al., 1985). However, correlations with peer preference measures were not provided, making it difficult to determine which dimensions contribute uniquely to peer liking and disliking.

The Taxonomy of Problem Situations (TOPS; Dodge, McClaskey, & Feldman, 1985) took the task-focused assessment approach one step further by drawing on the research literature to identify a set of socially challenging tasks (critical events) that would differentiate peer-rejected from peer-accepted children. The resulting 60-item inventory asks teachers to rate how likely a particular child is to respond inappropriately in various situations (each item is rated on a 5-point scale, from "never" to "almost always"). Eight subscales define child skill at the following social tasks: (1) Peer Group Entry ("when a group of peers have started a club or group and have not included this child"); (2) Response to Provocation ("when peers call this child a bad name"); (3) Response to Success ("when this child has won a game against a peer"); (4) Response to Failure ("when a peer performs better than this child in a game"); (5) Ability to Meet Peer Expectations ("when a peer tries to start a conversation with this child"); (6) Ability to Meet Teacher Expectations ("when the teacher is trying to speak to the whole class"); (7) Reactive Aggression ("when this child has been teased or threatened, he gets angry easily and strikes back"); and (8) Proactive Aggression ("when this child threatens or bullies others in order to get his own way"). The original research on this measure demonstrated strong internal-consistency and test–retest reliabilities, and showed that younger children received lower scores on all scales than older children, reflecting the scales' sensitivity to aspects of developmental competence (Dodge et al., 1985). A subsequent study by Volling, MacKinnon-Lewis, Rabiner, and Baradaran (1993) demonstrated that children who were sociometrically rejected had significantly more inappropriate scores on all scales than did children who were popular, neglected, or average in sociometric status. Interestingly, children who had controversial status obtained scores similar to those of rejected children on all scales except for the Ability to Meet Teacher Expectations and Ability to Meet Peer Expectations scales.

Although, intuitively, assessments that tap child competence in reference to specific social tasks are consistent with the conceptualization of social competence as an organizational construct, thus far research has not supported the idea that the TROSS-C or TOPS approach to classifying children has predictive validity or can inform intervention. This approach may share the fate of measures that attempted to assess discrete behavioral skills. In contrast, the developmental literature does provide evidence that classifying children based upon their social behavioral profiles (e.g., aggressive, inattentive, anxious/withdrawn) has predictive significance. For example, children who are both aggressive and withdrawn are at more risk for stable problems and peer rejection than aggressive, nonwithdrawn children (Ledingham & Schwartzman, 1984); aggressive, hyperactive, and inattentive/immature behaviors each make unique contributions to children's risk for peer rejection (Flanagan, Bierman, Kam, & CPPRG, in press; Pope et al., 1991). Hence, currently, the teacher measures that provide the capacity to assess child profiles across behavioral domains appear more likely to inform interventions than those focused on social tasks. Nonetheless, additional research that directly examines the utility of these different approaches to assessment for the purpose of designing and evaluating social competence interventions is needed.

PARENT RATINGS

In addition to teacher and peer ratings, parent ratings can be used to describe children's social behavior. Although parents often have trouble estimating the overall quality of their children's peer relations (Graham & Rutter, 1968), they can provide useful information in several other areas relevant to child social adjustment. First, parent ratings can provide information about behavior problems in the home setting that may be interfering with social adjustment, including aggressive and noncompliant behaviors and anxious withdrawal (see McMahon & Wells, 1998). For example, Schwartz and colleagues (1999) found that peer-nominated social preference was significantly correlated with maternal ratings on the Child Behavior Checklist scales of Social Problems ($r = -.23$ to $-.26$), Attention Problems ($r = -.35$ to $-.31$), and Aggression ($r = -.25$ to $-.28$). Similarly, French and Waas (1985) found that maternal reports of externalizing problems, social withdrawal, and activities/social competence on the Child Behavior Checklist differentiated children who were rejected by peers from children who were average or popular in status. These results suggest that a number of rejected children have behavior problems in both home and school settings, and that maternal reports can be useful in identifying home-based behavioral difficulties that may be associated with peer problems.

In addition, several teacher rating forms have parallel versions designed for parents to report on the aspects of social competence they observe in their children, including the TROSS-C (Clark et al., 1985) and the MESSY (Bell-Dolan & Allan, 1998). Bell-Dolan and Allan (1998) report correlations between parent and teacher ratings on the MESSY ranging from $r = .32$ (for the Appropriate Social Skills scale) to $r = .39$ (for the Total score)—levels of association that are equivalent to the expected degree of cross-situational consistency in children's behavior (Achenbach, McConaughy, & Howell, 1987). At the same time, identification of extreme groups of children with social dysfunction in the Bell-Dolan and Allan (1998) study resulted in nearly nonoverlapping groups when parent and teacher ratings on the MESSY were compared.

A 12-item Social Competence Scale was developed by the CPPRG (1998) to complement parent ratings of child behavior problems. This measure includes two factorially derived subscales—one assessing prosocial behaviors (e.g., "helpful to others," "shares things with others," "listens to others' point of view"; alpha = .82) and one assessing self-regulatory behaviors (e.g., "accepts things not going his/her way," "controls temper in a disagreement," "can calm down when excited"; alpha = .78). Parent ratings were significantly correlated with concurrent teacher ratings of social competence ($r = .32$), and were also significantly correlated with peer positive and negative nominations (r's = .29 and –.30, respectively).

In addition to standardized ratings, parents may provide information about the number of peer contacts their child has outside school and the characteristics of those peers, which may facilitate intervention planning. In this area, parents may provide a unique source of information, as teachers and classroom peers may have little knowledge of a child's social contacts or behavior outside of the school. Parents are often the only source (other than the child him-/herself) who can describe the social opportunities available to the child outside school, including the child's social interests and leisure time pursuits, and the characteristics of the child's social affiliates—information that can guide intervention efforts.

SUMMARY

Accessing the perspectives of members of the child's social community at school, including peers and teachers, provides a critical first step in an assessment of peer relations. Peer nomination and rating methods establish the degree to which a child is liked and disliked, provide information about reciprocated friendships, and identify a child's social status. These methods can also be used to provide descriptive information about behavioral factors contributing to peer difficulties, such as high levels of aggressive/disruptive, anxious/withdrawn, and inattentive/immature behaviors, and low levels of prosocial/cooperative behaviors. A number of teacher rating scales have been developed and validated for the specific purpose of assessing behavior problems and aspects of social competence that have a central influence on the quality of children's peer relationships. These measures focus on the behaviors that are easily observed in schools by teachers, and are empirically linked with peer liking and disliking. They also capitalize on psychometric strategies (multi-item scales, multipoint response formats) that produce more normally distributed scores, providing greater sensitivity to individual differences and change produced by intervention. Reflecting our developing understanding of social competence as an organizational construct, involving the capacity to regulate and organize behavior in social contexts, these teacher rating measures focus on functional dimensions of behavior rather than providing inventories of discrete social behavior.

Although parents often know less about the peer experiences their children have at school than peers and teachers, and are therefore less reliable assessors of child peer relation quality, parental perspectives can contribute to assessments in several key ways. Parents can provide information about child social behaviors at home. Although home behavior is often only mildly to moderately related to behavior at school (Achenbach et al., 1987), it broadens the cross-context understanding of the child's social adjustment. Parents can also provide important information about the quality and quantity of the child's interactions with peers outside the school context, which can guide intervention efforts.

8 Chapter 8

Observing Peer Interactions

Peer and teacher ratings establish the degree to which a child is liked and disliked by classroom peers, and provide information about general patterns of social behavior that contribute to peer difficulties. At the same time, both peer and teacher perspectives are subject to observer biases and can be colored by the child's social reputation (Hymel, Wagner, & Butler, 1990). Neither teachers nor peers typically have opportunities to systematically observe and analyze the specific characteristics of a child's social interaction sequences—information that can be helpful in formulating functional models of the stimuli and contingencies supporting problematic behaviors (Coie & Dodge, 1988). Observational methods can "fill in the gaps" existing in the broad-brushstroke assessments given by teachers and peers, allowing for a more specific, carefully quantified, and contextualized assessment of the child's social behavior.

Observations can play a particularly important role in the planning and evaluation of social interventions. Conceptually, observing children in challenging social situations provides an optimal opportunity to evaluate their capacity to organize their social behavior under conditions of affective engagement and arousal, and also to understand the specific patterns of reactivity and contingent responsivity that characterize their relationships with particular peers. As such, observations enable a case-specific functional analysis of a child's social interaction difficulties. Even among children who are rated by peers and teachers as rejected and behaviorally problematic (e.g., aggressive or avoidant), there is variability in the way in which their difficulties "play out" in their peer interactions. Observations can supplement peer and teacher ratings by providing specific details about the qualitative features of a child's interactive style that reflect his/her social competence and capacity to achieve peer acceptance. Observations also enable an assessment of the peer responses a child actually elicits, and the treatment the child receives from peers. In addition, observations including peers allow for an evaluation that is grounded in local norms, as the child's behavior can be evaluated in relation to other children of the same age, cultural group, and gender.

At the same time, observations can be time-consuming and difficult to code with reliability in field settings. Typically, researchers and practitioners have different goals in conducting observations. Developmental researchers often use observations of children with different social reputations (e.g., rejected vs. accepted, aggressive vs. non-aggressive) to understand how behavioral interaction patterns characterize and differentiate particular groups of children. Researchers evaluating social competence interventions often use observations to select groups of children with certain patterns of social skill deficits for intervention trials, and also use these observations to determine whether an intervention has had an impact on behavior change. In contrast, practitioners who are trying to tailor an intervention to meet the needs of a particular child are interested in the interactional experiences of that particular child in the context of his/her usual peer group.

This chapter relies heavily on the research literature to describe two sets of contexts for observational assessment: (1) the naturalistic settings of the classroom or playground; and (2) contrived contexts that simulate the interpersonal complexity of the naturalistic context, or provide analogue tasks designed to assess child capabilities in social challenge situations. At the end of the chapter, I consider the implications of observational research for practitioners, and describe observational strategies that may have utility in typical applied settings.

NATURALISTIC OBSERVATIONS

The school setting is the most common location for naturalistic observations. Classroom observations are often used, particularly at the pre-school level. In grade school, unstructured situations, such as recess, lunch, or transition periods in the classroom, provide a better opportunity to observe the quality of peer interactions than do structured classroom situations, although in the classroom one can assess inattentive and disruptive behavior (Foster & Ritchey, 1985). Examples of both types of observations are provided.

Classroom Observations

A good example of a classroom observation system comes from a study completed by Lewin, Davis, and Hops (1999). When the children in this study were in grades 2–5, classroom observations were conducted with a modified version of the Contingencies for Learning Academic Social Skills (CLASS) observational system (Hops & Walker, 1988). During 5-second recording intervals, four types of student behavior were counted: (1) appropriate peer social behavior, (2) inappropriate peer social behavior, (3) on-task behavior (appropriate academic or related tasks), and (4) off-task behavior (inappropriate or disruptive behavior). Four types of behavior directed by the teacher toward the target child were also observed: (1) approval (praise), (2) disapproval, (3) verbal (those comments other than approvals or disapprovals), and (4) attending (listening, watching, or viewing). Approximately 15 minutes of data were collected on each child. The CLASS observational system proved reliable (mean percentage of interrater agreement was 73%; mean kappas ranged from .89 to .97). When the behavioral codes were entered into a factor analysis along with multiple measures of prosocial, academic, and withdrawn behaviors, the on-task and teacher disapproval codes loaded on the Academic Behavior factor for both boys and girls, along with teacher ratings of academic performance and attentiveness. (As noted below, observations completed on the playground for this study loaded with factors representing Prosocial Behavior and Withdrawn Behavior, suggesting that observations in classroom vs. playground settings tap different dimensions of behavior.)

A second example regarding the utility of classroom observations comes from a study conducted by Gottman, Gonso, and Rasmussen (1975). In this study, observers began by picking a child, observing that child for ten 6-second intervals (using a clipboard with a 6-second light-emitting diode), and then moving to the next child on the list. A total of 14 different categories were observed, with an average interobserver agreement maintained at 85% throughout the study. Three of the classroom behavioral codes discriminated unpopular from popular children—off-task behavior (e.g., daydreaming instead of working or attending), and positive reinforcement given to and received from others (e.g., positive interaction, affection, conversation).

Thus classroom settings do afford the opportunity to assess on-task behavior. In some cases, differences in the social behavior of accepted and unaccepted children are also apparent during classroom observations (e.g., Gottman et al., 1975), but not reliably so (e.g., Lewin et al., 1999). Negative interpersonal behaviors are typically observed at such low rates in the controlled classroom setting that observations fail to differentiate between accepted and rejected children in rates of aggression (Foster & Ritchey, 1985).

One exception to this general rule may be the preschool classroom, where behavior is less constrained, and opportunities to observe more naturalistic peer interaction are available. A study by Vaughn and colleagues (2000) used classroom observations effectively to assess the social competence of preschool children, and the study also illustrates the utility of observer ratings. Observers worked in pairs and spent between 16 and 20 hours observing the children in a given classroom. They took notes on the behaviors and attributes of individual children over this period, taking care to observe each child on several different days and across a variety of activity settings (e.g., mealtimes, small groups, free play indoors, outdoor play, transition activities such as standing in lines, and cleanup). Following the observations, the observers completed Q-sort measures to describe the social behaviors they had observed, using a procedure established by Waters and Sroufe (1983): The Q-sort of each observed child was correlated with the Q-sort profile of a hypothetical child who exemplified social competence (generated by aggregating descriptions provided by social-developmental experts), to generate a score representing the child's overall level of social competence.

Playground Observations

As an alternative to the constrained social context of the classroom, investigators have observed children's social interactions in the more unstructured setting of the school playground. Examples are provided next of studies in which playground observations demonstrated their utility for identifying individual differences in prosocial, withdrawn, and aggressive behaviors, and also proved useful for the evaluation of an intervention. In the Lewin and colleagues (1999) study mentioned above, playground interactions were conducted with a modified version of the Peer Interaction Recording System (PIRS; Hops & Stevens, 1987). Observed behaviors were coded as verbal versus nonverbal, positive versus negative, and initiated by the target child versus received by the target child from a peer. Additional context codes included the following: alone, unoccupied, onlooking, or involved. Observers achieved high levels of reliability (mean percentage of agreement was 83%; mean kappas ranged from .78 to .95). In a multimethod factor analysis, positive interactions on the playground loaded with teacher ratings of positive social skills to represent a dimension of Prosocial Behavior. In addition, isolation observed on the playground factored with teacher ratings of withdrawal to represent a dimension of Withdrawn Behavior. Hence, relative to the CLASS classroom observations, the PIRS-V playground observations in this study revealed more information about the qualitative features of children's social behavior.

Rubin and his colleagues have also used playground observations effectively in a series of studies examining social withdrawal and peer relations (Rubin, 1985; Rubin, Daniels-Beirness, & Bream, 1984). The Play Observation Schedule developed by Rubin (1985) uses a continuous 10-second partial-interval coding system to classify children's free-play behavior into seven categories: unoccupied behavior, onlooker behavior, solitary activity, peer conversations, group interactions, conversations with teachers, aggression, and parallel play. Rates of sociable play (peer conversations + group interactions) and isolated play (unoccupied behavior + onlooker behavior + solitary activity) are stable across a 1-year period (Rubin et al., 1984) and correlate significantly with children's peer acceptance, social problem-solving skills, and internalizing and externalizing behavior problems (Rubin et al., 1984).

Evidence that playground observations can also reveal significant differences among children in aggressive behaviors comes from a study we conducted (Bierman, Smoot, & Aumiller, 1993). In that study, children were observed for 16 minutes at lunch and 16 minutes at recess during at least 2 nonconsecutive days. Trained observers used a time-sampling technique (observing for 6 seconds and recording for 6 seconds) and recorded the occurrence of six types of social behaviors (see Table 8.1 for coding category examples). Both child initiations and peer responses were coded. That is, coders recorded the number of intervals in which the target child exhibited any of the six types of social behaviors, and separately recorded the number of times peers directed any of these six types of behaviors toward the target child. Interrater reliability (kappa) averaged .75 across categories. Rates of observed negative behaviors were high enough to discriminate between physical and verbal aggression, which loaded on separate factors when combined with teacher and peer aggression ratings.

Ladd (1981) demonstrated that recess observations could serve effectively as a basis to identify children with skill deficits and to assess their responsivity to intervention. In his novel observational procedure, he asked teachers to schedule an "indoor recess," providing children with a variety of unstructured play materials (e.g., art supplies, wood crafts, construction supplies, etc.). Two 30-minute observation sessions were held in each classroom. By constraining the location of the recess, Ladd was able to observe children with more precision than might be available in the broad space of a playground. Observations were conducted with an instantaneous (scan) sampling

**TABLE 8.1. Coding Categories (with Definitions and Examples)
for Assessing Peer Interactions**

Physical aggression

Definition: This category is coded whenever a child physically attacks or attempts to attack another person. The attack must be intentional and of sufficient intensity to potentially inflict pain.

Examples: Hitting, kicking, slapping, taking an object roughly, swinging fists, throwing objects, destroying another's property.

Verbal aggression

Definition: This category includes verbal behavior that is intended to punitively control another person's actions, to express negative feelings toward another person, or to cause harm to the other person's feelings or reputation.

Examples: Negatively toned commands, yelling derisively, insults, taunting, cussing or swearing, mimicking another sarcastically, threatening, making negative insinuations.

Rough-and-tumble play

Definition: This category includes interactions that involve non-negative rigorous physical contact with others, or attempted rigorous contact. In contrast to physical aggression, the intent is to play rather than to harm.

Examples: Wrestling, playful restraint, carrying others, jumping on others in a playful manner, tackling or chasing others.

Prosocial/agreeable

Definition: This category includes verbal and nonverbal behaviors that are other-directed and prosocial in orientation, designed to help or please the other. Also included here are verbal and nonverbal behaviors that signal agreement with or acknowledgment of another's idea, suggestion, or command.

Examples: Helping behaviors, sharing, taking turns, compliance to suggestions, praise, invitations to play, affectionate physical contact, agreements.

Neutral interaction

Definition: This category includes other forms of verbal or play interactions that are neither clearly aggressive, rough play, or prosocial in nature.

Examples: Conversation, play behaviors, simple (non-negative) commands.

Solitary/unoccupied

Definition: This category refers to behavior that is solitary and unengaged. It does not include constructive solitary play, but refers to noninteractive and unengaged behavior.

Examples: Hovering onlooker behavior, unoccupied wandering, sitting on the sidelines and observing play.

Note. From Bierman and Welsh (1997, p. 349). Copyright 1997 by The Guilford Press. Reprinted by permission.

procedure. In this method, observers focused briefly (1–2 seconds) on a target child and immediately recorded his/her behavior, then focused on a second target child and immediately recorded his/her behavior, until all of the target children were observed. This cycle was repeated throughout the observation period. Coding categories were selected to map onto an intervention program, and included six categories: questions, leads, support, social negative, social other, and nonsocial. Observer agreement ranged from 75% to 97%, with a mean estimate of 87%. This method proved effective at identifying children low in conversation skills for intervention, and also documented posttreatment differences between children who received intervention and those who did not.

One additional, particularly innovative strategy to obtain naturalistic observations of children's peer interactions was utilized by Asher, Rose, and Gabriel (2001). They observed children in multiple school settings, including several lunch, recess, and physical education class sessions. In each of these settings, they used a wireless transmission system to record children's conversations with peers. A lightweight microphone was attached to a child's collar, and a transmitter was carried in a small pouch on the child's belt. The observer carried the receiver and taping equipment in a backpack. A video camera was used to obtain a visual record of the interaction, and this record was later synchronized with the audiotapes. This observational method allowed the research team to obtain highly detailed accounts of peer interactions, which could be coded into a finely differentiated account of the types of problematic peer transactions experienced by individual children (see Asher et al., 2001).

Similarly, Pepler and colleagues (Atlas & Pepler, 1998; Hawkins, Pepler, & Craig, 1999) used remote video and audio recordings to collect covert observations of bullying in the classroom. Bullying episodes are examples of "critical events," which occur relatively infrequently but have considerable negative impact on children. For example, Atlas and Pepler (1998) documented two episodes per hour (60 episodes occurring over 28 hours of videotape). It would have been difficult to capture these events through live observation, but the remote taping procedure allowed for their documentation and analysis.

CONTRIVED-SETTING OBSERVATIONS

Although naturalistic observations of children in school settings can be valuable, they can be quite time-consuming. Even in playground settings, which are considerably less structured than classrooms, the rate at which children (even very aggressive children) display aggressive behaviors is quite low. When they occur, hostile behaviors serve as "critical events" and have a strong negative impact on peer relations. However, the low base rates can make such behaviors difficult to observe naturalistically (Foster & Ritchey, 1985). For these reasons, a number of studies have supplemented or replaced naturalistic observations with observations conducted during contrived playgroups, utilizing social challenges to elicit interactive behavior (see Bierman & Welsh, 2000, for a review). Although one cannot get a realistic sense of base rate behaviors in contrived observations, the higher rate of social behavior makes it possible to assess qualitative aspects of a child's interpersonal behaviors in a relatively short period.

To elicit interaction, children are given tasks that require communication, cooperation, negotiation, emotion regulation, and problem-solving skills. For example, children may be asked to work on a cooperative art project, negotiate play with a limited number of toy choices, play with affect-arousing toys (such as toy soldiers or rescue squad figures), solve a group problem, or make a group decision. The success of the procedure rests on identifying a group of partners, setting, and task (or set of tasks) that will motivate a child to interact, and will elicit social behavior that is representative of the child's capacities for interpersonal interaction in natural social settings (Coie, Dodge, & Kupersmidt, 1990). To promote the social validity of contrived-interaction tasks, Sroufe (1996) suggests several guidelines for their design: (1) They should involve salient developmental challenges, tapping the skills and organizational capacities needed for age-relevant social interactions and requiring responses that are representative of naturalistic demands; (2) they should tax the integrative capacities of the individual, requiring the coordination of affect, cognition, and behavior; and (3) they should reveal the individual's capabilities to function effectively in the peer group, including interpersonal sensitivity and the ability to coordinate reciprocal interpersonal behaviors, solve social problems, and negotiate conflict. When designed in this way to incorporate the complexity of naturally occurring peer interactions, contrived-setting observations can be a cost-efficient and sensitive method of assessing social skill deficits and difficulties. Because they can be set up under controlled conditions, where more detailed coding (or videotaped coding) is possible, they allow for a closer examination of the more subtle aspects of children's interaction skills than do observations in naturalistic settings. Three kinds of contrived-setting observations illustrate the potential of this method for assessing children's social competence—playgroups, friendship interaction tasks, and social challenge tasks.

Playgroup Observations

The basic playgroup method involves observing children in small groups (usually four to eight members) engaging in various forms of play or cooperative activity. Group composition can be varied, allowing an investigator to observe differences when partners are familiar versus unfamiliar, or when partners vary in their social skillfulness or social characteristics. Group tasks can be arranged to provide a range of social challenges, and observations can be videotaped to allow for a careful examination of a child's social style, behavioral patterns, and social effectiveness (Guralnick, Gottman, & Hammond, 1996).

The playgroup method has been widely used at the grade school level, and has demonstrated its utility at identifying problem behaviors and social interaction patterns associated with peer rejection (Coie & Kupersmidt, 1983). For example, in a series of studies conducted by Coie, Dodge, and their colleagues (Coie, Dodge, Terry, & Wright, 1991; Dodge, 1983; Dodge, Coie, Pettit, & Price, 1990), small groups of boys were formed (group sizes ranged from four to eight) and observed over a series of sessions (number of sessions ranged from five to eight) for periods of 45–60 minutes each session. Groups met in rooms equipped with a variety of interactive toys (e.g., art materials, construction blocks), toys designed to elicit aggressive play (e.g., toy soldiers, boxing gloves), and a limited number of highly attractive toys (e.g., a single electronic toy). In most studies, children were observed during both structured interactions (e.g., adult-led activities and games) and unstructured interactions (e.g., free play, unsupervised time).

Within two to four sessions, children in these playgroups had established a social structure, indicated by the stabilization of sociometric status. Reflecting the validity of the group context for assessing a child's naturalistic social competence, playgroup status was significantly correlated with school-based sociometric status, with r's ranging from .50 to .74 (Coie & Kupersmidt, 1983; Coie et al., 1991). In the playgroup context, it was possible to identify individual differences in verbal aggression, physical aggression, reactive aggression, cooperative behaviors, and off-task behaviors that differentiated rejected from nonrejected boys (Coie et al., 1991; Dodge, 1983; Dodge, Coie, et al., 1990). The playgroup method also enabled the examination of interactional sequences of behavior, illustrating the tendency for aggressive–rejected boys (compared to their nonrejected peers) to initiate more instrumental aggression, to react aggressively without provocation, and to escalate aggressive exchanges by refusing to submit or negotiate. In contrast, children who were popular with their peers were distinguished in the playgroup setting by their high rates of prosocial behavior, cooperative interaction, social conversation, positive affect, and leadership behaviors (Coie & Kupersmidt, 1983; Dodge, Coie, et al., 1990). These studies suggest that the playgroup method may be a very efficient method of assessing individual differences in both positive and negative aspects of social behavior. In addition, playgroup observations have proven useful for the evaluation of intervention effects with grade school children (Bierman & Furman, 1984; Bierman, Miller, & Stabb, 1987)

With adaptations, the playgroup method has been used successfully to assess the social behavior of both preschool children and adolescents. Given that the characteristics of socially competent (and socially dysfunctional) children vary significantly across developmental levels, as do the nature of tasks that effectively assess age-appropriate social interactions, adaptations are needed in the structure, content, and coding systems used with children of different developmental periods.

For example, observing preschool children, Guralnick and colleagues (Guralnick, Connor, Hammond, Gottman, & Kinnish, 1996; Guralnick, Gottman, & Hammond, 1996) constructed a playgroup context that simulated a preschool/kindergarten setting, with a balance of structured time (circle time, music, art, snack, and story) and free play (at pretend-play and constructive-play centers, such as housekeeping, blocks, and books). Levels of social participation, verbal support, agreeability, and positive social orientation (e.g., leading and following peers, seeking and responding to peers, imitating or modeling peers) observed in the context of these groups predicted which children would successfully establish friendships. Levels of positive sociability in the playgroups differentiated children with communication disorders and developmental delays from their nondisordered peers, indicating the sensitivity of the playgroup method to detect meaningful individual differences in social competence (Guralnick, Gottman, et al., 1996).

At the other end of the developmental spectrum, Hops, Alpert, and Davis (1997) used a variation of the playgroup method to assess the social competence of adolescents. Reflecting developmental changes in normative types of social interaction, Hops and colleagues used an interaction task that focused on verbal behaviors and provided opportunities for conversation and discussion, rather than play. In addition, given the emergence of heterosexual interactions (and romantic interests) in adolescence, their observations included mixed-gender groups. In the Hops and colleagues study, groups of unfamiliar peers met for six sessions and were given a series of discussion tasks (e.g., solving problems involving parent–teen conflict, peer pressure, and dating;

planning a party; resolving moral dilemmas; and rank-ordering lists of musical groups, videos, and movie stars). "Facilitative behavior" during the group sessions (e.g., happy and caring affect, initiating and supporting conversation, active problem-solving efforts) predicted peer liking. Conversely, for both boys and girls, low rates of these behaviors contributed to peer ratings of "withdrawn." Youth who engaged in aversive behavior, displaying angry or hostile affect, and arguing with others were rated by peers as "aggressive/aversive." Group discussion tasks thus proved effective at eliciting patterns of social functioning associated with positive or negative reputations among adolescents (Hops et al., 1997).

Also working with adolescents, Englund, Levy, Hyson, and Sroufe (2000) used a group problem-solving observation task to assess social competence. First, adolescents at a day camp were divided into small same-sex groups (three to four youth) and were asked to come up with a plan for spending $150 on a group activity the last day of camp. Then these groups were combined into larger same-sex groups (six to eight youth) and were asked to discuss their ideas and come up with a group consensus regarding how to spend the money. Finally, the entire group of boys and girls was brought together to make the decision regarding how the money would be spent. Raters who were unaware of the adolescents' developmental histories coded videotapes of these group discussions and rated each adolescent on dimensions of task enjoyment, involvement, leadership, self-confidence, and global social competence. These observer ratings showed high concurrent validity, revealed in strong correlations with independent counselor ratings and peer sociometric measures; they also correlated with measures of the youth's social competence that had been collected earlier in the longitudinal study, when the children were in preschool and middle childhood.

Friendship Dyad Observations

Hartup, French, Laursen, Johnston, and Ogawa (1993) have suggested that "closed-field" situations, such as contrived observations of friendship dyads, can facilitate the assessment of friendship skills and friendship quality. Like the playgroup method, this method allows investigators to "stage" challenge situations that require friendship pairs to interact, discuss, negotiate, and solve problems. Observational studies of friendship pair interactions have provided useful information about the characteristics that promote positive relationships (at the preschool and grade school levels); they have also identified individual differences in friendship behaviors, as well as interpersonal dynamics within friendships associated with the escalation of antisocial behavior problems.

For example, Parker and Herrera (1996) demonstrated that they could detect differences in friendship intimacy and positive affect among children who had (or had not) experienced abuse. In their study, children and their best friends participated in a 90-minute laboratory session involving four tasks: (1) completing a consensual Q-sort describing the characteristics of their friendship, (2) preparing a snack, (3) playing a game that involved a Prisoner's Dilemma type of bargaining task, and (4) playing a puzzle game under cooperative and competitive rule structures. The friendship Q-sort discussion task proved most sensitive to dyadic differences in intimacy and positive affect; the competitive game task elicited the most conflict.

Also observing friendship pairs, Fonzi, Schneider, Tani, and Tomada (1997) gave dyads two tasks: (1) a negotiation task that required the children to decide how to divide and share a chocolate egg with a toy inside, and (2) a competitive car-racing task. These investigators found that the ability to negotiate sensitively and to resolve conflicts in this lab-based task predicted the longevity of the friendship during the subsequent school year.

Friendships undergo significant changes across development; they become more salient and more influential as children move into preadolescence and adolescence. However, even at the preschool level, observations of friendship dyads have proven useful as a means of assessing child social competence. For example, in one study, Gottman (1983) compared the audiotaped interactions of 13 preschool children as they played with best friends or strangers during sessions at their homes. In a second study, Gottman audiotaped the interactions of 18 preschool children as they played with unfamiliar partners over three sessions, examining interaction characteristics that predicted dyads whose members did or did not "hit it off" and become friends. In both studies, communication clarity (indexed by the extent to which children attended to and clarified their messages effectively when queried by their partners) emerged as an important characteristic of successful friendships. Additional characteristics of successful friendships were information exchange (sharing information about themselves and their joint activities), reciprocity in play, and the ability to resolve conflicts. Furthermore, children who demonstrated the most skills in their existing friendships were most likely to "hit it off" with strangers. Thus the friendship observations enabled an assessment of friendship quality, as well as of individual skill that predicted success with friends outside that particular dyad.

Friendship observations have proven to be particularly enlightening with adolescents (Dishion, Andrews, & Crosby, 1995; Dishion, Spracklen, Andrews, & Patterson, 1996). The basic method used by these researchers was to ask adolescent boys and their friends to plan an activity together, solve a problem that each boy had with his parents, and solve a problem that each boy had with his peers. The entire session lasted 25 minutes. Delinquent and nondelinquent youth were differentiated in this session by their level of rule-breaking talk (e.g., talk about antisocial or inappropriate activities) and by their tendency to reinforce rule-breaking talk with laughter (in contrast to nondelinquent boys, who tended to reward normative topics with laughter). In this case, the friendship observation provided information not only about the target youth's social skills, but about aspects of the friends' behavior that were linked with the likelihood of later escalations in antisocial behavior and drug use.

Social Challenge Tasks

Finally, a third approach to contrived observations has involved the construction of performance tasks to assess skills for specific social challenges, such as entering a group and communicating effectively to solve a social problem. These observations seek to examine a child's ability to organize cognitions, affect, and behavior in "critical event" situations. Assessments of the ability to enter a peer group, for example, have shown this task to discriminate effectively between popular and unpopular children. For example, Putallaz and Gottman (1981) and Dodge, Schlundt, Schocken, and Delugach (1983) both observed grade school children trying to enter an ongoing peer group activity. Putallaz and Gottman compared the strategies used by popular and unpopular children, and Dodge and colleagues evaluated the success of various strategies by assessing peer responses (favorable or unfavorable). Skillful entry strategies (those likely to elicit favorable responses) were undertaken more often by popular than by unpopular children; they included making group-oriented statements and engaging in the same behavior as the group, and waiting for an appropriate moment in the ongoing group interaction to request an opportunity to join in. In contrast, unsuccessful and unpopular children often used self-referent or other attention-getting behaviors, such as talking about themselves, stating their feelings or opinions, and criticizing or arguing with other children.

Researchers have also designed referential communication tasks to assess children's capacity to take the perspective of others and adjust their communications accordingly. In one such example, Whalen, Henker, Collins, McAuliffe, and Vaux (1979) compared hyperactive and nonhyperactive boys in the context of a game called Mission Control. In this game, children simulated landing a space capsule. One child acted as the "sender" of a message (giving directions to the astronaut), while the other acted as "receiver" (landing the space capsule). Observed behaviors on this task discriminated hyperactive from nonhyperactive children; hyperactive children exhibited less task focus, lower levels of sensitivity to the differential roles of "sender" and "receiver," and elevated rates of irrelevant conversation.

Finally, the task of carrying on a conversation has proven useful as an assessment device. In this technique, an adult engages a child in conversation and offers a series of scripted interview prompts (e.g., "I went to see a great movie last night," "What kind of music do you like to listen to?") (Bierman & Furman, 1984; Hansen, St. Lawrence, & Christoff, 1988). Responses given by the child are coded for verbal fluency, appropriateness of responding, and variety (e.g., range of self-disclosures, questions, and leads expressed). This observation method has proven effective in differentiating conduct-disordered youth from their normative peers (Hansen et al., 1988) and in documenting the effects of intervention (Bierman & Furman, 1984). The risk associated with contrived social challenge observations is that they will lack the complexity and regulatory demands associated with naturalistic interaction; at the same time, they may be useful when the goal is to assess a set of skills relevant to a particular social situation or event (e.g., group entry, conversation), and they may be quite sensitive to focused intervention efforts.

INTERVENTION APPLICATIONS

Observations serve two critical roles in intervention research: (1) They provide a basis to screen and select unaccepted children with specific performance deficits or excesses for interventions focused on those target areas, and (2) they serve as an index of the behavioral impact of such an intervention. Given the behavioral heterogeneity that exists among children with peer relation difficulties, behavioral observations provide an effective method for identifying subgroups of those children who share particular behavioral characteristics. For example, if an intervention is designed specifically to improve child conversation skills, it is likely to be most effective for those children whose peer difficulties are related to deficient conversational abilities (see Bierman, 1986a). A behavioral observation serves as a screening device that allows the clinician to match child needs with interventions targeting those needs. In addition, behavioral observations provide an important objective index of the degree to which an intervention has produced behavior change. In understanding how an intervention is working, observations allow the practitioner to determine whether the intervention has successfully changed its focused behavioral targets. Separate questions are whether teachers and peers have noticed those behavioral changes, and whether those behavioral changes have resulted in revised peer evaluations.

In intervention research, decisions about selecting children for an intervention and evaluating the intervention's impact are usually based on relative differences in the rates of various social behaviors displayed during observations, rather than standardized scores or "cutoff" scores designating clinical significance. Indeed, the specific rates of various behaviors in any dyadic or group interaction are affected by the context and interactional partners, and hence do not lend themselves well to scoring along the lines of absolute levels of behavior or the establishment of clinical cutoffs (DeRosier, Cillessen, Coie, & Dodge, 1994). If practitioners are working with individuals or small groups of children, it may be difficult to collect enough observations to provide for relative scoring of children within the larger peer group. However, in this case, observations can still be useful for understanding the qualitative features of a child's social behavior and the contingencies affecting it, as well as examining changes in a child's behavior from pretest to posttest.

Practitioners often work in contexts in which the resources for formal group observation and coding are limited. In this situation, Bijou, Peterson, and Ault (1968) suggest using a narrative observational method to describe the social interactions of individual children. Their system involves a four-column format for continuous recording. Each child's social behaviors are recorded, along with information about the setting and antecedent events, the child's responses, and consequent events. Collecting information in this kind of temporal sequence makes it possible to describe the social behaviors shown by a child, and also to examine and form hypotheses about how antecedent conditions/ events and interpersonal consequences may be eliciting and supporting those social behaviors.

Subtle qualitative differences in the way peer interaction problems "play out" for different children with similar teacher/peer-rated problem profiles become apparent in such observations. For example, consider the differences in these excepts from observations of playgroup behavior of AG and JK, two boys who were both rejected by their peers and rated as highly aggressive and disruptive by their teachers.

AG

AG was observed in a playroom with four other boys from his class during an indoor recess. When the boys first entered the room, AG stood
aloof from them and busied himself with putting on lip balm, while the
others went to the shelves to pick a game. The boys decided on a game
of Chutes and Ladders and sat down to play, and AG joined them at
the table. However, he fidgeted in his seat and continued to play with
his lip balm as the game started. The other boys began to talk about the
Pinewood Derby cars they were making for Boy Scouts. AG did not
comment or look at the others during this conversation, and seemed to
be more interested in his lip balm than he was in the game, but he took
his turn when the time came. After a few turns, AG landed at the top of
a large "chute," which would have caused him to fall back in the game,
well behind the other boys. He moved his piece ahead instead, skipping
over the "chute"; this elicited complaints from the other boys, who told
him he had to go back and go down the "chute." AG refused and raised
his voice, calling the other boys "cheaters." The other boys quickly decided to "just forget it" because AG was "being such a jerk," and left
AG at the table with the Chutes and Ladders game while they went to
the shelf to find something else to do.

Even during this relatively short (15-minute) observation, several
key aspects of AG's difficulties with peers became evident. AG appeared uncomfortable, anxious, and awkward with his classmates, and
frequently "hovered" around peer activities, focusing his attention on
something else (such as when he played with his lip balm while the
other boys looked over the games and decided what to play). When he
did engage in play, AG seemed unwilling or unable to follow standard
rules and protocol. The other boys appeared to ignore AG's "odd" behaviors (such as playing with the lip balm during the game), but had no
tolerance for his age-inappropriate lack of fair-play skills. Evidence that
they considered him "hopeless" as a play partner emerged as they routinely ignored him or excluded him from their play during the observation period.

JK

JK was also observed during an indoor recess, along with four other
boys from his classroom. JK was the first one into the room; he rushed
over to the toy shelves, calling the other boys' attention to several toys
as he thrust them off the shelves onto the rug area. As the other boys
joined him, he declared that the rescue squad toys would be the best
thing in the room to play with, and took the bin (containing police cars,

fire engines, emergency vehicles, figures, building blocks, and associated paraphernalia) over to the table. Two of the boys joined him there, while the other two continued to look through the options on the shelves. JK dug into the rescue squad toy bin and began to hand out play figures and vehicles. At first, JK kept all of the police vehicles to himself, exclaiming, "I'm going to play Cops!" When the other boys complained that it wasn't fair for him to keep all of the police cars, he threw some cars at them, telling the boys that they should just take them "if you're going to be babies about it." The group started to set up buildings, and the boys began to make suggestions about the scenarios they could create. JK finished taking everything out of the bin and fiddled with his set of toys for a few minutes, beginning to look bored. As the other boys were still setting up their figures, he gave them a sly smile and took one of his police cars. Making a machine-gun sound, he ran his police car into some of the figures set up by the other boys, calling out "Watch out! It's a raid!" The other boys yelled at him, "Stop it!" JK got up from the table, shrugged, and went back to the shelves to look for something else to do.

Like AG, JK had trouble joining in with other boys and sustaining positive interactions. Both boys seemed inattentive and insensitive to their playmates during the play session, and both behaved aggressively toward others. It is not difficult to see why teachers rated each boy as aggressive and disruptive, and why both were rejected by peers. Nonetheless, observations revealed some key differences in the ways in which their social interaction problems unfolded with peers. Whereas AG appeared anxious and awkward around peers, JK appeared excited and impulsive. AG avoided direct eye contact with peers, focusing his attention on his lip balm and the game. In contrast, JK attempted to direct and dominate peer play, bossing others and controlling the play materials. Both boys reacted to mild conflict with negative escalation. For example, AG raised his voice and called his partners "cheaters" when they told him he had to go back in the game; JK threw the cars and made a disparaging remark when his partners told him they wanted some police cars. In this case, observations confirmed the social behavior problems and skill deficits identified in teacher and peer ratings, but also provided additional qualitative information about the boys' social behavior and peer responses.

SUMMARY

Observations can play a useful role at the second step in assessments of children's social relationships. Whereas teacher and peer ratings provide the best starting point in assessments—providing information about multiple dimensions of peer relations, including group status and behavior, close friendships, peer group treatment, and peer network affiliations—observations enable more in-depth and objective analyses of the specific interaction processes contributing to children's relationship difficulties. Observations enable an assessment of a child's behavior, as well as an analysis of antecedent conditions and of the peer responses a child elicits. In addition, observations of a variety of peers permit the evaluation to be grounded in local norms, as the child's behavior can be compared to that of other children of the same age, cultural group, and gender.

Observations in naturalistic settings can be useful, particularly in situations that offer opportunities for unstructured social interaction, such as recess, lunch, transition periods, or indoor play periods (Foster & Ritchey, 1985). However, naturalistic observations can also be time-consuming, as children (even very aggressive children) display problematic behaviors at relatively low rates. Low base rates can make such behaviors difficult to observe naturalistically (Foster & Ritchey, 1985). Observations of children in contrived settings provide an alternative. Designed to simulate the complex interpersonal demands of naturalistic peer interactions, playgroup and friendship interaction tasks involve the "staging" of critical events, and allow investigators to complete careful microanalyses of child behaviors, affect, and interactional sequences. The success of these observational procedures rests on identifying a combination of partners, setting, and task(s) that will cause a child to interact, and that will elicit social behavior reflecting the child's capacities for interpersonal interaction in natural social settings (Coie et al., 1990). Specific social challenge tasks, such as entering a group and communicating effectively to solve a social problem, also show some promise; however, the social validity of these approaches requires more study.

In addition to the "objective" assessments describing children's peer relations and social behavior provided by peers, teachers, and observations, the child's perspective warrants attention. Self-perceptions and social reasoning may contribute to problematic social relationships, and hence should be considered in assessment and intervention planning. Assessments of these self-system processes are discussed in the next chapter.

Chapter 9

Assessing Self-System Processes

Teacher/peer ratings and direct observations of a child's social behavior are valuable because they reflect the perspectives of school community members. At the same time, because teacher/peer ratings and observations focus on overt behaviors, they are more useful in identifying the behavioral manifestations of a child's social difficulties than they are at elucidating the kinds of feelings, regulatory difficulties, or thought processes that may contribute to problematic behaviors. Behavioral descriptions are critically important to intervention design, as they identify target behaviors that require suppression (such as aggression) or promotion (such as cooperation). However, in order to foster sustained and generalized changes in these behaviors, interventions need to attend to the underlying thoughts, feelings, beliefs, and associated "relational schemas" that affect a child's display of problem behaviors and their reactions to various social contexts.

Social competence requires the capacity to coordinate adaptive responses flexibly to various interpersonal demands, and to organize social behavior in different social contexts in a manner beneficial to oneself and consistent with social conventions and morals. For this reason, a child's social-cognitive capabilities and affect regulation skills, which foster the child's ability to select and enact social behaviors in a way that is contextually sensitive and responsive, play an important role in determining his/her social competence (Bierman & Welsh, 2000; Dodge & Murphy, 1984; Rubin, Bukowski, & Parker, 1998; Sroufe, 1996).

Self-system variables, including social-cognitive and affect regulation processes, function prominently in theoretical models of social–emotional development. For example, children are believed to develop relational schemas based upon their social experiences; these schemas assist them in their social perceptions and interpretations, allowing them to navigate the complex social world with efficiency, familiarity, and comfort (Crick & Dodge, 1994; Dodge & Murphy, 1984; Lochman & Dodge, 1994; see Chapter 4). In relational schemas, conceptions of the outside world and others are intertwined with conceptions of oneself and one's ability to influence or act on the social world in effective ways (Baldwin, 1992; Skinner, 1995). They also include stored information about social patterns and sequences in the form of scripts, tagged affectively with the expectations, feelings, goals, and motivations children associate with different situations (Abelson, 1981; Fiske & Taylor, 1984). Under positive circumstances, relational schemas support adaptive social functioning (Cairns, 1991; Epstein, 1991). However, these schemas can also promote resistance to change, as children settle into habitual patterns of social responding that were functional in previous relationships and have become part of their affective, cognitive, and behavioral orientation toward their social world and sense of self. Self-protective motivations can prove socially maladaptive, particularly when they encourage "fight-or-flight" reactivity to a social world perceived as dangerous or difficult to control.

Unfortunately, relative to assessments of observable behaviors, much less is known about how to assess self-system variables with validity and how to link these assessment results with intervention strategies. It is not even clear which aspects of the self-system deserve attention in assessment or intervention. For example, a number of studies have focused on the accuracy of children's self-perceptions regarding their social behavior and peer status. In general, however, research suggests that such self-perceptions do not correlate well with the perceptions of teachers or peers. As discussed in Chapter 4, the perceptions of aggressive–rejected children appear particularly vulnerable to positive biases, so that they often perceive themselves to be better liked by their peers than they actually are (Zakriski & Coie, 1996).

However, "accuracy" (i.e., correspondence between self-perceptions and others' reports of social relationships) may not be as important for children's well-being as the degree to which their self-systems are functioning adaptively. From a theoretical perspective, self-systems serve different functions than do perceptions of others, and consequently emphasize and weigh information in different ways. Conceptually, self-systems, particularly the schemas children construct concerning their social world and their relation to it, serve three important functions: (1) They provide a basis for the prediction and control of the outside world; (2) they preserve a system of internal synchrony or consistency in the sense of self; and (3) they promote self-protection, maintaining a favorable sense of self to motivate action and adaptive problem solving

(Cairns, 1991; Epstein, 1991). Correspondingly, in assessments of children's self-system processes for the purpose of intervention, the most important questions may involve the degree to which their perceptions of and reasoning about others support adaptive peer interactions, and the degree to which their interrelated perceptions of and reasoning about themselves provide a favorable basis for feelings of social comfort and adaptive social coping. In this chapter, I first examine the basis for anticipating differences between self-perceptions and others' perceptions. Then I address the assessment of child perceptions and reasoning about peers (their social cognitions and social information-processing biases); this is followed by an examination of measures for assessing children's perceptions of themselves (including feelings of distress regarding their peer relations) and their attributions and control beliefs regarding their capacity to influence their social outcomes.

SELF-VIEWS VERSUS PEER AND TEACHER RATINGS

When researchers have compared self-ratings of social behavior and social status with peer and teacher ratings on similar measures, notable differences emerge. Peer and teacher ratings tend to be moderately correlated, usually in the range of $r = .50–.70$ for overt behaviors, revealing convergence in the views of these two kinds of "observers" (Landau, Milich, & Whitten, 1984; Ledingham, Younger, Schwartzman, & Bergeron, 1982).

Correlations between child self-views and teacher or peer views tend to be considerably lower, usually in the $r = .20–.35$ range (Ledingham et al., 1982; McKim & Cowen, 1987). Self–other agreement is usually higher for ratings of overt behaviors (such as aggression) than for ratings of inferred or subtle characteristics (such as popularity, withdrawal, likability, or emotional distress) (Achenbach, McConaughy, & Howell, 1987; Ledingham et al., 1982; Stanger & Lewis, 1993). This probably reflects the fact that aggressive acts are more salient and easily classified, for both the self and the observer, than are other aspects of social adjustment. In general, however, linkages between self and others show considerable divergence when social behaviors and adjustment are being described. Indeed, the agreement among sources outside the self—whether ratings are derived from peers, teachers, or direct observations—is consistently greater than agreement between the self and any of these "outside" sources (Achenbach et al., 1987; Cairns, Cairns, Neckerman, Ferguson, & Gariepy, 1989). Self–other discrepancies are usually greatest for children at an extreme of a continuum, such as those rated by teachers as particularly high in aggression or low in popularity (Cairns, Cairns, et al., 1989; Ledingham et al., 1982).

The tendency for aggressive youth to report positive self-views has been described in terms of distorted perceptions or inflated self-esteem; it has even been labeled "narcissism." Indeed, researchers have documented positive biases in the evaluations of peer relations made by many aggressive–rejected children (Hughes, Cavell, & Grossman, 1997; Zakriski & Coie, 1996). It is possible that these positive biases result in a lack of motivation to change and/or difficulty accepting new information and performance feedback in the context of intervention (Hughes et al., 1997). However, it is also possible that positive biases serve a useful purpose, by protecting these rejected children from the low levels of self-regard, perceived incompetence, and depressed affect that trouble other aggressive–rejected children (Rudolph & Clark, 2001). In general, the tendency for individuals to perceive and understand their own behavior in a manner different from the perspective of others is a common human characteristic—as is the tendency for individuals to explain their behavior (including negative behavior) as a justified reaction to situational factors, rather than reflecting stable personal traits or characteristics (Jones & Nisbett, 1972).

Actor–Observer Differences in Social Perception

A body of research in social psychology has documented reliable differences between self (actor) and other (observer) in accounts of behaviors. In general, self-descriptions tend to emphasize contextual factors in such accounts, whereas others tend to see those behaviors as reflections of the actor's dispositions and motivations (Jones & Nisbett, 1972). Even under experimental circumstances, when observers viewed actors behaving under clear external constraints, they failed to accommodate to these conditions and assumed that the behaviors reflected the actors' stable dispositions (Jones & Harris, 1967). In this research, similar to studies of child self-ratings versus peer ratings of social behavior, ratings by self and by others show the highest agreement when they are describing overt behavior or environmental outcomes (e.g., the behavior that occurred and the outcome that ensued)—areas in which the self and others have equivalent information (Jones & Nisbett, 1972). Significant discrepancies emerge, however, when self and others are asked to describe motive, affect, and cause. In these cases, actors and observers have different kinds of information available to them, as well as different orientations for information processing and interpretation.

Jones and Nisbett (1972) describe observer–actor differences in orientation in the following ways. First, consider the perspective of an observer. The observer is interested in recognizing and understanding consistent patterns in the behaviors of people around him/her, and forming stable and coherent perceptions of those people. This information will facilitate the observer's task of predicting interactions with those people, allowing him/her to make decisions about whether and how to approach and respond to those people in the future. Hence the environment is relatively unimportant for the observer, as his/her focus is on identifying consistent and predictable patterns in the behaviors of others. In contrast, that environment takes center stage for the actor who is interacting with the environment him-/herself, as he/she is focused on perceiving and interpreting the environmental cues (including interpersonal cues) that elicit and require behavioral responding. In other words, the actor is focused on detecting and responding to variations in environmental and social cues. Correspondingly, people tend to explain the behavior of others in terms of consistent patterns and behavioral dispositions, whereas they tend to explain their own behavior in terms of situational contingencies, and view their own behavior as more flexible and varied than do observers.

In addition, self-system processes are organized in a way that preserves a system of internal synchrony and promotes self-protection. Hence, to some extent, positive self-functioning is characterized by a self-protective bias in self-perceptions (Cairns, 1991).

Self-Protective Biases in Self-Perceptions

The tendency to view one's own behavior in a positive light, and to view negative social behaviors as justified under the circumstances, appears to be a normative and generally healthy feature of human functioning (Cairns & Cairns, 1991). In their study of school-based conflicts, for example, Cairns and Cairns (1991) found high levels of agreement concerning the identities of children involved in various conflicts and the consequences of those conflicts. However, when respondents were asked to describe who started the conflict and what their intentions were, agreement was much more spotty. With regard to self-protective biases, it was notable that fewer than 10% of the children in their normative sample stated their own culpability when asked, "Who started it?" Conversely, children who fail to show a self-protective orientation, and who experience chronic bad feelings and self-blame regarding their behaviors and problems, tend to show high levels of depressed mood and social anxiety (Boivin & Begin, 1989; Quiggle, Garber, Panak, & Dodge, 1992; Williams & Asher, 1987).

Children who are struggling socially may be particularly stressed in terms of their capacity to sustain a self-protective frame of mind, which is needed to fuel the motivation to engage in social coping efforts. Certainly some rejected children express high levels of distress about their social situation, report feelings of social anxiety and depressed mood, and blame themselves for their difficulties (Boivin & Begin, 1989). In contrast, other rejected children do not report feeling distressed about their situation; instead, they focus on their friendships or other evidence they have that they are included or accepted by peers. Similarly, although aggressive children generally tend to rate themselves slightly lower than average in areas of popularity and social competence, their self-ratings appear inflated when compared to teacher and peer ratings, on which they score quite low (Cairns & Cairns, 1991). This outcome is consistent with the thesis that the self-system functions to buffer the private self from discordant public evaluations, even when a child is unloved and unloving. This buffering function may be even more important for rejected children than for likable ones.

Hence the "accuracy" of children's self-perceptions, defined as correspondence with teacher and peer perceptions, may not be a critical issue for assessment or intervention. Instead, perhaps the critical issues should be the degree to which a child's self-system supports (1) social-cognitive reasoning about others that promotes adaptive functioning with peers, (2) positive self-evaluations and associated feelings of social comfort versus distress, and (3) attributions and control beliefs that motivate active social engagement and coping.

SOCIAL-COGNITIVE REASONING ABOUT OTHERS

The idea that children's mental representations of their social relationships might contribute to maladaptive functioning with peers was documented in developmental research and had a strong influence on the design of initial coaching programs in the 1980s. The central focus was on the ways in which children's social cognitions and social information-processing skills (i.e., their social knowledge, social goals, social problem-solving skills, and reasoning about relationships) influenced social behavior and, thereby, affected their capacity to form positive relationships with their peers. As reviewed in Chapter 4, a substantial body of research has linked social information processing with both aggressive behavior and peer rejection. For example, compared to non-aggressive children, aggressive youth more often select instrumental than social goals, focus on aggressive cues in the environment, interpret the ambiguous behavior of peers as hostile, generate fewer prosocial and more aggressive responses to social situations, express more confidence in their ability to use aggression effectively, and expect aggression to produce more desired outcomes (Crick & Ladd, 1990; Dodge, 1986; Dodge, Asher, & Parkhurst, 1989; Dodge, Murphy, & Buchsbaum, 1984; Gouze, 1987; Lochman & Dodge, 1994; Perry, Perry, & Rasmussen, 1986). Compared with peer-rejected children, peer-accepted children produce more prosocial solutions to hypothetical social problems and fewer aggressive or inappropriate strategies (Asarnow & Callan, 1985; Ladd & Oden, 1979; Rabiner, Lenhart, & Lochman, 1990; Richard & Dodge, 1982).

Despite evidence of their association with problematic peer relations, and the importance of the underlying processes, it remains unclear how useful the currently available measures of social knowledge, social information processing, and related social cognitions are to social competence assessments and interventions. Although they have sometimes been used as "proxy" measures to represent children's behavioral tendencies, existing social-cognitive measures do not have adequate concurrent or predictive validity to replace teacher/peer ratings or observational measures in the assessment of peer relation or social behavior problems. Given the current database, it would be difficult to justify providing intervention to a child simply on the basis of a social-cognitive measure that indicated deficiencies in social knowledge or response generation, if peer and teacher ratings of that child revealed positive peer relations and socially competent behavior. Conversely, if peer and teacher ratings indicated peer rejection and high levels of aggressive behavior, one would want to intervene, even if an interview with that child revealed a high level of social knowledge and prosocial strategies. In other words, available measures of social cognition do not share the validity of the measures described in Chapters 6–8 for identifying the degree to which a child's social-cognitive reasoning is supporting adaptive functioning with peers.

However, given a situation in which problematic peer relations and negative social behavior have been documented, social-cognitive measures may provide a basis for hypothesis generation concerning the role that the child's reasoning about others (particularly his/her social goals, social knowledge, social perceptions, hostile attributions, and response generation and evaluation processes) may be playing in supporting behavioral and relationship difficulties (Crick & Dodge, 1994). In the next sections, I describe research-based methods used to assess child social cognitions, and discuss their utility for intervention planning.

Assessing Social Cognitions with Hypothetical Stories

Several standardized measures have been developed that use hypothetical social problem prompts described in stories, followed by questions regarding the social goals, attributions, response possibilities, and outcome evaluations children would make if they were faced with those situations. For example, the Home Interview with Child (HIWC; Dodge, Bates, & Pettit, 1990) was designed by Dodge and his colleagues in the Child Development Project to assess multiple components of children's social information processing. This measure consists of eight short vignettes, which describe peer entry or interpersonal problems involving ambiguous provocation. Pictures accompany the vignettes, which are described to children in individual interviews. Children are asked to listen to the story and imagine themselves as the protagonist. Children are then asked several questions about the story. Attributions are assessed by asking children why they think the protagonist in the story did what he/she did. Response generation is assessed by asking children to list different ways that they might respond in the same situation. In more recent renditions, children are also asked to rate how they would feel in the situation, what their goals would be, and how effective they believe their solution would be at solving the problem.

Examples of HIWC stories follow:

Ambiguous provocation: Pretend that you are standing on the playground playing catch with a kid named Todd/Jessica. You throw the ball to Todd/Jessica and he/she catches it. You turn around, and the next thing that you realize is that Todd/Jessica has thown the ball and hit you in the middle of the back. The ball hits you hard, and it hurts a lot. (A) Why do you think that Todd/Jessica hit you in the back? (B) What would you do about Todd/Jessica after he/she hit you?

Peer group entry: Pretend that you see some kids playing on the playground. You would really like to play with them, so you go over and ask one of them, a kid named Alan/Leah if you can play. Alan/Leah says no. (A) Why do you think that Alan/Leah said no? (B) What would you do about Alan/Leah after he/she said no?

In order to increase the realism of the social situations described in the hypothetical stories, and to better model the complexity of the social perception process, investigators have also explored the use of videotaped prompts. For example, Dodge and his colleagues (Dodge & Coie, 1987; Dodge, Murphy, & Buchsbaum, 1984) developed videotapes to assess intention cue detection skills, hostile attributional biases, and response tendencies. Their measure involved a set of twelve 30-second vignettes, each showing a situation involving some form of peer provocation or conflict (e.g., a peer knocks down another's block tower; a peer takes a child's toy). Vignettes display a variety of affect and intentions on the part of the provocateur, including hostile, ambiguous, or positive intent. Children watch each videotaped vignette, and are then asked to give their interpretation of the intentions displayed by the provocateur and to state how they would respond in the situation. (For more information about the impact of different presentation methods on the assessment of social cognitions, the reader is referred to a meta-analysis conducted by de Castro, Veerman, Koops, Bosch, & Monshouwer, 2002).

Although both theory and research support the importance of attending to social-cognitive processes in interventions, the utility of social-cognitive measures (such as those described above) to inform intervention design for individual children remains questionable. It remains somewhat doubtful whether these kinds of interviews provide a valid enough assessment of individual child social-cognitive deficits or biases to serve as a basis for either tailoring or evaluating intervention impact. Effect sizes based on group data are mild to moderate, as are correlations between social-cognitive measures and measures of social behavior and peer status (Dodge, Pettit, McClaskey, & Brown, 1986). Children may show improvements in social-cognitive measures without corresponding improvements in social behavior, raising questions about the validity of interviews as intervention outcomes (Beelmann, Pfingsten, & Losel, 1994).

In part, the limited utility of social-cognitive interviews for intervention design and evaluation may reflect the considerable gap that exists between our theoretical understanding of the way social-cognitive reasoning functions to influence social adjustment in real life (i.e., as affectively charged information processing informed by past experiences and situational contexts, often operating below the level of consciousness) and the way social cognitions are assessed in interviews (i.e., as children's verbal reports of their appraisals of unknown peers in hypothetical situations, under conditions of "cold cognition"). For intervention planning and evaluation, a child's social-cognitive reasoning about familiar peers may be of particular importance if these are the peer relations being targeted for improvement, rather than the child's more abstract reasoning about peer relations in general.

Assessing Social Cognitions via Review of Videotaped Interactions

In a creative attempt to access a more realistic assessment of children's *in vivo* social information processing, Putallaz (1983) interviewed children about videotaped interactions they had actually experienced. In her study, Putallaz first videotaped children as they attempted to enter a new group situation. She then reviewed the tape with each child individually, stopping the tape periodically to question the children about their social perceptions, their goals, and the cues to which they were attending. This method, although more time-consuming than techniques employing analogues, may be particularly valuable for intervention planning because it assesses a child's cognitions in the context of his/her own behavior and relationships. Certainly the review of a child's videotaped interactions with his/her naturalistic peer group warrants further investigation as a method for assessment and intervention focused on children's social perceptions and reasoning about their interactions with peers.

SOCIAL SELF-CONCEPTIONS AND EXPERIENCES OF SOCIAL DISTRESS

Self-reports appear to be the only reliable method of assessing the degree to which a child is experiencing negative self-appraisals, feelings of loneliness, anxious or depressed affect, and low levels of perceived social efficacy—all of which deserve attention in intervention (Hymel & Franke, 1985; Parker, Rubin, Price, & DeRosier, 1995). Self-reports of psychological distress have face validity, whether or not they correspond with ratings by teachers or peers, and feelings of social distress warrant attention and intervention efforts.

Although there are individual differences, many children who experience peer difficulties view themselves as less socially competent than higher-status children, express lower levels of perceived self-competence and social worth, and indicate greater loneliness (Asher, Parkhurst, Hymel, & Williams, 1990; Boivin & Begin, 1989; Bukowski, Hoza, & Boivin, 1994). Investigators have postulated that children who feel socially incompetent and lonely are at high risk for depressed mood and social anxiety (Boivin, Hymel, & Bukowski, 1995; Bukowski et al., 1994). These feelings of psychological distress warrant assessment and are important targets of intervention, as they can play a role in fostering continued social difficulties as well as continued discomfort for a child. Low levels of perceived competence and associated emotional distress may lead to socially avoidant behaviors, thereby impeding improvements in peer relations (Bukowski & Hoza, 1989). In addition, the tendency for individuals to perceive and store information that is consistent with their established set of self-expectations can contribute to stability in social orientation and behavior (Markus & Wurf, 1987). Individuals who have a positive sense of their social competence and self-worth tend to construe events and process information in a way that promotes the maintenance of these positive self-perceptions (Taylor & Brown, 1988). Conversely, individuals with more negative self-perceptions tend to encode, store, and retrieve information in a way that focuses on the schema-consistent negative information about the self, and that filters out or deemphasizes schema-inconsistent positive information (Quiggle et al., 1992; Taylor & Brown, 1988). In this way, negative self-perceptions can fuel continuing peer difficulties, both by inhibiting adaptive social coping attempts and by biasing social information processing in negative ways. Below, I describe measures that assess several key dimensions of social self-appraisals and social distress: loneliness, social anxiety, and perceived social competence.

Loneliness

The Loneliness Scale, developed by Asher, Hymel, and Renshaw (1984), is a self-report measure of loneliness and social dissatisfaction for children. It consists of 16 items that assess loneliness at school (e.g., "I have nobody to talk to," "It's hard to get other kids to like me," "I feel left out of things") and 8 filler items (e.g., "I like to read"); each item is rated on a 5-point scale. In addition to strong internal consistency, the measure has demonstrated stability among grade school children, with a reported 1-year test–retest reliability coefficient of .55 (Asher et al., 1984). As noted above, rejected children show elevated scores on the Loneliness Scale (Asher et al., 1990). In addition, high scores on this scale appear associated with a generally negative pattern of self-perceptions, including low perceived competence, internal attributions for social failure, and negative expectations for future social exchanges (Hymel & Franke, 1985).

Social Anxiety

Guided by adult self-report measures of social anxiety, which tap a number of different dimensions, Hymel, Franke, and Freigang (1985) developed a scale to assess three aspects of social anxiety: Social Anxiety, Social Avoidance, and Negative Peer Attitudes. Although all three subscales evidenced good internal reliability and consistency, a 1-year follow-up study revealed considerably higher levels of stability in Social Anxiety ($r = .61$) and Social Avoidance ($r = .38$) than in Negative Peer Attitudes ($r = .12$). Hence, in the final scale, only the first two subscales were retained. Each subscale consists of six items, each rated on a 5-point scale (1 = "not at all true about me," 5 = "always true about me"). Sample items include "I worry a lot about what other kids think of me" (Social Anxiety) and "If I had a choice, I'd rather do something by myself than do it with other kids" (Social Avoidance). Additional research with this measure has revealed some gender differences (i.e., girls scoring higher than boys), as well as associations of self-reported social avoidance with loneliness and low perceived competence (Hymel et al., 1985).

La Greca, Dandes, Wick, Shaw, and Stone (1988) developed the Social Anxiety Scale for Children. This 10-item measure includes two subscales—Fear of Negative Evaluation ("I worry about doing something new in front of other kids," "I worry about being teased," "I worry about what other kids think of me") and Social Avoidance and Distress ("I feel shy around kids I don't know," "I get nervous when I talk to new kids," "I only talk to kids that I know really well"). Items are rated on a 3-point scale, from "never true" (0) to "sometimes true" (1) to "always true" (2). The scale showed good internal consistency (alphas of .83 and .63 for the two subscales, respectively, and .76 for the full scale). Some gender differences emerged, with girls reporting greater fear of negative evaluation than boys. Evidence of concurrent validity was also provided. Significant correlations emerged between this scale and the Revised Children's Manifest Anxiety Scale. In addition, sociometrically rejected children reported higher levels of social anxiety than average, popular, or neglected children (La Greca et al., 1988).

Perceived Social Competence

The most widely used measure of children's perceived competence is the Perceived Competence Scale for Children (Harter, 1982). This scale taps perceived competence in the social domain in one subscale ("have a lot of friends"); it also includes subscales assessing cognitive competence ("good at school work"), physical competence ("do well at sports"), and general self-worth ("happy the way I am"). On each item, the child is asked to select between two statements to indicate the one that is more like him/her, and then to indicate whether the statement is "sort of" true or "very true" for him/her. Items are scored along a 4-point response scale (from 1 = "really true, negative" to 4 = "really true, positive").

Based on Bandura's (1977) conceptualization of self-efficacy, which focuses on the individual's perceptions of his/her capacity to perform behaviors that lead to positive outcomes, Wheeler and Ladd (1982) developed the Children's Self-Efficacy for Peer Interaction Scale. The scale consists of 22 items assessing children's perceptions of their ability to enact prosocial verbal persuasive skills in specific peer situations. Each item consists of a statement describing a social situation (e.g., "You want to start a game"), followed by an incomplete statement requiring the child to evaluate his/her ability to perform a particular verbal skill ("Asking other kids to play is ____ for you"). For each item, children circle one of four response choices: (1) "HARD!", (2) "hard", (3) "easy", or (4) "EASY!". Twelve items depict conflict situations (e.g., intervening in an argument, confronting a child who has taken your turn or pushed into line), and 10 items depict nonconflict situations (e.g., asking to play a game, initiating a game). In Wheeler and Ladd's empirical evaluation, the scale demonstrated good internal consistency (alpha = .85) and good test–retest reliability (r = .80–.90 over a 2-week period). Correlations with positive sociometric nominations were mild to moderate (ranging from r = .08 to r = .36 across grade levels).

In addition to these measures that assess children's affective and cognitive appraisals of their social comfort, support, and capability in peer relations, children's perceptions of the causal links between their characteristics/behaviors and their social outcomes warrant attention, as these attributions and control beliefs affect their level of psychological distress and influence their motivation for and engagement in active coping attempts.

ATTRIBUTIONAL STYLE AND CONTROL BELIEFS

The way that children interpret the causes of their social experiences, particularly negative social events, may determine what impact experiences of rejection or victimization have on their self-conceptions and associated feelings of distress. In normative samples, children tend to attribute social failure to external causes, whereas success is attributed more often to internal or neutral causes (Ames, Ames, & Garrison, 1977). Children who attribute social failures to internal and stable causes are at elevated risk for depression, anxiety, and feelings of low self-worth, as well as reduced attempts at adaptive social problem solving and goal-directed behavior (Goetz & Dweck, 1980; Graham & Juvonen, 1998; Quiggle et al., 1992; Vitaro, Tremblay, Gagnon, & Boivin, 1992). Although relatively few studies have examined standardized measures to assess causal attributions in social situations, a few examples exist. Hypothetical vignettes have been used to elicit reasoning, followed by rating scales or open-ended coding.

For example, Quiggle and colleagues (1992) used hypothetical vignettes such as those used to assess social information processing among children in grades 3 through 6. In addition to asking about the intentions of the others, what they would do, and how well their strategies would work, they asked children why they thought the problem might occur. On this measure, depressed children, like aggressive children, showed a hostile attributional bias; however, they were also more likely to attribute negative situations to internal, stable, and global causes.

Sobol, Earn, Bennett, and Humphries (1983) presented children with a series of hypothetical vignettes that varied with regard to outcome (successful or unsuccessful) and initiator (self or other). They then asked children for their spontaneous explanations of the outcome. For example, a vignette describing a self-initiated interaction with a successful outcome was this: "You ask a child to go to the movies with you and he does. Why do you think this would happen?" Causal responses were coded along the dimension of locus of control (internal, mutual, or external), stability (stable or unstable), and controllability (controllable, intermediate, or uncontrollable). The majority (90%) of the causes children gave could be categorized into six types: luck (37%), others' assessment of self (17%), others' motives (14%), personality interaction (10%), third-party intervention (10%), and others' personality (5%). Reflecting the validity of this method of assessment, rejected children were more likely to suggest that luck was the cause of their social outcomes than popular children were. Children who identified stable causes for their failures expected future failures in their social relationships, whereas children who endorsed controllable causes had higher self-esteem.

More recently, investigators have explored the use of rating scales with hypothetical vignettes. Such rating scales have less flexibility than other measures, but provide greater ease of administration and scoring. Exploring this measurement technique, Graham and Juvonen (1998) presented middle school students with hypothetical vignettes describing incidents of victimization, and then asked them to rate the extent to which they felt different causes might contribute to these events. Two vignettes were used. In one, students were asked to imagine being the target of peer humiliation at school; in the other, they were asked to imagine being the target of physical threat from peers. For each scenario, respondents rated how much they agreed with 32 statements describing potential thoughts, feelings, and behavioral reactions. Attributions included stable, internal causes ("If I were a cooler kid, I wouldn't get picked on"); unstable, internal causes ("I should have been more careful"); and external attributions ("These kinds of kids pick on everybody, no one is safe in this school anymore").

These research-based measures have proven useful in documenting links between attributional style and psychological distress in the domain of peer relations. However, their utility for intervention assessment and evaluation remains questionable. Like measures of social information processing, these measures rely on children's responses to hypothetical incidents. For intervention planning and evaluation, it may be more useful to have measures that reflect children's attributions and control beliefs regarding their actual relationships with peers, since their personal experiences and beliefs about their own relationships may have a more proximal and important impact on their capacity to engage in and sustain behavior and attitude changes toward their peers than their more general peer orientation may.

IMPLICATIONS FOR INTERVENTION PLANNING AND EVALUATION

In Chapter 4, I have argued that self-system processes deserve more attention in social competence interventions designed to promote positive peer relations. Research has accumulated to suggest that multiple features of the self-system affect and are affected by children's peer experiences, particularly their social cognitions (beliefs and reasoning about others) and self-appraisals (affective and cognitive assessments of their comfort and capability in peer relations). Yet little is known about the optimal ways to assess these features of self-system processes for the purposes of intervention design and evaluation.

Social-cognitive measures that assess children's social perceptions, interpretations, response generation, and outcome evaluations in hypothetical peer situations differentiate children who do and do not have social behavior and peer relation problems in research studies. However, the correlations are not strong enough to support these measures as valid indices for either planning social competence interventions or evaluating their effectiveness. Instead, teacher/peer ratings and observations provide more valid indices of child social behavior and peer relationship problems for both these purposes.

Children's responses to hypothetical peer problems may be of limited utility for intervention planning, because they do not include information about the child's actual social-cognitive processes in their naturalistic peer relationships. Measures that provide more information about how children are actually thinking and reasoning about their "online" peer interactions, such as the videotape review interview method used by Putallaz (1983), may hold more promise for informing interventions directed toward improving children's functioning in those peer relationships. Certainly more research is needed to address this important area of assessment and evaluation.

Of the self-system process measures reviewed in this chapter, children's self-reports of their social distress show the greatest promise and validity for intervention assessment and evaluation. In particular, children's feelings of loneliness, social anxiety, and perceived competence have demonstrated good psychometric properties and reflect children's appraisals of their current state of affective comfort or distress in their peer relations. Measures of attributional style and control beliefs in social interactions are of considerable importance from a theoretical perspective, but available research measures focus on child responses to hypothetical situations; hence they suffer from the same limitations as the research measures of social-cognitive processes described above, in terms of their utility for intervention planning and evaluation.

SUMMARY

In 1985, Hymel and Franke noted that we know very little about how self-system processes influence subsequent social behavior and the effectiveness of intervention programs. This statement is still true today, although progress has been made in identifying the multiple facets of self-perceptions and social reasoning that appear associated with peer relations. For example, we know that children with problematic peer relationships often show evidence of thoughts and feelings that contribute to their interpersonal difficulties—making it difficult for them to experience security or intimacy in their friendships, to balance their autonomy striving with interpersonal sensitivity, or to approach social environments with confidence and well-regulated coping. We also know that teacher and peer ratings, which provide critical information about the nature and degree of children's social difficulties, are not particularly accurate in their assessment of the kinds of feelings or thought processes that may contribute to a particular child's problematic behaviors. Feelings of psychological distress (e.g., loneliness, social anxiety, depressed mood, perceived victimization) often accompany peer problems, and these appear to contribute to, as well as result from, social maladjustment (Egan & Perry, 1998). Social reasoning—including the way in which social information is encoded and interpreted, and the ways in which possible responses are generated and evaluated—also has an impact on social behavior (Crick & Dodge, 1994). Causal cognitions, particularly attributions regarding the control of positive and negative social outcomes, affect both motivation for social coping and the accompanying feelings of self-worth (Graham & Juvonen, 1998; Skinner, 1995).

As important as these self-system constructs are to our developmental models, their assessment and treatment remain less well understood than observable social behaviors. That is, much less is known about how to assess self-system variables with validity and how to match these assessment results with intervention strategies than about how to assess observable behaviors.

Children's reports regarding their feelings of loneliness, social anxiety, and depressed mood certainly have face validity and deserve attention in intervention (Hymel & Franke, 1985; Parker et al., 1995). Research is needed to identify the ways in which attention to these feelings can be embedded within interventions creating interaction and relationship opportunities that a child can realistically feel good about.

Determining how to assess and address child social-cognitive processes in intervention (e.g., social goals, attributions, and response generation and evaluation processes) also requires more study. Although research has linked children's responses to hypothetical vignettes with their peer status, it is not clear that the general perceptual and attributional frames captured in these measures are the optimal targets for intervention. Theoretical models suggest that "online" social-cognitive processing is affected by the complexity of the social situation, the child's affectively charged cognition of the child, and the child's personal orientation toward and past relationship history with the others in the social setting (Baldwin, 1992; Crick & Dodge, 1994). Hence assessments that focus on discrete components of hypothetical scenarios lacking in personal reference, and that are conducted in "cold-cognition" settings, may fail to capture the types of thinking and social information processing that are proximal and functional in children's everyday interactions with peers. It may be that for the purposes of intervention, these factors are better assessed and addressed in the context of *in vivo* interactions, via interviews and process comments during the course of naturalistic and therapeutic peer interactions. This idea is explored further in the discussion of intervention strategies.

Part III provides a consideration of intervention strategies. First, Chapter 10 presents a review of the empirical literature, as well as a consideration of the features of intervention programs that appear linked with improvements in child social competence and positive peer relations. Chapters 11–13 then delve into pragmatic considerations associated with the design and management of social competence interventions. In addition to intervention strategies that target aspects of a rejected child's social competence, I discuss strategies focused on "preparing the environment" and creating more supportive contexts for promoting positive social development at school and home.

PART III

INTERVENTION METHODS

Chapter 10

Approaches to Intervention

The idea that interventions could be designed to remediate problematic peer relations and promote social competence first emerged in the late 1930s and early 1940s. As noted in Chapter 1, Chittenden (1942) designed a set of lessons for preschool children who often had conflicts with peers. She used dolls to depict positive strategies for getting along with others, and recorded positive changes in children's behaviors as a result (see Renshaw, 1981). In this chapter, I take a historical look at developments in intervention design that emerged during the 20th century, particularly during the past 50 years. I track the key changes in the conceptual models that have guided social competence interventions across the years, as well as the empirical findings that support the effectiveness of modern techniques. The review begins in the 1960s, when emerging behavioral management techniques were applied to the promotion of positive social behavior. It then moves to the mid-1970s, when—informed by a growing base of developmental research on peer relations—interventions became more instructional, using modeling, instructions, and multicomponent coaching strategies to teach social skills. I then describe the expansion of coaching techniques that occurred in the 1980s, as investigators struggled to better address the behavioral heterogeneity of children with poor peer relations, and attempted to improve the generalization and maintenance of treatment effects. Finally, I describe developments that have characterized recent years, as well as key questions that remain.

This chapter focuses on intervention research that identifies effective strategies and techniques for promoting the social competence of children with problematic peer relations, including both "lessons learned" and continuing issues and challenges for intervention design. Chapters 11 and 12 use this research, as well as experience and theory,

161

to frame issues that require attention during the design of social competence coaching interventions; these include the organizational structure and content of social competence coaching programs (Chapter 11), and the potential impact of different types of coaching processes on child self-system change (Chapter 12). In this chapter, I concentrate specifically on interventions designed to improve the peer relations of identified children with peer problems. "Universal" programs, delivered by teachers and designed to promote the social competence of all children in the classroom, are described in Chapter 13, as are recent efforts to embed social competence interventions in multicomponent and multilayered prevention and intervention programs.

OPERANT STRATEGIES: MANIPULATING ANTECEDENTS AND CONSEQUENCES

Although the historical underpinnings of social competence interventions consist of a few studies conducted in the 1930s and 1940s (Renshaw, 1981), there was a long hiatus in peer relations research between the mid-1940s and the 1960s. Hence this review begins with intervention designs conceived in the 1960s and the programmatic development in social competence training techniques that followed.

During the 1960s and early 1970s, a technology for behavior change based on the manipulation of antecedents and consequences emerged and was applied to changing the rates of children's social behavior. Reinforcements (such as contingent attention, token reinforcement, or primary reinforcements) were manipulated to increase positive social behaviors, whereas time out, response cost, and differential reinforcement programs were applied to reduce negative social behaviors (for reviews, see Elliott & Gresham, 1993; Gresham, 1981). Contingent reinforcement proved to be a highly effective method of increasing rates of peer interaction among socially isolated children. For example, when Allen, Hart, Buell, Harris, and Wolf (1964) instructed a preschool teacher to attend to and praise a withdrawn boy whenever he interacted with peers but to ignore him when he was playing alone, the child's rate of social interaction increased dramatically from 10% to 60%. Similarly, investigators asked teachers to selectively praise the cooperative behaviors displayed by aggressive children, and documented corresponding increases in the children's cooperative peer interactions and reductions in aggressive exchanges (Brown & Elliott, 1965; Hart, Reynolds, Baer, Brawley, & Harris, 1968; Pinkston, Reese, LeBlanc, & Baer, 1973). Peer attention, as well as contingent teacher attention, proved effective at increasing positive social behavior and decreasing disruptiveness (Solomon & Wahler, 1973).

Focusing on antecedent conditions rather than consequences, a number of researchers explored the effects of providing children with more cued opportunities to play (see the review by Gresham, 1981). In a series of studies, Strain and his colleagues demonstrated that they could increase the social interactions of withdrawn preschoolers in several ways: by (1) coaching peer confederates to initiate invitations to play (Strain, 1977); (2) prompting the isolated children verbally and physically to interact (Strain, Shores, & Kerr, 1976); and (3) involving the children in structured sociodramatic play, acting out well-known stories (Strain & Weigerink, 1976).

Although providing opportunities and reinforcement effectively promoted rates of social interaction, these tactics had only a limited impact on the long-term quality of children's peer relations, for several reasons. First, increasing the quantity of peer interaction did not always result in improved quality. For example, when Kirby and Toler (1970) used primary reinforcement to increase the rates of peer interaction for a socially withdrawn boy, aggressive behaviors increased along with positive interactions. Second, effects appeared dependent on extensive teacher monitoring and continued delivery of reinforcement, resulting in high-demand interventions with little generalizability across contexts or time (Gresham, 1981). Third, as illustrated by research accumulating during the later 1970s and early 1980s, rates of social interaction appeared only weakly related to positive peer relations; quality of social interaction was a far more powerful predictor than quantity (Asher, Markell, & Hymel, 1981).

Operant techniques, designed to increase social interactions by manipulating antecedents or consequences, were ill suited to teaching new social skills that were not already part of a child's repertoire (Gresham, 1981; Ladd & Mize, 1983). The behavioral approaches assumed implicitly that children were not performing skillful behaviors because those behaviors were not elicited and reinforced in their social environments, or because other competing responses took precedence (La Greca, 1993). As such, these intervention strategies assumed that poor peer relations stemmed from performance deficits, rather than skill deficits (Gresham, 1981).

Meanwhile, research on children's peer relations was leading investigators to conclude that peer acceptance required more sophisticated interaction skills than initiating positive acts or refraining from hitting others. For example, it was becoming clear that being a positive social partner required behavioral flexibility and social responsivity—the capacity to adapt behavior to various interpersonal contexts and in response to interpersonal cues (Asher et al., 1981). Operant techniques alone appeared inadequate to promote this kind of behavioral flexibility. Hence investigators turned their attention to intervention strategies that could teach children new social skills involving more complex and flexible behavioral responding. During the early 1970s, two instructional approaches were developed; one focused on the use of modeling techniques to teach positive play behaviors, and the other focused on the use of instructions, discussion, and role-play techniques to teach social problem-solving skills.

INITIAL INSTRUCTIONAL APPROACHES: MODELING AND SOCIAL PROBLEM SOLVING

Conceptualizing poor peer relations as the result of social skill deficits, modeling strategies assumed that children who lacked the social behaviors that they needed to interact effectively with peers could learn those behaviors via modeling (Bandura, 1969; Gresham, 1981). A series of studies demonstrated that the social interactions of withdrawn preschool children could be increased by exposing the children to filmed models portraying positive peer interactions (Evers & Schwarz, 1973; O'Connor, 1972). The impact appeared greatest when the models had characteristics that were similar to the target children, when a variety of examples and models were used, when first-person narration was used, and when children were explicitly instructed to model the behaviors and reinforced for doing so (Gresham, 1981). Although some investigators were able to document maintenance of the effects for weeks after film exposure (Evers & Schwartz, 1973; Evers-Pasquale & Sherman, 1975), others found limited maintenance and a nonsignificant impact on peer acceptance when modeling was used alone (Gottman, Gonso, & Schuler, 1976). This research suggested that modeling could be an important technique for promoting change in social behaviors, but that sustained impact on children's peer relations was not likely if the technique was used in a limited way.

A different approach to teaching social skills, which focused on teaching social problem-solving skills, emerged parallel to (but was distinct from) interventions using modeling techniques. This approach focused on improving the social competence of all children in a classroom, rather than targeting the skill deficits of children with identified peer problems (see Chapter 13). It is mentioned here briefly, as the social problem-solving instructional model influenced and in some cases was incorporated into later social competence coaching interventions.

Introduced by Spivack and Shure (1974), this approach differed from earlier, behavior-focused programs, both in terms of the instructional techniques used and in the focus of intervention efforts; it relied primarily on verbal instruction to enhance children's social knowledge regarding social problem-solving strategies. Unlike behavioral management or modeling approaches, the social problem-solving method emphasized the importance of the thinking skills that provided the foundation for effective social interaction. The premise was that children's cognitive capacities to recognize and accurately assess social problems, as well as their ability to generate and evaluate multiple potential responses, to set goals, and to self-monitor their behavioral performance in light of those goals, provided the critical building blocks for flexible, socially responsive, and adaptive behaviors (Allen, Chinsky, Larcen, Lochman, & Selinger, 1976; Weissberg & Allen, 1986). Research on this approach is reviewed in Chapter 13, which describes systemic approaches designed to promote positive peer relations at the classroom level. Critical to later interventions focused on children with poor peer relations was the emphasis on thinking skills, which, in combination with traditional behavioral approaches, informed the development of expanded coaching programs.

By the mid-1970s, the empirical literature on social skills training approaches was large enough to support a number of reviews (see Asher, Oden, & Gottman, 1977; Combs & Slaby, 1977). Generally, the conclusion at that point was that these approaches (including manipulating antecedents and consequences, modeling, and instructions) showed promise in terms of effects on immediate social behavior, but lacked evidence of long-term maintenance and positive impact on children's peer relations. A critical issue raised by some reviewers involved the social validity of the change efforts, as well as their overall effectiveness (Gresham, 1981). The late 1970s and early 1980s thus witnessed the emergence of coaching techniques, designed to strengthen the impact of social skill training methods. These techniques included an expanded set of instructional methods, as well as increasing emphasis on sociometric measures for participant selection, target skill identification, and program evaluation.

INITIAL COACHING STRATEGIES

Like modeling and social problem-solving instructional programs, the coaching programs developed in the late 1970s were based upon the premise that unaccepted children lacked the requisite skills to develop and maintain positive peer relations, and that acquisition of these social skills would promote their peer acceptance (Asher & Renshaw,

1981; Furman & Gavin, 1989). However, coaching programs introduced changes in intervention design that distinguished them from
earlier intervention approaches in three ways: (1) They utilized an
expanded set of instructional methods, including opportunities for
guided practice and feedback; (2) they identified participants and evaluated program effectiveness via socially valid sociometric ratings; and
(3) they selected target skills based on empirical evidence of linkages
between particular behavioral skills and peer acceptance.

    First to emerge was the use of an expanded set of instructional
procedures that included structured and comprehensive attention to
the teaching of skill concepts, the development of behavioral competence, and the promotion of self-monitoring and responsivity to social
feedback (Ladd & Mize, 1983; Furman & Gavin, 1989). To establish a
conceptual basis for skill development, coaching programs began with
a presentation of the target skill(s); this presentation typically employed
a combination of modeling, instruction, and discussion, often with exposure to both positive and negative examples. The objective was to
enhance children's skill knowledge and understanding by providing information about the purpose, form, and functional value of the target
skills (Ladd & Mize, 1983). Next, to promote children's abilities to
perform the skills comfortably and flexibly, children were given opportunities for behavioral rehearsal with peer partners under supportive
conditions. Finally, children received performance feedback and reinforcement. In addition to helping the children adjust their social behavior, the purpose of this feedback was to strengthen the children's attention to their own behavior and its interpersonal impact. Through
enhancing children's self-monitoring and social awareness, the goal was
to promote socially responsive behavioral flexibility.

    In one of the first attempts to use this kind of formalized set of
coaching techniques to improve social behavior, Cooke and Apolloni
(1976) used a combination of instructions, live modeling, and praise to
increase the positive social behaviors (e.g., smiling, sharing, positive
physical contacting, and verbal complimenting) of four students with
learning disabilities. Classroom observations suggested that these social
behaviors, learned in coaching sessions, generalized to the classroom
and were maintained at a 4-week follow-up assessment. Bellack and
Hersen (1977) also used coaching techniques, including instructions
and demonstrations, to promote more effective communication skills
(loudness and duration of speech), and added a criterion-referenced
period of behavioral rehearsal. That is, children were required to engage in supervised practice until they could perform the trained skills
proficiently, matching a performance standard identified to represent
skill mastery. Although these two studies suggested the potential effi-

cacy of the multifaceted coaching approach in changing behavior, it remained unclear whether or not these approaches enhanced the quality of child peer relations.

Gottman and colleagues (1976) introduced sociometric ratings as a source of socially valid information about peer relations, to be used for the selection of participants and evaluation of effectiveness of coaching strategies on peer relations. Working with two girls who received low sociometric ratings, Gottman and colleagues used coaching techniques to target four social skills: (1) greeting, (2) asking for and giving information, (3) extending an offer of inclusion, and (4) effective leave taking. The two children who received coaching showed improvements in "play with" and "work with" sociometric ratings, relative to two children in a control comparison condition, who played games with an adult.

These three studies represented important explorations of the coaching method, illustrating the potential of the technique. However, each included only a few participants, providing little information about the potential impact of coaching strategies on a larger group of children. In addition, the basis for target skill selection was highly variable across the studies.

In 1977, Oden and Asher designed a larger-scale coaching trial, with randomly assigned coaching, peer pairing, and no-treatment control groups. In this study, they emphasized the important concept of identifying target skills based upon evidence of empirical association with peer ratings. Prior to the Oden and Asher study, the skills targeted in operant, modeling, and early coaching studies showed wide variability across studies; they often represented specific discrete behaviors that, based on face validity, appeared related to positive sociability, such as maintaining eye contact, smiling, and speech duration. Described as "molecular" skills by La Greca (1993), these types of skills lacked evidence of social validity and did not always reflect the complex nuances of effective social interaction. In contrast, Oden and Asher took a "molar" approach to skill identification, targeting four broader domains of social behavior that were correlated with sociometric measures—participation, cooperation, communication, and validation support. This strategy represents the "competence correlates" approach to skill identification (La Greca, 1993). During coaching sessions, children are taught multiple specific behavioral examples of broadly defined social interaction strategies (e.g., taking turns and sharing as examples of cooperation). The goal is to teach children general strategies for social interaction, with multiple behavioral examples, in order to enhance their behavioral flexibility in domains relevant to peer acceptance (Ladd & Mize, 1983). Oden and Asher also formally introduced the concept of including peers into social competence coaching programs, in order to provide target children with "real-life" opportunities for skill practice, and to promote positive changes in peer perceptions of the target children.

The Oden and Asher (1977) study focused on the four skill domains noted above: participation, cooperation, communication, and validation support. Third- and fourth-grade students, selected on the basis of low "play with" and "work with" sociometric ratings, were randomly assigned to participate in coaching, peer pairing, or no treatment conditions. In the coaching condition, students participated in five 30-minute sessions, each consisting of three parts. First, students met individually with a graduate student who provided verbal instructions, examples, and demonstrations of the target skills, presented as strategies that might make playing games more fun. Next, the children had the opportunity to practice the skills as they tried out various games with rotating classroom partners. In the last 10 minutes of each session, the coach met with each child individually, reviewing the child's use of the target skills and his/her assessment of their efficacy. Children in the peer-pairing condition also played games with classroom partners, but did not receive preplay or postplay coaching. Behavioral observations collected during the game-playing sessions revealed no differences between children in the coaching and peer-pairing conditions in their use of the target skills. However, children in the coaching condition showed significant increases in their "play with" sociometric ratings at posttreatment, with a trend that suggested sustained intervention effects at a 1-year follow-up assessment.

The Oden and Asher (1977) findings were exciting, but a replication study conducted by Hymel and Asher (1977) with unaccepted third- to fifth-grade children revealed inconsistent patterns of impact. In that study, the coaching procedures were similar to those used by Oden and Asher, but Hymel and Asher compared the impact of standardized coaching (all participants were coached on the same skills) and individualized coaching (after presentation of the four basic skill concepts, later sessions emphasized skills identified to be of greatest relevance for a particular child). However, in contrast to the earlier findings, neither coaching condition produced significant gains in sociometric ratings compared to the peer-pairing condition; nor did behavioral observation data show significant coaching effects. In terms of raw scores, all three groups improved, so the failure to show a positive impact for coaching may have resulted in part from the positive influence of the peer-pairing condition, which served as the attention placebo control. Unfortunately, however, due to the lack of a no-treatment control group, the potential effects of peer pairing with or without coaching could not be determined by this study.

Two additional studies conducted in 1980 warrant review. Each involved a strong randomized trial design, participant selection based upon sociometric "play with" and "work with" ratings, and the evaluation of coaching effects on both social behavior and sociometric ratings. Gresham and Nagle (1980) worked with third- and fourth-grade students, and compared the impact of coaching procedures used alone, modeling procedures used alone, a combination of coaching and modeling procedures, and a no-treatment control condition. Children in the coaching-only condition met in dyads or triads for six 20-minute coaching sessions, with each session organized into the three segments defined by Oden and Asher (1977)—skill presentation, skill practice, and performance feedback and review. In addition to targeting the skills of participation, cooperation, communication, and validation/support (in sessions 1 and 2), further skills were taught in later sessions. Friendship-making skills of greeting others, asking for and giving information, extending an offer of inclusion, and effective leave taking were taught in sessions 3 and 4, and initiating and receiving positive and negative interaction were taught in sessions 5 and 6. The modeling condition consisted of viewing videotapes of targeted social skills (e.g., participation, cooperation, friendship making) during the six sessions, and the combined group received an abbreviated sequence of modeling and coaching. All three instructional conditions proved equivalent in their capacity to significantly increase children's display of positive social behaviors and their sociometric "play with" ratings; however, the two coaching conditions had a stronger impact on reducing rates of initiating and receiving negative social interaction than the modeling alone did.

A second randomized trial (La Greca & Santogrossi, 1980) evaluated the impact of coaching on unaccepted third through fifth graders. Eight skill areas were targeted (smiling, greeting, joining, inviting, conversing, sharing and cooperating, complimenting, and grooming), and the effects of coaching were compared to an attention placebo and a waiting-list control group. Relative to children in the two control groups, coached children demonstrated higher rates of the trained skills in a role-play situation, and higher rates of social initiations with peers during free-play sessions at school. However, no significant treatment effects were found on sociometric ratings.

These coaching studies demonstrated promising but mixed findings in regard to sociometric impact, with some studies producing significant improvements on peer ratings (Gottman et al., 1976; Gresham & Nagle, 1980; Oden & Asher, 1977) and others reporting no significant impact (Hymel & Asher, 1977; LaGreca & Santogrossi, 1980). Behavioral changes were more consistent, with significant effects demonstrated by a number of studies (Bornstein, Bellack, & Hersen, 1977;

Gresham & Nagle, 1980; LaGreca & Santogrossi, 1980), but not all (Hymel & Asher, 1977; Oden & Asher, 1977). Even in the behavioral domain, the changes were not always consistent with the coaching predictions. For example, neither La Greca and Santogrossi (1980) or Gresham and Nagle (1980) witnessed increases in positive social behavior, although the former study produced increased rates of social initiations and the latter study found decreased rates of negative social behavior among coached children. To some extent, the divergent findings may reflect measurement issues and the lack of sensitivity of some of the measures used to intervention impact. Overall, the pattern of findings promoted feelings of confidence about the capacity of the coaching approach to improve children's peer relations, but also suggested that coaching programs needed further development and refinement.

COACHING PROGRAMS OF THE 1980s

Based on accumulating basic research on children's peer relations, two major hypotheses emerged regarding factors that might affect the impact of coaching. First, it was becoming clear that children who were unaccepted by peers (i.e., those who received low scores on "play with" and "work with" sociometric ratings) were a heterogeneous group. Depending upon the severity of the rating cutoff score used to identify unaccepted children in coaching studies, some proportion of these children were probably neglected (not liked by children, but not disliked), whereas others were probably rejected (actively disliked by their peers). In addition, unaccepted children showed wide variations in the behavioral bases for their peer difficulties. It was possible that coaching programs were differentially effective with children who were neglected or rejected, and that different kinds of coaching strategies or target skills might be needed by different subgroups of unaccepted children, particularly those who were aggressive rather than simply withdrawn. Thus coaching programs that identified children on the basis of low "play with" or "work with" preference ratings alone, like those described above, were likely to recruit participants who varied significantly—both in the severity of their peer problems and in their behavioral characteristics and patterns of skill deficits. These differences could well create variability in their responsivity to the coaching interventions.

The second major hypothesis was that to increase the sustained impact of coaching, it might be necessary to focus on the mastery of a smaller set of skills (including more extensive practice in more naturalistic settings), rather than on brief exposure to a larger set of skills (e.g., simply introducing and reviewing skills for one or two sessions). In addition, the role of peers in the generalization process gained attention. Coaching programs assumed that once unaccepted children learned and displayed more positive social behavior, peers would respond positively and improve their evaluation of those children. Unlike the earlier operant programs, which were dependent upon reorganizing the contingencies in a child's social environment to achieve behavior change, the premise in coaching programs was that didactic training in social skills would allow children to transfer improved behavior to their naturalistic environments without any focused attention on the alteration of those social contexts (Gresham, 1985; Schneider, 1992). However, the resistance to change in peer sociometric ratings even in the context of documented improvements in unaccepted child behavior (La Greca & Santogrossi, 1980) suggested that greater attention to generalization issues in general, and peer responding and reputational biases in particular, might strengthen the impact of coaching programs.

A coaching program designed by Ladd (1981) included modifications to address each of these issues. For example, Ladd introduced the idea of a dual-screening system for the identification of target participants. First, he used sociometric "play with" ratings to identify third-grade children who were unaccepted by peers. Then he conducted behavioral observations of the unaccepted children during free-play periods (indoor recess), in order to identify those who exhibited low rates of the skills targeted by his intervention. This screening process determined that the unpopular participants who entered the coaching program demonstrated deficiencies in the skills to be taught; it thus increased the likelihood that training in those skills would address the behavioral needs associated with peer difficulties. In earlier studies where screening was based on sociometric ratings alone, participants did not necessarily have skill deficiencies in the targeted area, which may have reduced the programs' impact. For example, in the Hymel and Asher (1977) study that failed to produce behavioral gains, the sociometrically unaccepted target participants did not, as a group, show lower rates of the target skills than their peers in pretreatment classroom observations. This made it less likely that the particular source of low peer acceptance involved deficiencies in the target skills for a number of the participants (and/or it reflected a failure of sensitive behavioral measurement).

To strengthen the sustainability of skill training, and to allow for more practice and consolidation, Ladd (1981) focused on a small set of skills and extended the training to allow for almost twice the amount of instructional time as Oden and Asher (1977) provided. He also built upon the peer-pairing idea introduced by Oden and Asher, and included two sessions focused on promoting skill generalization to interactions with classmates. Ladd's program focused on three communication skills associated with peer acceptance—asking questions, offering useful suggestions and directions, and making supportive statements. During the first six 45-minute sessions, pairs of socially isolated children met with a coach and received instruction in basic skill concepts, opportunities for behavioral rehearsal, and review of their skill performance. Then, in the last two sessions designed to promote skill maintenance and generalization, two new classmates joined the groups, and children were encouraged to try out their new behaviors during structured games with these additional classmates. At the end of each of these sessions, children received performance feedback and had the opportunity to discuss strategies to improve future interactions. Compared to children in an attention control group and a no-treatment group, the coached children improved significantly in asking questions and offering suggestions, and decreased their nonsocial behavior during classroom observations. Both the coached and attention control group improved in "play with" sociometric ratings collected immediately after the intervention, but only the coached children showed sustained improvements at the 4-week follow-up assessment.

A colleague and I (Bierman & Furman, 1984) used a dual-screening assessment process similar to the design used by Ladd (1981) to identify preadolescents who were unaccepted by peers (low friendship ratings) and who showed low rates of conversation skills during playgroup observations. We also used coaching procedures similar to those used by Ladd to teach three conversation skills—self-disclosure (sharing information about oneself), questions (asking others about themselves), and leads (offering suggestions, help, or invitations to others). In addition, our study was designed to carefully evaluate the inclusion of nontarget peers in the intervention as a method of increasing generalization of effects and improving sociometric ratings. The Bierman and Furman design included four conditions: (1) individual coaching, (2) coaching in a peer group context, (3) peer group experience without coaching, and (4) a no-treatment comparison. The purpose and method of including nontarget peers in the intervention were based on research suggesting that reputational biases represent challenges to the generalizability of coaching programs, so that changing target child behavior may be insufficient to change peer reputations and peer responding. Instead, direct intervention procedures may be required to change reputational biases, particularly for preadolescent and older youth. Based on the research of Sherif, Harvey, White, Hood, and Sherif (1961), we (Bierman & Furman, 1984) postulated that opportunities to interact with peers on tasks characterized by superordinate goals might promote positive changes in peer liking. Research suggests that when children have successful experiences working on super-ordinate goals, and are able to attain goals by coordinating their efforts and energies, within-group cooperation and liking improve (Bryan, 1975; Sherif et al., 1961).

In the Bierman and Furman (1984) study, the effects of providing unaccepted children with opportunities to engage in positive interactions with classroom peers were examined directly. In the two peer group conditions, each unaccepted target child was put into a group with two randomly assigned, same-gender, peer-accepted classmates. Triads were told that their help was needed to make instructional videotapes for college students, illustrating the kinds of things that grade school friends talked about and did together. In a series of ten 30-minute sessions, triads engaged in cooperative activities designed to help the members get to know one another better; then they planned and rehearsed a series of videotapes. In the final session, each triad produced a friendship videotape. In the group coaching condition (coaching plus peer experience), the triads received coaching in conversational skills as part of their planning and rehearsal sessions; the coaching procedures were very similar to those of Ladd (1981). In a second condition (peer experience only), triads engaged in similar activities and made videotapes, but did not receive any specific social skills training. In a third condition (individual coaching), students received skills training and made videotapes of themselves conversing with the adult coach.

The results suggested that coaching and peer involvement had complementary effects. Coached children (in both the individual and group coaching conditions) showed increases in conversation skills relative to noncoached children (those receiving peer experience only or no treatment). In contrast, children who participated in a peer experience condition (with or without coaching) received higher sociometric ratings at the posttreatment assessment, rated themselves as more socially competent, and showed higher rates of lunchtime peer interaction than children who did not experience peer involvement (e.g., those who were coached individually or were in the no-treatment control group). However, only children who received both types of interventions (i.e., coaching with peer involvement) showed enduring gains in skill concept acquisition, effective social interaction, and improved peer acceptance at the 6-week follow-up. Interestingly, however, peer acceptance improved only among the peer partners who participated in group activities with target children, and not among the broader set of classroom peers. This finding suggested that direct exposure to the improved behavior of unaccepted children and opportunities for cooperative interaction may be needed to change negative reputational biases and improve peer status.

An analysis of the videotapes made by children in the group coaching and group experience conditions revealed that coached target children showed low levels of conversational skills in the early treatment
session videotapes and increased their skill performance in later sessions, whereas target children in the peer experience condition showed
no change over time (Bierman, 1986a). Hence, as postulated, group
coaching promoted skill acquisition in a way that simple involvement
with peers did not. In addition, peer partners showed a higher rate of
contingent positive responding to the positive behaviors of target children in the group coaching condition than in the peer experience
condition, suggesting that group coaching increased the saliency of
positive social behaviors for the nontarget peer partners. Given the
likelihood that peers' contingent responding is an important factor affecting the generalizability of behavior change, this finding suggests
that involving peers in coaching sessions may promote sustained behavior change via its impact on peer responding.

The Ladd (1981) and Bierman and Furman (1984) studies suggested that the impact of the coaching method developed in earlier
studies could be strengthened in several ways: (1) by using a dual-
screening system to identify unaccepted children with the specific skill
deficits targeted in the intervention, (2) by extending the length of intervention and focusing more training time on a smaller set of skills,
and (3) by including peers in the intervention. These refinements in
coaching program design appeared to enhance the intervention's impact on behavioral and sociometric gains for socially withdrawn children who were unaccepted by peers.

At the same time, developmental research on peer relations was
accumulating to suggest that socially withdrawn, unaccepted children
did not represent the highest-risk group in terms of problematic peer
relations. Rather, children who were actively rejected by their peers
were most distinctively characterized by elevated levels of aggressive
and disruptive behavior (Coie, Dodge, & Coppotelli, 1982). It wasn't
clear how coaching programs for unpopular, socially withdrawn children would meet the needs of aggressive–rejected children. A study
conducted by Tiffen and Spence (1986), which suggested that neglected children might be more responsive to coaching programs than
rejected children, increased interest in reconsidering the design of
coaching programs to improve the impact on rejected children. Similarly, in their meta-analytic review, Schneider and Byrne (1985) concluded that withdrawn subjects responded better than aggressive young-
sters to social skill training programs, further spurring interest in
adapting coaching programs to meet the needs of aggressive–rejected
children.

ADAPTING COACHING PROGRAMS
FOR AGGRESSIVE–REJECTED CHILDREN

Although aggressive–rejected children often show prosocial skill deficits (Bierman, 1986b; Coie, 1990), their social problems are exacerbated by their behavioral excesses. For example, aggressive children typically show a learned propensity to use coercive behaviors to control their interpersonal relations (Patterson, 1986). In conflict situations, aggressive children escalate quickly to use verbal or physical aggression to get what they want or to terminate another child's aversive behavior (Asarnow, 1983). Their impulsive and intrusive behavior alienates others over time, but because it is often effective in the immediate interaction, it is reinforced and becomes functional for them. In addition, aggressive–rejected children often show school adjustment problems, including elevated rates of attention problems and academic difficulties (Coie, 1990). In the mid-1980s, investigators began to supplement coaching procedures focused on promoting positive play skills with additional intervention components designed to reduce aggressive responding and/or to address other deficits contributing to the problematic school adjustment of aggressive–rejected children.

Coie and Krehbiel (1984) examined the impact of combining academic skills training with social skills training to enhance the peer relations of aggressive–rejected children who had academic delays. Their study compared the effects of (1) academic skills training alone (30 sessions consisting of individual tutoring in reading and/or math); (2) social skills training alone (12 sessions focused on participation, cooperation, communication, and validation/support); (3) the combination of academic skills and social skills training; and (4) a no-treatment comparison condition. Children who received academic skills training improved in multiple domains, showing higher rates of on-task behavior in the classroom, higher achievement scores, and higher social preference scores than untreated children. In contrast, social skills training alone produced only transitory improvements in sociometric ratings and no changes in classroom behavior. Coie and Krehbiel hypothesized that academic delays fueled student frustration and high rates of disruptive, off-task behaviors in the classroom, which in turn alienated peers. Hence promoting academic skills fostered improved classroom behavior, which, along with coaching in prosocial skills, enhanced the peer relations of the aggressive–rejected target children. In addition, tutoring was conducted in the context of positive, one-to-one relationships with adults; this may have provided children with a source of social–emotional support in the school setting, positively influencing their affect and social behavior.

Mize and Ladd (1990) identified preschool children who were poorly accepted by peers (either neglected or rejected sociometrically) and who also showed evidence of behavior problems during classroom observations. Children qualified for the intervention if their behavior involved elevated aggressive behavior and/or low levels of communication skills (e.g., leading, asking questions, commenting on ongoing play, and supporting peers). In this intervention—in which puppet modeling was used to present skills, and sociodramatic play provided a context for skill practice and reinforcement—coached children showed increases in their performance of the target skills after intervention, compared to children in the control condition. However, coaching did not have a significant impact on levels of aggressive behavior observed in the classroom, or on sociometric "like most" or "like least" nominations. Similar to the Coie and Krehbiel (1984) study, this study raised questions about whether a coaching approach that focuses solely on the promotion of prosocial skills can substantially decrease aggressive behavior and improve the peer acceptance of aggressive children, and it suggested the need to add program components designed to address excessive levels of aggressive behavior.

Responding to this need, we (Bierman, Miller, & Stabb, 1987) examined the utility of adding prohibitions and behavioral control strategies to reduce negative behavior to a coaching program that utilized instructions, practice opportunities, and performance feedback to increase positive social behavior. We assigned aggressive–rejected boys in grades 1–3 to one of four treatment conditions: (1) instructions and coaching in positive behaviors (helping and cooperating in play, asking questions, sharing); (2) prohibitions and response cost for negative behavior; (3) both instructions and prohibitions; and (4) a no-treatment comparison group. Prohibitions with response cost for negative behaviors resulted in immediate and stable declines in negative behavior and led to temporary increases in positive responses received from peers, whereas instructions, coaching, and reinforcement of positive social skills promoted sustained positive peer interactions 6 weeks after treatment. Only the combination of coaching and prohibitions led to improved sociometric ratings, and these were limited to reductions in the "like least" nominations given to target boys by their nontarget treatment partners.

Interestingly, the effects of coaching on the positive social skills of the targeted aggressive–rejected boys in the Bierman and colleagues (1987) study differed from the impact of coaching on withdrawn children demonstrated in the Bierman and Furman (1984) study (see also Bierman, 1986a). At the beginning of the school year, when pretreatment observations were conducted, the aggressive–rejected target boys did not show lower than average levels of positive peer interaction. However, over time, positive behaviors were observed less frequently in noncoached boys, resulting in deficient levels of prosocial skill performance (relative to their peers) by the posttreatment and follow-up assessments. Coaching did not increase the prosocial behavior of coached boys; rather, it protected boys against this decline in positive interactions, thus serving to maintain their prosocial behavior at normative levels.

These studies suggest that coaching in positive play skills can be one useful intervention component for aggressive–rejected children. However, they also suggest that coaching in positive interaction skills alone may be inadequate to meet the needs of these children, who often exhibit multiple behavioral and social difficulties. In addition to using contingency management strategies to reduce aggressive behavior and coaching to promote prosocial skills, a number of researchers began to explore the impact of social-cognitive intervention strategies that targeted self-control, anger management, and social problem-solving skills as methods for reducing aggressive, impulsive, and disruptive social behavior.

SOCIAL-COGNITIVE INTERVENTIONS TO REDUCE AGGRESSION

The design of social-cognitive intervention strategies to reduce aggression was based on research suggesting that aggressive social behavior is associated with certain distinct patterns of social-cognitive information processing. Specifically, asocial goals, negatively biased social perceptions or interpretations, and a reliance on domineering approaches to social problem solving were often observed in the social-cognitive processing of aggressive children (Dodge, 1989; see Chapter 4). Hence social-cognitive intervention programs were designed to reduce aggression by teaching children to inhibit their initial responses and to think more carefully about the causes and effects of their social behavior. The goal was to foster self-control and thoughtful interpersonal problem solving (Lochman & Lenhart, 1993). The majority of these interventions were focused on improving behavioral adjustment rather than increasing peer acceptance, with the expectation that decreased aggression would lead to improved peer acceptance. For example, Lochman and his colleagues developed the Anger Coping program (Lochman, Burch, Curry, & Lampron, 1984; Lochman & Curry, 1986). This 12-session group program included coaching in self-control procedures, strategies for coping with anger, and interpersonal problem-solving skills. In addition, teachers monitored classroom behavior, providing contingent reinforcement for the inhibition of aggressive behaviors and the display of positive behaviors. Several studies demonstrated this program's effects on the reduction of aggressive behavior (reported by parents) and antisocial behavior (reported by participants). However, peer reputations (peer ratings of aggression) were not affected by the program, and peer sociometric status was not measured (Lochman et al., 1984). The results suggested that cognitive-behavioral interventions designed to reduce aggression were not sufficient to improve the peer relations of aggressive–rejected children, but might contribute to this goal.

In a review paper, Weissberg and Allen (1986) suggested the logical step of integrating programs focused on coaching children in positive peer interaction skills with social-cognitive programs focused on social problem solving and related self-control skills. Weissberg and Allen noted that coaching and social problem solving interventions shared a similar instructional approach to promoting skill acquisition and behavior change; they both targeted mediating cognitions and adaptive interpersonal behavioral outcomes. Furthermore, these authors argued that the content foci of the two programs were quite complementary— with coaching programs promoting specific prosocial interaction strategies, and social problem-solving programs emphasizing the covert thinking processes (e.g., generating alternative solutions, anticipating consequences) that allow children to make good choices in interpersonal conflict situations.

Indeed, by the end of the 1980s, programs that included coaching in positive interaction skills along with self-control and social problem-solving skills began to emerge (see the review by Beelmann, Pfingsten, & Lösel, 1994). For example, Plienis and colleagues (1987) applied a multiple-baseline design to evaluate the effects of a combined intervention on three students in a special education class for emotionally disturbed students. The program included a combination of conversation skills and social problem-solving skills training, and generated case study evidence for improved social-cognitive skills (e.g., ability to generate appropriate solutions to hypothetical social problems) and social behavior (e.g., teacher ratings of adjustment, ratings of increased quality and quantity of social interactions during informal class parties).

Using a stronger group comparison design, however, Schneider and Byrne (1987) found only tentative support for the power of a coaching program that included four skill clusters (i.e., social perception skills, social cognition, coping with conflict, and forming friendships). Relative to children in a waiting-list control group, children who received individualized combinations of these four skill training components showed higher rates of cooperative play during recess. However, coaching produced no significant declines in observed aggression, and peer sociometric data were not gathered.

Also using a strong randomized control group design, Lochman, Coie, Underwood, and Terry (1993) tested the effects of a comprehensive coaching program for aggressive–rejected fourth graders. They used an extended period of individual sessions (26 sessions lasting 30 minutes each), followed by eight small-group sessions designed to promote practice of adaptive social behavior in naturalistic peer interactions. Sessions focused on both positive skills (cooperative play skills and group entry) and self-regulatory social-cognitive skills (dealing effectively with negative feelings and social problem-solving skills). Multiple intervention strategies were used to support both social-cognitive and behavior change, including modeling videotapes, discussion, role playing, instruction in self-talk, cooperative activities (including making a group videotape), feedback, and goal setting. Postintervention and 1-year follow-up data showed reductions for treated aggressive–rejected children in both observed aggression and peer-rated rejection, compared to the no-treatment group. The length and structure of the program— with multiple instructional strategies, graduated and extended opportunities to practice and consolidate skills, and the dual focus on prosocial interaction strategies and self-regulatory skills—may have contributed to the effectiveness of this program for aggressive–rejected children.

MOVING INTO THE 21ST CENTURY: WHERE ARE WE?

Two large meta-analytic reviews were completed in the 1990s summarizing the effects of social competence interventions. In each of these meta-analyses, a wide variety of interventions was included; these differed in participant characteristics, intervention content and structure, outcome measures, and general strength of the evaluative design. Given this mixing of "apples and oranges," the results of these meta-analyses must be interpreted with caution, but they do give some sense of the cross-study consistency and strength of findings.

In his review of 79 controlled studies, Schneider (1992) described the overall short-term effectiveness of social skill training programs as "moderate," with a mean effect size r of .40 (corresponding to an average success rate of 70% for experimental subjects, compared with 30.2% for controls). Follow-up assessments were reported for only 26 of the 79 studies they reviewed and indicated a decline in impact over time (follow-up effect size of $r = .35$). Two years later, Beelmann and colleagues (1994) conducted a meta-analytic review of 49 studies con-

ducted between 1981 and 1990. They suggested the term "social competence training" to describe the more comprehensive social skill and
social-cognitive skill training programs that had emerged during the
1980s to modify behavioral, cognitive, and affective components of social behavior. Echoing Schneider, they concluded that social competence training interventions were moderately effective, although their
estimates of intervention effectiveness were slightly lower than those
made by earlier reviewers. Beelmann and colleagues noted that although interventions had become more complex and multimodal during the 1980s, and thus more effective, they also tended to use outcome measures that were more socially valid and difficult to change
(e.g., teacher ratings, behavioral observations in naturalistic settings,
and sociometric measures), rather than "proxy" measures (e.g., role-
play estimates of social skills). In addition, programs in the 1980s were
more likely than earlier programs to target participants with severe
problems in social behavior, increasing the challenge to improve their
adjustment. Overall, the studies reviewed by Beelmann and colleagues
produced effect sizes of .47, meaning that the average score of the
treated group following treatment was higher than the average score
for about 68% of the control group. These authors concluded that as
social competence intervention programs were becoming increasingly
sophisticated, their effects appeared stronger and better sustained over
time. However, the generalizability of treatment effects remained a major challenge, in terms of the capacity of intervention programs both to
sustain effects over time and to affect broad indices of social adjustment—an issue reinforced in other reviews conducted at about the
same time (Gresham, 1994; La Greca, 1993).

Interestingly, Beelman and colleagues (1994) noted a decline in
the number of studies evaluating social competence interventions during the 1980s, with 30 studies conducted between 1981 and 1985, and
only 19 conducted between 1986 and 1990. Since 1990, this decline has
continued. To some degree, research has shifted away from a focus on
the evaluation of "stand-alone" social competence interventions, and
toward evaluating multifaceted prevention and intervention programs
that include social competence coaching as one intervention component.

For example, several large prevention trials were mounted during
the 1990s, testing the effectiveness of multifaceted programs that included social competence training along with parent-focused and
school-based interventions. For example, Tremblay and his colleagues
(1992) created a comprehensive prevention program designed to improve the behaviors and social adjustment of aggressive boys by combining behavior management training for parents with social compe-

tence training for the boys. Similarly, social competence coaching was embedded (along with parent training, medication, and academic support) in the Collaborative Multisite Multimodal Treatment Study of Children with Attention Deficit Hyperactivity Disorder (the MTA Study; see MTA Cooperative Group, 1999a, 1999b; Richters et al., 1995). In addition, two large-scale preventive trials focused on community-based samples of children at risk for the development of conduct problems—the Fast Track program (Conduct Problems Prevention Research Group, 1992) and EARLY ALLIANCE (Dumas, Lynch, Laughlin, Smith, & Prinz, 2001; Dumas, Prinz, Smith, & Laughlin, 1999)—included classroom-level social competence interventions and small-group social competence coaching sessions, along with parent training and academic support programs. (The MTA and Fast Track programs and research findings are discussed in more detail in Chapter 13.)

The shift in research focus away from "stand-alone" social competence coaching programs, and toward multicomponent prevention and intervention programs targeting children at high risk for serious behavior disorders, has been both beneficial and (in some ways) detrimental to the understanding and treatment of peer rejection. On the positive side, accumulating research has made it apparent that many of the children who experience chronic and severe peer relation difficulties have concurrent behavioral, cognitive, and/or emotional difficulties that reduce their capacity to sustain positive peer relations. For example, aggressive–rejected children typically show a range of conduct problems, including disruptive, hyperactive, and disagreeable behaviors as well as physical aggression. Many show concurrent inattention and social anxiety (Bierman, Smoot, & Aumiller, 1993). Conversely, many children with significant mental health difficulties (particularly conduct problems, attention-deficit/hyperactivity disorder [ADHD], depression or other mood disorders, and anxiety disorders) have serious peer relation difficulties (Dodge, 1989). Social competence coaching programs, when used alone, have not demonstrated a capacity to produce sustained reductions in conduct problems and improvements in peer acceptance among aggressive–rejected children; they are especially unlikely to be effective as a single intervention approach when child peer problems are embedded in a broad set of behavioral and emotional difficulties, such as those represented by ADHD and conduct problems, which require more intensive and multifaceted intervention (La Greca, 1993). In such cases, coaching interventions may make an important contribution, but additional intervention components are needed to address behavioral and emotional problems, family contexts, and concurrent adaptational difficulties (e.g., academic difficulties) (Coie & Koeppl, 1990).

At the same time, the negative impact of this new research direction has been a concurrent decline in empirical attempts to further develop and strengthen intervention techniques designed specifically to improve the social competence and peer acceptance of rejected children. That is, the research focus has emphasized importing existing coaching strategies into multicomponent programs, at the cost of further research devoted to developing social competence interventions themselves. There are two major reasons why further research devoted to the development of social competence programs is needed.

First, longer-term, multicomponent intervention programs have focused on children with severe, often clinically significant levels of social–emotional and behavioral disturbance, such as children with ADHD or high levels of conduct problems. These children are over-represented in the group of children who are rejected by peers, and hence prevention and intervention programs targeting them have relevance for the treatment of peer rejection, just as social competence coaching programs have relevance for multifaceted intervention programs designed to meet their needs. At the same time, peer-rejected children are a heterogeneous group. Not all rejected children have the multiproblem profile that includes serious acting-out behavior problems. Although much has been learned in the last 50 years about the design of effective such coaching programs, the technology of such coaching still requires attention. Issues such as tailoring coaching programs to meet the needs of children with different problem profiles and skill deficits; the optimal structure and content of coaching sessions; processes and mechanisms of promoting social competence; and strategies designed to enhance positive peer responding and improved peer relations all require further attention and development. In addition to supplementing social competence coaching interventions with other intervention foci (e.g., parent training, academic tutoring) for children with multiple needs, it is important to continue to examine and develop social competence intervention techniques themselves, and to further our understanding of the ways in which different intervention designs foster improved peer relations.

The second major reason why research focused on developing and evaluating social competence interventions is needed is that current coaching programs are outdated in terms of their attention to and incorporation of central aspects of peer relations that have emerged in developmental research. In the first four chapters of this book, I have reviewed research describing the multiple aspects of children's peer relations, including peer group liking and disliking, friendships, social networks, and experiences of victimization. I have described research illustrating the contributions of children's social behaviors and self-system processes, along with peer influences, including peer respond-ing and negative reputational biases to their peer status. (Figure 5.1 in Chapter 5 summarizes all of these factors.) Current social competence coaching programs address some pieces in this model, but have not yet expanded to include others. Coaching programs have been designed to promote behavior change, particularly increases in prosocial skills and decreases in problematic social behaviors. As described in this chapter, the technology for promoting behavior change has been developed and refined. Since the 1980s, coaching programs have attended to so-cial cognitions, have begun to incorporate some emotion focus (e.g., anger coping), and have explored the inclusion of peers in various ways in order to enhance generalization and improve peer responding and reputations. However, important work remains to be done. We under-stand little about how variations in peer inclusion or group experiences of different kinds may promote positive changes in the peer context or generalized changes in child social functioning. Little is known about the mechanisms or processes of change underlying effective treatment processes, particularly with regard to factors that promote positive changes in child self-system processes. Intervention strategies that may be integrated with coaching to improve friendship quality, to address social networks and social niche opportunities, and to decrease victim-ization require attention. In general, a broad area in need of further research and development is the technology for involving peers effec-tively in the intervention process and providing vulnerable (and some-times difficult-to-like) children with opportunities for positive peer interaction and support.

SUMMARY

The past four decades have witnessed the extensive development and refinement of interventions to promote positive peer relations and so-cial adjustment. Fueled by developmental research elucidating the behavioral, cognitive, and affective characteristics associated with prob-lematic peer relations and the dynamics of rejection processes, social competence interventions have become increasingly multifaceted in their focus. The technology for producing improvements in social rela-tionships has expanded in notable ways—moving from a single focus on the manipulation of antecedent conditions and consequences for behavior change to a comprehensive set of instructional techniques de-signed to promote an expanded repertoire of social skills, along with the social sensibilities needed for flexible and sensitive social respond-ing. Across studies, there is substantial evidence for the effectiveness of social competence training, with moderate size of effects. Social competence interventions have become broader in focus, with adaptations designed to enhance their effectiveness with children who have serious social–emotional and behavioral problems. Multifaceted intervention programs have begun to include social competence training components, combining them with parent-focused interventions and nesting them within universal school-based social competence promotion efforts.

At the same time, there is more work to be done. Interventions continue to show mixed patterns of effects across studies, with the production of sustained improvements on socially valid measures of social behavior and sociometric measures a continuing goal. Three issues warrant close attention in future research and intervention development:

1. Further attention to the characteristics of the children being treated; the range of social–emotional, cognitive, and behavioral skills they need to attain positive peer relations; and the corresponding combinations of intervention components that may be needed to produce lasting effects.
2. A better understanding of the mechanisms underlying effective treatment processes, as well as the intervention features associated with changes in child self-system processes and improvements in various types of outcomes for various types of children.
3. Development of the technology for involving peers effectively in the treatment process; creating opportunities for positive peer interaction; and addressing friendships, network affiliations, and niches of positive social opportunity for vulnerable children.

Next, in Chapter 11, I turn to a discussion of pragmatic issues regarding the structure and organization of coaching sessions, and provide examples of program content and session activities. In Chapter 12, I discuss the process of change during coaching sessions, describe issues in coach–child relationships, emphasize the need for coach attention to emotional issues and group dynamics during sessions, and describe strategies for behavior management designed to enhance children's self-regulation of their social relationships. In both of these chapters, the research base is utilized when possible; however, I also rely heavily on theory and personal experience, since many of the issues discussed await close empirical examination.

Chapter 11

The Design of Social Competence Coaching Programs

Developmental research has clarified the complex nature of the problems faced by unaccepted children, including the interplay of behavioral, cognitive, and emotional factors that affect their social competence, as well as the negative peer transactions associated with rejection processes. Intervention research has documented the effectiveness of a skill training approach, and identified strategies for producing improvements in social relationships. As such, the research base provides guidelines for the design of effective social competence interventions, both as "stand-alone" programs and as components in multifaceted prevention or intervention programs.

This chapter draws from the previously reviewed research literature evaluating intervention strategies, as well as from my own personal experiences and observations, to describe some of the "nuts and bolts" of coaching program design (Bierman, 1986a; Bierman & Furman, 1984; Bierman, Greenberg, & Conduct Problems Prevention Research Group [CPPRG], 1996; Bierman, Miller, & Stabb, 1987). The research base provides a solid basis for recommendations with regard to some of the issues discussed—notably the components of effective coaching sessions and strategies for promoting prosocial skill acquisition, as well as the identification of target skill domains that represent core social competence correlates. Other issues (including decisions about intervention design, such as context, length, organization, and staffing) have varied across studies, but have not been explored systematically with regard to their impact on program outcomes. Hence, in these areas, I note issues and make recommendations based on my colleagues' and my experience.

The chapter begins with a consideration of guiding principles for program design, followed by a discussion of session structure and core intervention components, which are well grounded in the available research base. Program content is then discussed, including the selection of target skills, and skill presentation and practice activities. Finally, pragmatic issues in program design are identified, such as group size and composition, program length, staffing, and recommended rules and routines for session management. Recommendations reflect the assumption that best practices should incorporate empirically supported programs and principles whenever possible, and should utilize our knowledge of social development and behavior change processes.

GUIDING PRINCIPLES

This section identifies guiding principles for the design of effective social competence coaching programs—lessons learned from past research on this topic, as reviewed in Chapter 10. From this literature, I distill three key design features that have characterized effective coaching programs: (1) they focus on training social skills (social competence correlates), using a variety of instructional techniques and practice activities; (2) they include components to address the specific social needs of children involved in the program; and (3) they incorporate components designed to enhance the generalization and maintenance of social skills and improved peer relations.

Focus on Training Social Skills

Past research provides strong evidence linking child behavior problems with peer relation difficulties. That is, most of the children who experience chronic peer rejection display problematic behaviors, in the form of social awkwardness, insensitivity, intrusiveness, and/or aggressiveness (Coie, 1990). Hence the first guiding principle for effective interventions is that they must target child behavior change. In addition, research suggests that behavior change efforts should focus on skill domains of effective social interaction (the "competence correlates" approach to selecting target skills), rather than specific discrete behaviors. In the competence correlates approach, general strategies of social interaction are selected for training based upon empirical evidence of their association with peer acceptance. It is recognized that child social competence extends beyond discrete behaviors and involves the capacity to organize behavior in a manner that is sensitive and responsive to situational contexts and social cues, and in line with social conventions.

The overall intervention goal is to help a child become a more positive and interpersonally sensitive social partner who has the capability to adapt behavior flexibly to fit into varied social situations, respond sensitively to others, and handle social conflicts with fairness.

Research has demonstrated that with coaching, children can develop the capacity to inhibit inappropriate behaviors and interact with peers in an interpersonally sensitive and responsive fashion. Coaching appears most effective when it utilizes an expanded set of instructional techniques to teach social skills, including modeling, verbal instructions, positive and negative examples to clarify the social concepts, and opportunities for guided practice and feedback. Consistent with early conceptions of social skill learning (e.g., Goldstein, Sprafkin, Gershaw, & Klein, 1986; Ladd & Mize, 1983), research has validated the importance of four components of coaching programs: (1) skill presentation, (2) opportunities for skill practice, (3) performance feedback, and (4) generalization programming (see Table 11.1).

Recognizing and Addressing Heterogeneous Child Needs

Developmental research has made it clear that unaccepted children have difficulty gaining peer acceptance for different reasons. Coaching programs appear most effective when they focus on unaccepted children who display behavioral deficiencies in the skills targeted by the coaching program (Bierman, 1986a; Ladd, 1981). Many disliked children are characterized by aggressive and intrusive social behavior, as well as low rates of prosocial interaction. Hence their skill deficits may include poor emotion regulation, poor impulse control, and poor social problem-solving skills. Because of this heterogeneity and complexity of skill deficits among children with peer problems, effective coaching programs need to address multiple skill domains, including behavioral features (e.g., promoting prosocial behaviors and promoting the self-regulation of negative social behaviors), emotional issues (e.g., addressing negatively biased relational schemas and associated feelings of interpersonal discomfort), and cognitive features (e.g., improving interpersonal problem-solving skills) (Coie & Koeppl, 1990).

Programming for Generalization and Maintenance

Past research has indicated that among the greatest challenges for coaching programs are attaining generalized and sustained behavior change, and improving peer responding and evaluations. The "train and hope" method, in which one assumes that a child who has been trained in new social skills during intervention sessions will use those

TABLE 11.1. Components of Effective Social Competence Coaching Programs

Intervention component	Why?	What?
Skill presentation	Promote children's understanding of the form, importance, and use of each skill	Modeling, instructions, discussions, presentation of multiple examples
Skill practice	Help children learn to implement new skills with external prompts, support, and reinforcement	Role plays, structured activities
Performance feedback	Help children to adjust and improve skill performance, as well as to self-monitor behavior and interpersonal responses	Discussions, self-evaluations, feedback from social partners, videotape review
Generalization programming	Gradually help children to implement skills under increasingly autonomous and naturalistic conditions	Homework assignments, practice in naturalistic peer interactions, provision of new niches of social opportunity

skills in naturalistic settings to elicit peer acceptance, has proven inadequate (Stokes & Osnes, 1989). The behaviors of others (peers, teachers, siblings, parents) influence child behaviors in reciprocal transactions, and social interaction problems often become overdetermined, embedded in a system of relationship histories and established social network patterns (Hymel, Wagner, & Butler, 1990; Price & Dodge, 1989). Hence generalized improvements in social relationships require attention to the interpersonal contexts in which social behavior and peer interactions take place, with focused efforts to involve peers in intervention to change their attitudes and behavior toward rejected children (Price & Dodge, 1989).

One strategy to facilitate generalization involves techniques applied during the course of intervention sessions, such as the use of multiple role plays and homework assignments. A second strategy involves the use of naturalistic practice games and activities within sessions.

In addition to using coaching techniques that maximize generalization, and structuring sessions to prepare children better for naturalistic peer interaction contexts, research suggests that preparing the peer environment can foster generalization. For example, one advantage of including peers in the intervention process may be that they are trained to be more sensitive and positively responsive to the skill performance

of target children (Bierman, 1986a). Contingent positive peer responding to skillful behavior may be a critical factor affecting the degree to
which new skills become used to replace existing behaviors, which here-
tofore have proven "functional" in the peer environment. Specific efforts to prepare the peer environment to support the skillful behavior
of target children and to create new niches of social opportunity for
them are explored further in Chapter 13. With these general principles
in mind, let us now consider the basic components of coaching sessions—the core building blocks of effecting coaching programs.

COMPONENTS OF COACHING SESSIONS

Typically, each coaching session includes elements focused on skill presentation and concept building, structured practice, and skill consolidation and generalization training, with opportunities for feedback, self-
monitoring, and self-reward.

Skill Presentation Strategies

Sessions begin with instructions, modeling examples, and discussion
activities designed to provide children with a conceptual understanding
of the target skill. Behavioral examples of the skill (positive and negative) are given, and a sense of its functional form and value is conveyed.
Skill concept building is often aided by posters or handouts that label
each skill and define behavioral examples. For example, Goldstein and
colleagues (1986) hand out cards (Skill Cards) listing the name of each
skill and its behavioral steps. Guevremont (1990) recommends the use
of a blackboard to define skills and identify behavioral "dos" and
"don'ts." In the Fast Track program, illustrated posters define the core
skills and provide pictorial examples (Bierman et al., 1996).

Modeling can include live role plays or videotaped examples that
demonstrate skillful behaviors in action. To maximize effectiveness,
modeling should provide examples that are similar to those encoun-
tered by the children, presented in a way that elicits their attention and
motivation to learn. Through narration and discussion, group leaders
highlight the key characteristics of the model's behavior to illustrate the
skill, and point out the cause–effect linkages between the model's
behavior and the social consequences. Multiple examples are useful, so
that participants see models showing the behavior in a variety of relevant settings.

A good example of the use of modeling is provided in the coaching program designed and evaluated by La Greca and Santogrossi

(1980). For each of the eight skills in that program, group leaders presented videotapes of peer models demonstrating the skill. Each modeling tape was about 4 minutes in length and contained multiple models of both sexes demonstrating target social skills in a variety of settings with positive social consequences. Following the videotapes, children reviewed the content of the tapes with the coaches, and discussed the ways in which they might use the skill in their daily peer interactions.

To maximize attentional engagement and learning, it is useful to vary the specific methods used to present skills within and across sessions. For example, skill presentation can include posters, picture–word matching games, quiz show games, and cue cards. The group leaders should use a variety of media and methods to help children understand the characteristics, use, and importance of each skill. Modeling can include coach role plays, videotaped examples, modeling stories, or (with younger children) puppet demonstrations.

Structured Opportunities for Skill Practice

The process of learning complex social skills is sometimes compared with that of learning complex physical skills (e.g., riding a bike). During the early phases of skill acquisition, it is important to have the opportunity to practice the skill under supportive conditions. For example, an adult teaching a child to ride a bike might schedule initial practice sessions with assistance available (e.g., with training wheels attached and the adult's supportive hand) and on easy surfaces (e.g. a flat, smooth driveway). As the child's ability increases, these supports are gradually withdrawn and the contextual challenge is increased, giving the child the opportunity to practice bike riding under increasingly difficult and more naturalistic circumstances (e.g., without training wheels, on bumpy surfaces with hills).

Similarly, in learning new social skills, initial practice opportunities should include adult support and a low level of difficulty. As the child's skill level and confidence increase over time, adult support should decrease and the level of social complexity should increase, to move toward the level of challenge that exists in naturalistic peer interaction settings.

Initial practice activities are typically brief structured or scripted interactions that allow each child to practice the target skills with clear external direction, support, and reinforcement. One such commonly used practice activity is role playing, in which the group leader and group members discuss and then act out the use of the skill in situations that represent potential real-life skill utilization opportunities. The group leader elicits from the members ideas about when, where, and how the skill might be useful to them, and then sets the stage for role playing by defining a physical setting, set of preceding events, and assigned roles. The group discusses specific behaviors that could be used in that setting prior to the actual role play, and key behaviors or cues are often listed on paper to provide structure for the role-play participants. Following the role play, the group discusses how it went. Sometimes positions in the role play are reversed to allow children to experience a social situation from multiple perspectives. Various hypothetical situations are included, to enable skill practice across multiple settings.

Typically, initial role-play activities are very brief, highly structured, and dyadic. As each child's skill increases, the challenge level of role-play scenarios is increased gradually by increasing the number of children involved, expanding the length of the role plays, and introducing some stumbling blocks (e.g., peer nonresponse or mild provocation).

In addition to (or in place of) role plays, structured activities or games can be used to provide supportive opportunities for behavioral rehearsal and skill practice. For example, Strain and Weigerink (1976) used sociodramatic play as a context for skill practice, encouraging preschool children to act out familiar nursery stories. The use of sociodramatic play with developmentally appropriate materials can both increase positive social involvement and provide a fun, structured opportunity to practice various social skills (e.g., appropriate emotional displays, group participation, turn taking, and following rules). Behavioral rehearsal can also be embedded within games, as illustrated by the practice opportunities used in the Oden and Asher (1977), Ladd (1981), Bierman and Furman (1984), and Bierman and colleagues (1987) programs. Later in this chapter (and, in greater detail, in the book's Appendix), illustrations are given of specific games and other activities that provide structured opportunities for the practice of commonly targeted social skills.

Opportunities for Skill Consolidation and Generalization Training

Practice in the context of supportive and structured activities, such as role plays and simulated peer interaction activities, enables children to exhibit and refine skillful behavioral performance. However, these tasks alone do not adequately prepare children for naturalistic social contexts, which tend to be more complex; they require responses to subtle social interaction cues, as well as the flexible manifestation of skillful behavior. Hence, to promote the generalization of skills trained in coaching sessions to real-life settings, it is important to include intervention components that are designed to bridge this gap.

One way to promote generalization is through the use of homework assignments, in which children are encouraged to use targeted skills with their peers outside the intervention setting, and then to review their experiences with the group in subsequent sessions. For example, Goldstein and colleagues (1986) and Guevremont (1990) emphasize the importance of using multiple exemplars drawn from real-life scenarios for practice role plays during intervention sessions to enhance generalization of learning. They also use self-monitoring discussions during sessions and homework assignments to encourage youth to use their new skills in real-life settings, with both self-reward and group reward to reinforce attempts at generalized skill use.

Although homework assignments may be useful, they do not reduce the gap between the amount of structure and support in the skill training context of the intervention and the amount available in naturally occurring settings. An additional strategy is to include in group sessions activities that are designed to mimic more directly the sorts of naturalistic interactions children face with peers. These may include cooperative work activities, cooperative and competitive play, and unstructured play opportunities that tax the children's ability to use new skills in a consolidated way under naturalistic, social challenge settings.

For example, in the Fast Track project's first-grade program, each Friendship Group session includes a snack activity, which provides opportunities for children to practice cooperative planning, problem solving, and communication skills in the "real-life" context of preparing, serving, and consuming food (Bierman et al., 1996). The structure of the snack is varied across sessions, to increase its challenge level. For example, during initial sessions, children practice reciprocity and turn taking as they make group decisions about who will pass out cups and napkins, pour juice, and clean up. In later sessions, more elaborate snacks are prepared, providing opportunities for group communication, helping, sharing, and problem solving.

Over time, the group composition can also be structured to provide a scaffold for gradually increasing the degree of naturalistic challenge in the training situation, in order to provide practice under conditions that better approximate the "real-life" settings. For example, both Ladd (1981) and La Greca, Stone, and Noriega-Garcia (1989) incorporated a set of graduated peer interaction experiences into their intervention design. In the latter case, intervention began with individual sessions (4 sessions), then moved to training in the context of dyadic interactions (6 sessions), and then went on to training in the context of a small peer group (26 sessions).

In general, to enhance the gradual acquisition and mastery of social skills, activities designed to foster the consolidated and generalized use of skills should be built into the program systematically, so that children move from structured opportunities that provide maximal support for skill acquisition to activities that gradually increase the level of difficulty and naturalistic challenge.

Performance Feedback and Self-Monitoring

Performance feedback serves two goals: (1) to promote improvements in skill performance; and (2) to encourage children to self-monitor, so that they can become more adept at assessing the ongoing impact of their social behavior on the responses of others and adjusting their skill performance accordingly. Hence one aspect of feedback involves recognition, praise, and sometimes rewards that reinforce positive skill performance, and motivate future efforts. This includes both immediate praise for positive behavior, and delayed praise that occurs after an interaction (to avoid interrupting ongoing interaction). For example, in the Fast Track program, each session ends with a "compliment circle." Coaches lead the compliment sharing by offering comments on skillful behaviors observed by each child during the session, and then eliciting from the group members compliments that specify positive behaviors they have observed and appreciated during the session. Children are also asked to give themselves compliments. Some sessions also include ribbons, medals, or certificates to denote achievements, as well as the distribution of a one-page handout for parents describing the key skills learned in the session that allow for follow-up praise from parents. Useful feedback identifies the presence or absence of specific, concrete behaviors that have made social interactions mutually rewarding for all social partners involved.

Corrective feedback that allows a child to identify problems in skill performance (and competent alternatives) is also important, as it fosters the child's ability to improve his/her competence and efficacy for skillful social behavior. Eliciting the child's involvement in self-evaluation is important, to assure that improved social behavior is not dependent upon adult structure and feedback, but becomes part of the child's personal goals and self-monitoring system (Ladd & Mize, 1983). One strategy that fosters the child's self-monitoring ability is to videotape interactions for later review. For example, in both the La Greca and Santogrossi (1980) and Bierman and Furman (1984) studies, group leaders videotaped child role plays and led the group members in identifying positive aspects of the role plays and areas in which improvements could be made. A second strategy involves the elicitation of feedback from both children themselves and their peers in the context of social challenges. For example, after children engage in a negotiation task, the coach can ask each of them how it went for them, underscore positive features of the interaction, and elicit (and give) suggestions about things that might improve the negotiation in future activities.

PROGRAM CONTENT

The competence correlates approach to target skill selection emphasizes the value of focusing intervention on social interaction strategies that are associated empirically with peer acceptance or rejection (La Greca, 1993). In addition, theorists have noted the importance of considering intervention goals broadly. That is, in addition to reducing rejection and promoting peer acceptance, interventions may seek to foster friendships and reduce victimization (Asher, Parker, & Walker, 1996; Furman & Robbins, 1985). Based upon the competence correlates approach, seven skill domains are most frequently selected for training, and are presented in Table 11.2: social participation, emotional understanding, prosocial behavior, self-control, communication skills, fair-play skills, and social problem-solving skills. These skill domains incorporate the research-based movement away from defining social skills as a finite set of discrete behaviors, and toward defining them as domains of behavioral options that children can use in flexible ways across varying social contexts.

Variations exist across programs in the specific ways in which skill domains are defined (particularly the number and breadth of domains), and in the specific language used to describe each skill. Some skill domains may be separated into several discrete units, in order to facilitate the design of an intervention for children with specific types of social difficulties or to match the developmental level of the participating children. For example, when my colleagues and I are teaching social problem-solving skills to children with oppositional and disruptive behavior problems in the Fast Track program, we present separate skill training units on self-control ("Stop and think"), emotional understanding and problem definition ("Say the problem and how you feel"), and negotiation skills ("Make a deal") before presenting the unit on social problem solving, which incorporates all three steps. The goal is to train children in the more discrete skills they need as prerequisites for adaptive social problem solving before presenting the more comprehensive model. In addition, we present skills in order of their level of developmental sophistication, in units that occur at different points in the program. For example, basic social participation skills ("Join in, pay

TABLE 11.2. Seven Competence Correlate Social Skill Domains

Skill processes	Skill components
Social participation	Joining with peers in play and activities Attending to peers Feeling comfortable in peer interaction contexts Initiating interactions and entering ongoing activities
Emotional understanding	Identifying others' feelings accurately Expressing one's own feelings appropriately Responding appropriately to the feelings of others
Prosocial behavior	Playing cooperatively Taking turns, helping, and sharing Showing kindness toward others
Self-control	Inhibiting reactive responding Coping effectively with frustration, anxiety, and anger Setting and working toward goals
Communication skills	Appropriate self-expression Listening respectfully to others' viewpoints Asking and answering questions Extending invitations and suggestions
Fair-play skills	Following rules Good sportsmanship
Social problem-solving skills	Identifying problems Generating and evaluating solutions Making and executing a plan Negotiating and supporting good ideas Evaluating and reconsidering strategies

attention, cheer for your friends") are presented as the first set of skills in the program. Group entry skills, which are more complicated and involve assessing the group, selecting the right timing to ask for entry, and handling rejection gracefully, are not introduced until later in the program, because these are viewed as developmentally more complex skills. Similarly, self-control ("Stop and think") is presented relatively early in the program, whereas the more advanced skills of handling provocation (anger management) and avoiding retribution are presented later. With this kind of organization, there is some recycling through skill domains over the course of the program, with the level of developmental sophistication of the specific skills in the domain increasing over time.

Sequencing Skills for Coaching

In general, decisions about the order in which skills will be trained in an intervention program can be as important as the selection of the target skills themselves, because the intervention program is designed to help children gradually accumulate and internalize greater social competence. Usually the first session provides a general orientation to the group, including introductions of participants, discussion of the purpose and goals of the group, and review of the rules and routines. In groups designed for grade school children, the rationale is usually fairly basic, focusing on the goals of having fun, making friends, and learning to solve problems so that being together is fun for everyone.

When group leaders are organizing skills into a sequence, it is useful to keep two principles in mind. First, children are developing relationships with other group members as they learn about how to develop and sustain relationships; their affective and interpersonal experiences with peer partners in the intervention context are as much a part of their learning experience as the didactic skill material presented by the coaches. Hence organizing skills in an order that follows the natural flow of relationship formation makes sense. For example, initial sessions might focus on basic social participation skills, self-disclosure, and question asking, which facilitate group engagement, establish common ground, and provide a foundation for the development of friendships among group members. Skills for interpersonal problem solving and conflict resolution come later in the program, as children who are forming relationships move into more involved interactions that require coordination and negotiation.

A second guiding principle for skill organization is that focusing on things to do in order to enjoy being with someone (e.g., learning new strategies for positive initiation and engagement) is generally more interesting and rewarding for children than learning how not to do something (e.g., behavioral inhibition). Hence combining topics that have a primary focus on positive interpersonal exchange (e.g., cooperation) with skills that have a primary focus on inhibition (e.g., self-control, anger management) creates more balanced and engaging sessions than an extended focus on behavioral inhibition alone.

The next sections present the seven core skill domains selected as competence correlates and listed in Table 11.2. I describe approaches to skill presentation and give examples of activities that provide opportunities for practice and performance feedback. A summary listing of activities for each domain is provided in Table 11.3; detailed descriptions of the activities are given in the Appendix.

TABLE 11.3. Activities for Practicing Skills in Seven Competence Domains

Skill domain and type of activity	Activity description
Domain of social participation	
Naming games	Name and Favorite Food Memory Game Friend, Friend, Chase Who Ate the Cookies?
Self-disclosure activities	Hot-Potato Friendship Discovery Discovery Posters
Friendship team activities	Naming the group Designing a group logo Painting group hats or T-shirts
Domain of emotional understanding	
Recognizing and labeling feelings	Feelings Collages Paper Plate Feeling Masks Name That Feeling
Role-play feelings display	Feelings Charades Feelings Treasure Hunt Sociodramatic play Feelings Hot Potato
Domain of prosocial behaviors	
Cooperative activities	Cooperative art projects Cooperative play
Negotiation activities	Sharing Snacks Cracker Stackers
Partner activities	Blindfold Partners Partner Interdependent Tasks
Domain of self-control	
Role-play practice	Obstacle Course Fortune Noodle Hunt
Self-control games	Red Light, Green Light Simon Says Pass the Bell
Domain of communication skills	
Interview games	TV Talk Show Twenty Questions
Partner challenges	Partner Puzzles Partner Picture Challenge Partner Design Challenge

(continued)

TABLE 11.3. (*continued*)

Skill domain and type of activity	Activity description
Domain of fair-play skills	
Competitive games	Carnival games with Decision Wheel
	Simple board games
Coordinated play	Rescue squads
Domain of social problem-solving skills	
Role plays	Common conflict situations
Team challenges	Line Up
	Crossing the River
	Maze

Social Participation

The skill domain of social participation involves joining in group activities, paying attention to other members of the group and to the game or activity, and sharing positive affect in the context of joint play or conversation. This skill domain includes the behavioral components of proximity seeking and sustained on-task behavior, and also includes affective and motivational features. The goal is to enable children to participate in interactions with others comfortably and with enjoyment. Basic social participation skills are often the first ones targeted in intervention programs, as they provide a context for discovering common ground and a foundation for additional skills. Activities that underscore the "togetherness" and joint "team" identification of group members can foster feelings of social bonding and comfort. Later sessions may include the skills of initiating social interactions and entering ongoing group play.

In the Fast Track program, this skill domain is identified by a poster entitled "Good Teamwork," which lists "joining in," "paying attention," and "cheering for your friends." A modeling tape drawn from the *Reading Rainbow* TV series is used to illustrate the importance of and strategies for participating as a team member; it includes interviews with and videotapes of a dance troupe and a firefighting unit. Discussions are used to help children generate example of things that are more fun to do by participating with others than by oneself (Bierman et al., 1996). Practice activities include games that support social participation and encourage children to self-disclose in a way that promotes the discovery of common ground. For example, the Hot-Potato Friendship Discovery and Discovery Posters activities encourage children to tell about themselves, learn about others, and identify areas of shared interests. (Again, see the Appendix for detailed activity descriptions.)

Emotional Understanding

The abilities to recognize and label one's feelings and the feelings of others are key skills providing a foundation for self-control and successful social interaction. Particularly important may be the capacity to recognize the difference between internal feeling states and voluntary behaviors that affect others. In the Providing Alternative Thinking Strategies (PATHS) curriculum (Greenberg & Kusche, 1993; Kusche & Greenberg, 1995), for example, children are taught that "All feelings are OK. Behaviors can be OK or not OK." Lessons focus on helping children differentiate feelings from behaviors, emphasizing that "You can't always control how you feel, but you can control how you behave." Being able to recognize, label, and talk about their feelings provides children with a language for self-control, problem identification, and the exploration of different behavioral strategies to cope with emotional arousal. This skill domain includes the capacity to (1) recognize the differences between feelings and behaviors, (2) label one's own feelings and express them appropriately, (3) understand other's feelings, (4) communicate effectively with others about their feelings, and (5) express concern about and empathy for the feelings of others.

The PATHS curriculum (Kusche & Greenberg, 1995) includes a number of presentation strategies designed to help children understand and label emotions. These include presenting illustrations and photographs of children with different emotional expressions, and discussing the feeling label, the associated internal and behavioral cues, and the kinds of situations or events that might elicit each feeling state. Modeling stories provide contextualized examples of characters' experiences of different feeling states, and discussions are used to help children identify the salient features of the situation and emotional experience of the story characters. The *Reading Rainbow* series includes a videotaped illustration of different feelings. In addition, in the PATHS curriculum, feelings are depicted on individual cards. Children collect a set of "feeling face" cards as different emotions are discussed, and can use these cards to display and discuss their feelings. In the Fast Track program, the PATHS feeling faces are used, and children are encouraged to display their feelings in a chart. Each session as children enter the group, they are asked whether they would like to display a feeling face, and they are encouraged to talk about how they are feeling. During group sessions, particularly if there are conflicts, children are asked whether they want to change their feeling face. The process of going to the feeling face board, labeling the new feeling, and changing the feeling face provides children with a concrete method for inhibiting negative behavior and replacing it with a verbal description of the problem and how they feel.

Activities that provide children with opportunities to practice emotion recognition include Feelings Collages (making drawings or pictures of different feeling expressions), Paper Plate Feeling Masks (making masks to illustrate different feeling expressions), and games such as Name That Feeling or Feelings Charades (in which children mime and guess feelings expressed during role-played interactions). Sociodramatic play also provides an opportunity for practice in the display and labeling of feelings, as do games such as Feelings Hot Potato, when children take turns telling about times when they felt happy, mad, sad, or scared.

Prosocial Behaviors

Prosocial behaviors include friendly, kind, and caring behaviors, such as taking turns, sharing, helping, and cooperating with others. They involve the capacity to function effectively as a team member, negotiate reciprocal roles, and support each other. Behavioral exemplars include (1) treating others with kindness; (2) sharing, helping, and taking turns; (3) inviting others to play; (4) cheering others on and supporting them; and (5) cooperating with others and taking reciprocal roles.

Skill presentation activities are designed to emphasize the importance of treating others with kindness and caring, and of sharing, helping, and cooperating with others in order to make friends and enjoy spending time together. In addition to providing positive exemplars of prosocial behaviors, it can be useful to illustrate this concept by providing demonstrations of negative examples of the skill (e.g., refusing to share, ignoring others who want to play) and asking children to identify the problem and solution. Having children role-play negative examples of a skill is a somewhat risky procedure, as it can be hard to control the level of arousal and to maintain a clear differentiation between the role play and the reality of negative child behavior. A safer alternative is to have the adult coaches role-play the problem behavior, and have the children serve as the audience. For example, in the Fast Track program, a Kid's Court model for role plays has proven quite engaging for children. In this method, the adult coaches describe a problem and ask the children to watch them enact the situation and raise their hands when they see a problem emerge. Then children are asked to identify the problem and the feelings of the coaches, and to suggest alternative positive behaviors. For younger children in particular, it is important to use examples of typical peer interactions as role-play problems, representing situations the children may actually encounter, rather than examples of adult problems the coaches may have actually experienced. The adults need to feel comfortable role-playing an argument over sharing the chocolate cookies at lunch or taking turns in a game.

Cooperative art projects and activities that require children to plan together, to share limited materials (such as one pair of scissors, one glue stick, or a few attractive stickers), and to work on a shared goal or joint product all create naturalistic opportunities to discuss each other's desires and ideas, take turns, share materials, and negotiate plans. Cooperative play can also provide opportunities for practicing prosocial behavior, particularly when it is structured to require substantial sharing, turn taking, and negotiation. Variations in snack procedures can also provide an engaging opportunity to practice cooperation and negotiation. In the Sharing Snacks activity, for example, children are provided with the ingredients for a snack (e.g., a trail mix) and must talk with each other to put together and distribute the snack.

Games and other activities that create interdependence between partners also promote prosocial interaction. For example, Blindfold Partners and Partner Interdependent Tasks create situations of dyadic interdependence, in which children must work together to reach a shared goal; these activities thereby elicit and reinforce prosocial and cooperative interactions.

Self-Control

In order to maintain organized and goal-directed social behavior, it is important for children to be able to inhibit reactive responding in the face of heightened emotional arousal. The capacity to exert self-control in the context of peer conflict or provocation is particularly useful for children, as it gives them the opportunity to engage in thoughtful problem solving and to select a strategic behavioral response that might solve the problem without aggravating the social partner. Effective communication and problem solving to resolve conflicts cannot take place when children are highly aroused—very angry or very upset. Hence the capacity to inhibit or divert behavioral reactivity in the face of high arousal allows children time to calm down.

Concrete imagery can be helpful in teaching young children about the concept of self-control. For example, Robin, Schneider, and Dolnick (1976) developed what they called the "turtle technique" to help young children control anger. Children are taught to play "turtle" when angered or upset by "going into their shells" and protecting themselves from verbal assaults. Depending upon the age of the children, "going into their shells" may involve physical retreat (putting their heads down or closing their eyes) or a figurative cue (stopping and retreating mentally from the interaction to focus themselves, and then deciding what to do). Relaxation training procedures can be taught in conjunction with visual imagery. Izard (2002) suggests that a physical action (e.g., clenching fists, crossing arms) can help children redirect emotional arousal and refocus cognitively.

In the PATHS curriculum (Kusche & Greenberg, 1995), as in several other social problem-solving programs, a traffic light model is used to cue organized responding in the face of emotional arousal. At the Red Light, children are taught to inhibit behavioral reactivity ("Tell yourself to stop"), divert arousal energy ("Take a long, deep breath"), and use language to label their feelings and problem ("Say the problem and how you feel").

Skill presentation strategies may include posters or signs representing the Red Light steps; a discussion and listing of strategies to calm down when upset; modeling stories, role plays, or puppet shows illustrating the use of the Red Light steps; and Kid's Court modeling exercises, in which the children give the coaches advice about when and how to use the Red Light steps in their conflicts. Discussions about temper problems can be useful to children, including discussions of conditions under which tempers arise, and strategies for effective coping and self-regulation. In this conceptualization, self-regulation ("going to the Red Light") enhances a child's ability to cope with everyday frustrations and conflicts.

Several programs also include skill training in anger management that is particularly focused on maintaining control under conditions of peer provocation, such as teasing or name calling (Hinshaw, Henker, & Whalen, 1984; Lochman, Burch, Curry, & Lampron, 1984). Hinshaw and colleagues (1984) focus on "stress inoculation," which involves the capacity to identify external events (being teased) and internal events (thoughts, tension) associated with negative emotional arousal, and to use coping strategies to reduce tension. Lochman, Coie, Underwood, and Terry (1993) integrate a similar focus on anger management with social problem solving. In group discussions, children discuss the feelings associated with anger, and describe incidents that evoke anger. They then discuss strategies to reduce feelings of anger and stress, and practice using them as they imagine events in which they feel angry.

Coie and Koeppl (1990) suggest that with older children, it is important to recognize the value many children put on "saving face" and not backing down in conflict or situations involving peer provocation. Rather than simply focusing on calming down and walking away from peer provocation (which could be perceived by children as a show of weakness), Coie and Koeppl recommend focusing skill presentations and discussions on the idea of developing personal power—demonstrating how "keeping your cool" and being in control represent a display of power, which prevents others from getting the best of children or manipulating them.

Role plays can be embedded within game-like activities to help children practice the steps of self-control in a structured setting. For example, in the Fast Track program, children work in dyads or triads to role-play going through the steps of the Red Light in hypothetical problem situations. To make this task more engaging, the role plays are sometimes set in the context of games, such as Obstacle Course or Fortune Noodle Hunt. Games that require self-control also provide a good context for the naturalistic practice of self-control skills. For younger children, games like Red Light, Green Light; Simon Says; or Pass the Bell require organized behavioral inhibition.

Some programs include role-play practice in which children are subjected to peer provocation (see Guevremont, 1990). In a carefully constructed context, children in the group take turns demonstrating their ability to "keep their cool" as other members of the group tease or provoke them. Although many programs have demonstrated that this kind of practice activity can be useful to children, it is a somewhat risky practice in terms of group cohesion and support. Unless carefully constructed and monitored, the children who are role-playing provocateurs or victims can lose sight of the role-play limits of the game, and iatrogenic effects are possible. It may be a similarly effective and less risky intervention practice to use modeling stories or videos about others who are subjected to victimization as a basis for group discussion and role play of regulatory skills, rather than involving children in a more personalized role play. Research comparing the effectiveness of these different techniques is needed.

Communication Skills

Effective communication skills include the capacity to express one's point of view and feelings clearly (self-expression and appropriate self-disclosure); to listen to others' points of view and respect their perspectives; to ask questions to elicit information; to join in and maintain a conversation; and to extend suggestions or invitations regarding joint activity. Coaching programs for withdrawn children, such as the Ladd (1981) and Bierman and Furman (1984) programs, have focused on three core communication skills: self-expression, questions, and leads (invitations and suggestions).

Guevremont (1990) uses the TV Talk Show game to give children structured opportunities to practice communication skills. In this game, one child serves as a TV "host" whose job is to interview a "guest" (see the Appendix for more details). Other structured games that foster practice in conversation skills include the Partner Puzzles, Partner Picture Challenge, and Partner Design Challenge activities, which involve referential communication. That is, one partner has information needed to guide the other partner toward a goal, so that each partner must take the other's perspective and communicate with the other in order for the pair to accomplish that goal together (again, see the Appendix).

Fair-Play Skills

Team games, board games, and other organized play activities require the willingness and ability to abide by general norms of reciprocity, rules, and fair play. Fair-play skills include the capacity to participate and regulate oneself in rule-based games with peers, including following rules, demonstrating good sportsmanship, refraining from teasing or boasting, and coping effectively with frustration or losing at a game. In addition, the capacity to negotiate and compromise in game situations is important, including negotiating with peers about the choice and rule structure of shared activities.

Deciding when to introduce competitive play into an intervention program requires consideration. Whereas cooperative play provides opportunities for team building and practicing cooperation, negotiation, and problem-solving skills, competitive play provides a context for practicing emotion regulation and self-control, and for learning to balance autonomy striving with social sensitivity.

In the Fast Track program, this skill domain is taught using a "Fair Play" poster that identifies the key components as "Take turns," "Follow rules," and "Don't tease or boast." Kid's Court role plays by the coaches are used to illustrate fair-play problems, which serve as a basis for group discussions and illustrations of appropriate fair-play behaviors. Specific discussions focus on key concepts and behavioral examples: (1) identifying fair versus unfair behaviors in play situations; (2) identifying put-downs, including teasing and boasting, and thinking of alternatives; and (3) discussing good ways to express feelings when one is winning or losing at a game.

Specific behavioral cues are developed during group discussions and activities to help children cope with difficult situations. For example, children construct a Decision Wheel, on which they list six different fair ways to decide who goes first. They are encouraged to use the wheel in situations where they can't decide who should go first. Children also help construct cue sheets that list "Good Things to Say When You Lose" and "Good Things to Say When You Win." These specific examples are designed to give children appropriate expressions to use when they are emotionally disappointed or frustrated (i.e., when they lose) or excited (i.e., when they win). For example, expressions that help children cope effectively with losing include "I guess it's your lucky day," and "Let's play again."

In addition, the Fast Track program includes specific skill presentation focused on the importance of negotiating with friends in play situations. Children are taught to "make a deal" with their friends by following three steps: "Give an idea," "Check it out," and "Say 'yes' to good ideas." This concept provides a basic foundation for more expanded social problem-solving skills, which are presented later in the program.

Coaches should consider carefully the choice of competitive games for initial practice. Games that are moderately interesting (but not highly arousing) and have simple rules and procedures are desirable. Games that are fairly quick and allow children the opportunity to "try again" are preferred during initial practice trials, whereas more extended board or card games or physical competitive play (e.g., kickball) represent heightened regulatory challenges that should be used for practice only after children have demonstrated competence with less challenging competitive games.

During initial practice activities, it is useful to provide cue sheets (e.g., the Decision Wheel or lists of good things to say) as children play, and to encourage them to use these prompts as needed. In addition, clear reward structures for fair play, such as a score sheet for fair-play behaviors, can enhance children's skill performance during initial trials. The goal is to reduce children's reliance on these external supports over time as they become more competent at generating and maintaining positive competitive play behaviors.

In addition, as discussed more thoroughly in Chapter 12, the statements the coach makes during the game process can provide important feedback and support. For example, if a child taunts another with a boast such as "I won, ha, ha," the coach can reframe and reword the boasting, with feedback such as the following: "You're proud that you've played so well. Let's think of a way to say that without hurting other people's feelings. You could say, 'This is my lucky day.' "

Among grade school children, fair-play skills are also needed to sustain coordinated toy play. For example, coordinated play with firefighter and police squads, or toy soldiers and jeeps, requires the equitable distribution of different play pieces (e.g., characters and vehicles) and the definition of rules of play (e.g., the themes of play and reciprocal roles). In some cases, such as skillful play with toy soldiers, children need to make some agreements about when, where, and how battles will be allowed (e.g., "You can't knock anything down until we say 'start'). Although some might advocate that interventions should avoid play involving aggressive themes, developmental research suggests that pretend play represents an important context in which children learn to regulate their aggressive impulses (Hartup, 1983). The use of coordinated, affectively charged pretend play activities can thus provide a useful naturalistic context for the practice of self-regulatory negotiation and fair-play skills.

Social Problem-Solving Skills

To deal effectively with conflicts that inevitably arise in social interactions, children need social problem-solving skills. This skill domain builds upon the domains presented earlier (e.g., emotional understanding, self-control, fair-play skills), and it includes not only the cognitive capacity to generate alternatives, but also the organizational capacity to employ skills sequentially to deal with interpersonal conflicts *in vivo*. The skill sequence includes the capacity to (1) identify the problem and associated feelings with words, (2) express one's own viewpoint and listen to others, (3) generate and consider a set of alternative solutions, (4) anticipate the personal and interpersonal consequences of different choices, (5) plan and execute a response, and (6) evaluate the impact of one's actions. Theoretically, these social problem-solving skills provide a critical foundation for children to sustain long-term positive interpersonal relationships (Lochman & Curry, 1986; Spivack & Shure, 1974; Weissberg & Allen, 1986).

A number of programs have been developed to teach children social problem-solving skills. Here I describe a three-step sequence for problem solving (an expanded traffic light model), which is used in the young elementary version of the PATHS program (Kusche & Greenberg, 1995). First, children are taught to go to the Red Light to calm down and define the problem. As in self-control, this step includes "Tell yourself to stop" (behavioral inhibition), "Take a long, deep breath" (relaxation), and "Say the problem and how you feel" (problem and feelings identification). Older children are taught to use I-statements to describe the problem, and to use active listening techniques in respectfully considering the viewpoints of the other party. Then children are taught to move on to the Yellow Light to consider possible solutions and their potential consequences. Prompts at the Yellow Light include the questions "What could you do?" and "How would that work?" Because negotiating can be particularly difficult for some aggressive–rejected children, my colleagues and I also include the three-step "make a deal" target skill, described above in connection with fair-play skills ("Give an idea," "Check it out," and "Say 'yes' to good ideas"). Once a good solution is identified, children are prompted to go to the Green Light, try out their plan, and see how it works. At more advanced levels, children may also be instructed in the steps of making plans, anticipating roadblocks, and considering alternatives.

Role-play activities are commonly used to practice social problem-solving skills. For example, Guevremont (1990) recommends that coaches prepare a large number of vignettes and scenarios containing common social conflict situations, writing them on index cards. Group members are also encouraged to identify actual conflicts that they have experienced with their peers. Initially, group coaches may model each of the problem-solving steps as they role-play finding a solution to one of the identified conflict situations. Then children are involved in role playing through the problem-solving steps, by defining the problem, generating alternatives, discussing potential consequences, and planning a course of action. Role plays can be videotaped for later review and performance feedback.

In addition to role-play exercises, team challenge activities can be constructed to elicit problem-solving skill practice in more naturalistic contexts. A number of team challenge activities are described in the Appendix, such as the Line Up, Crossing the River, and Maze games. In each case, children are encouraged to work through the traffic light steps in order to identify their problem, generate alternative problem solutions, and create and follow a problem-solving plan to master the challenge. Following the completion of this group challenge, the coach encourages children to reflect on their process ("Did you solve the problem?," "How did you do it?," "How did you feel when you first started?," "How did you feel when you got it?"). This kind of discussion reinforces understanding of successful problem-solving processes, and also provides practice in interpersonal communication skills.

In addition, it is important for coaches to provide a scaffold for children to use these steps when conflicts emerge in the context of group interaction. The "online" application of social problem-solving skills in the course of naturalistic peer conflicts may be a critical learning experience, as this application occurs in the context of arousal and engagement, rather than in the "cold cognition" of a staged role play. Thus the application of the skill in actual conflicts better mirrors the organizational capacity needed to apply social problem solving effectively in naturalistic peer interactions outside the group setting.

Developmental Organization of Skills: The Fast Track Program Example

In addition to identifying the skill domains that will be included in a particular coaching program, it is important to consider the sequential organization. As noted earlier, skills are ideally presented in a developmental sequence, such that skills presented early in the program provide a foundation for later skills. Skill domains are thus integrated across time.

One example of the way in which skills might be organized in a developmental pattern comes from the first-grade Friendship Group program of the Fast Track project (Bierman et al., 1996; CPPRG, 1992). This program focuses on promoting positive social interaction and self-regulatory skills, with the parallel goals of increasing positive behaviors and decreasing negative behaviors. There are four units in the first-grade program, ordered developmentally. Recognizing that friendships begin with the identification of shared interests and common ground, the program begins with skills from the domains of participation, communication, and emotional understanding; the initial focus is on providing opportunities for joint activities that foster self-disclosure and the discovery of common ground, and that facilitate "togetherness" and "team" identification among group members. A presumption underlying this first unit is that shared positive affect, and feelings of trust and security (within the coaching context with the adult coaches, and in a group context with other children in the group), create an important foundation for child engagement and improvement in the intervention. Identifying feelings (one's own and others) is emphasized, to provide a foundation for interpersonal awareness and self-control. The second unit emphasizes cooperation and self-control skills. Sessions in this unit introduce relaxation and self-calming strategies, which are designed to empower children to self-regulate their behavior, inhibit reactive aggressive or destructive responding, and cope with uncomfortable feelings in socially appropriate ways. In addition, cooperation skills are introduced. The third unit of the program focuses on the understanding of reciprocity in relationships. Movement beyond parallel play into cooperative and organized play requires the division of labor, the taking of different roles by various group members, and the organization of activity so that the efforts of one child are complemented by those of others. Team games, board games, and other organized play activities require the willingness to abide by general norms of reciprocity, rules, and fair play. Finally, the more advanced skills needed to maintain friendships, including attending to feedback, giving feedback, avoiding retribution, and using interpersonal problem-solving skills to work through conflicts, are presented in the final program unit (see Table 11.4).

PROGRAM STRUCTURE AND ORGANIZATION

Prior research provides strong evidence for the effectiveness of the coaching techniques described in the previous sections (e.g., multifac-

TABLE 11.4. Developmental Skills in the Fast Track First-Grade Friendship Group Program

Unit 1: Establishing Common Ground (Sessions 1–6)
   Good Teamwork (participation)
   Tell about You (self-expression)
   Talk about Feelings (labeling and understanding emotions)

Unit 2: Caring and Controlled Behavior (Sessions 7–11)
   Share and Help (cooperation)
   Going to the Red Light (self-control)

Unit 3: Fair Play: Reciprocity and Negotiation Skills (Sessions 12–16)
   Fair Play (taking turns, following rules)
   Make a Deal (negotiation skills)

Unit 4: Attending to Feedback: Sustaining Friendships (Sessions 17–22)
   Taking Care of Friendships (conflict resolution skills, handling competition)
   Keeping Friends (apology and repair strategies)

eted skill presentation, opportunities for structured practice, performance feedback, and generalization planning that includes support for skill use in naturalistic peer interactions). Developmental research on the correlates of peer acceptance and rejection provides useful guidelines for the selection of skill domains around which coaching programs should be focused. However, little research exists to guide practitioners in the pragmatic decisions that must be made about program structure—issues such as the context for coaching, group size and composition, the number and length of sessions, the number and characteristics of group leaders, and the organization and structure of sessions. Research is needed to determine how variations in these dimensions of coaching programs may affect their impact. Below, I provide suggestions based upon my colleagues' and my own experiences, and upon recommendations made by other practitioners and researchers. In reality, some of these decisions will depend upon the goals and context of the particular coaching program. Here I simply identify key issues and provide available theoretical principles and working guidelines for making these decisions.

Context for Coaching Programs

At the outset, it is important to note that social competence coaching programs are undertaken in a variety of contexts. Many of the programs evaluated empirically have been run in school settings, with coaching sessions held during school hours as "pull-out" programs,

scheduled as indoor recesses, or held during other nonacademic periods. School-based programs have the advantage of providing easy access to the naturalistic peer group; this can enhance the inclusion of
peers in group programs and generalization programming, but it also
requires careful attention to program length, frequency, and timing.
Given the concurrent academic difficulties experienced by many rejected children, it is important to schedule school-based programs in
ways that complement and do not conflict with academic programming. At the same time, serious peer problems make it difficult for children to engage positively in the school setting, and can contribute to a
disruptive and nonsupportive learning community. Hence social competence coaching programs represent an appropriate part of school-
based programming and support.

Some research-based programs have identified child participants
through school-based screening, but have scheduled intervention sessions during extracurricular periods (after school or Saturdays; see, e.g.,
La Greca & Santogrossi, 1980, and CPPRG, 1992). Some coaching programs have been implemented in a summer camp context—for example,
the Collaborative Multisite Multimodal Treatment Study of Children
with Attention Deficit Hyperactivity Disorder (the MTA Study; see
MTA Cooperative Group, 1999a, 1999b). Finally, social competence
coaching programs are often scheduled in special education or mental
health clinic settings (see, e.g., Guevremont, 1990), serving children
with significant emotional or behavioral difficulties. Empirical research
suggests that coaching can be effective in each of the settings mentioned, but more research is needed to determine the impact of different scheduling protocols (e.g., brief sessions held during the school
day vs. intensive day-long programs held during specialized summer
camps).

In the following sections, I discuss a number of other pragmatic issues regarding program design. Again, some of these decisions will depend upon the particular context in which a coaching program is undertaken, and on the characteristics of the children being served in that
program.

Group Size and Composition

Social skills training can be conducted during individual sessions,
which have proven successful in increasing prosocial skills (Bierman &
Furman, 1984). However, group training is more often used, as it can
enhance the effects of coaching in several ways: by (1) providing social
partners for skills practice; (2) providing social support and, in some
cases, a context to initiate new friendships or strengthen existing ones;

and (3) enabling the intervention to target improvements in peer responding as well as in child behavior. A number of school-based coaching programs have used a combination of individual and group sessions, or have mixed the two formats during sessions. For example, Oden and Asher (1977) conducted the skill presentation and performance feedback parts of each session with individual target children, but included peer partners for the play practice portion of the session. Ladd (1981) ran a school-based program in which initial sessions were conducted with pairs of socially isolated children, and later sessions (designed to promote skill maintenance and generalization) included two additional classmates to form small groups of four. These strategies represent a balance between focused attention to the skill deficits of particular children (in individual or dyadic sessions) and opportunities to generalize skills with larger groups of nonproblematic peers (in small-group sessions). They also minimize time lost from normative school activities for the nonproblematic peer partners, who may not benefit from involvement in the entire coaching program. Other research-based programs have utilized small groups (usually of three to five members) for the entire coaching program, with some including nonproblematic peer partners throughout the program to serve as models and to build friendships (Bierman & Furman, 1984; Bierman et al., 1996), and others focusing on groups in which all members have peer relation difficulties (Gresham & Nagle, 1980; La Greca & Santogrossi, 1980). When one is designing a group coaching program, particularly if groups are composed of children who all have peer relation difficulties, it is important to consider the nature and severity of the children's social difficulties, in order to preserve a supportive peer context for positive social learning (Rose & Edleson, 1987). Children certainly learn from each other in the contexts of these groups, and this influence can be both positive and negative (Dishion, Poulin, & Burraston, 2001).

The size of the group, the characteristics of the social partners, and the tasks used in sessions all affect the skillfulness required to navigate the interactions successfully, as well as the degree of personal support and opportunities for involvement available to children during the interaction. For example, the social tasks become more difficult as groups get larger, as there are more social cues to monitor, more inhibitory control needed (e.g., waiting for one's turn in the mix of multiple interaction players), and less frequent opportunities for personal interaction and support (as group members are responding to each other, the frequency of interaction with any one group member is lower than in a smaller group, where conversational turns are more focused).

The characteristics of the children in the group also affect the degree to which the group context provides opportunity for interaction and support for each child. When a group contains members with well-regulated social behavior and a high rate of prosocial responding, it creates an ordered social context with predictable opportunities for social interaction, and a high rate of positive contingent responding. In contrast, a group that contains multiple members with high rates of socially domineering and intrusive behavior can be threatening and unpredictable. This kind of group climate elicits emotional arousal and reactive responding; it is prone to escalating conflicts as children react to perceived autonomy threats, or to disruptive behavior as they respond to the unpredictability of the social context and seek to increase peer or adult attention and contingent responding.

Finally, the tasks selected for group interaction also influence difficulty level. Tasks that are structured, with clearly defined reciprocal social roles (e.g., role plays, scripted sociodramatic play), provide more guidance and support for social behavior than do unstructured tasks (such as free play). Cooperative tasks, which require coordinated efforts, are more difficult than individual tasks; however, they are typically less difficult than competitive activities, which require regulation around rules and coping with the emotions of winning and losing, as well as the coordination of social behavior.

Group size, composition, and tasks can be altered systematically to create a smaller and more supportive session structure during the first phase of intervention, but expanded to include a gradual increase in the degree of naturalistic challenge as child skill acquisition progresses during the course of intervention. Most of the school-based coaching programs described in the empirical literature use small groups (two to three children) and one trainer. Programs run outside school settings often use larger groups (four to six children) with two trainers. Practitioners such as Goldstein and colleagues (1986) and Rose and Edleson (1987) suggest that skill training is most effective in groups with no more than three to eight children (optimally, five to six) and two trainers. Research examining the impact of group size and composition on intervention process and outcome is needed to provide better guidance in this area.

From a practical standpoint, decisions regarding the composition of an intervention group involves a tradeoff between two competing principles. On the one hand, coaching appears most effective when the participants are clearly deficient in the particular skills targeted in the intervention; this supports a selection strategy in which children with similar patterns of skill deficiency and social behavioral problems are grouped together (Goldstein et al., 1986). On the other hand, groups that contain multiple members who show reactive, aggressive, and impulsive styles of interpersonal interaction can create a group context characterized by frequent escalating conflicts (Guevremont, 1990) and deviant partnerships (Rose & Edleson, 1987). Groups composed of children who all have conduct problems have shown iatrogenic effects, fostering peer affiliations that increase the youth's risk for future anti-social activity (Dishion et al., 2001). In my own experience, effective coaching becomes very difficult in groups that contain many impulsive and reactive youth, because behavior management issues take prece-dence over skill training. That is, vigilant efforts must be expended to inhibit escalating cycles of peer reactivity that elicit and reinforce problematic social behavior. Although the use of behavior manage-ment techniques (e.g., rules, token systems, time out) can promote behavioral control within such a group, the focus of the group becomes one of management via external control, which detracts from opportu-nities to promote positive social learning in the context of supportive peer interactions (see Chapter 12 for a more complete discussion of this issue).

In some cases, complementarity rather than similarity in the social needs of group members may create a more therapeutic social context. Rose and Edleson (1987) suggest that children in a group need to have some common ground in terms of social skill deficits, but that variation in the behavioral manifestations of their social difficulties can be an ad-vantage. That is, group members may have in common deficits in coop-erative play skills or anger management, although some react with so-cial withdrawal and hostile avoidance, whereas others exhibit impulsive aggression. This kind of group may provide a common basis for skill training and may become quite cohesive, without creating a threaten-ing or resistant social dynamic in the intervention group that impedes the coaching agenda.

In addition, coaches must make decisions regarding the gender composition of the group. Grade school friendships are typically (though not always) same-sex partnerships, and most of the programs that have coached children in small groups (dyads or triads) have opted to use same-sex groups. However, larger coaching groups often include children of both sexes. Research is needed to compare the impact of same-sex versus mixed-sex coaching groups for children's peer rela-tions.

Number and Length of Sessions

The number of sessions needed depends upon the nature and severity of the child social problems targeted by the intervention (Rose & Edleson, 1987). Programs of 10–12 sessions have proven effective at promoting positive behavior change and improving sociometric ratings for unaccepted, socially withdrawn children (Bierman & Furman, 1984; Ladd, 1981). In contrast, effective programs for aggressive–rejected children, children with learning disabilities, or children with attention-deficit/hyperactivity disorder (ADHD) have typically been much longer, ranging from 18–22 sessions (Guevremont, 1990; Plienis et al., 1987) to 36 sessions (La Greca et al., 1989). Guevremont (1990) has argued that for children with more severe social relationship problems, additional time in treatment is needed to establish group cohesion, rules, and routines. Overlearning and consolidating the mastery of each skill are critical, and time to practice skills across multiple sessions fosters children's abilities to use positive skills with ease and automaticity.

Most programs involve sessions of 30–60 minutes in length, once or twice per week, with the exact length determined by factors such as the children's attention span, impulsivity, and verbal ability (Goldstein et al., 1986). Children's difficulties in maintaining attention and behavioral focus during sessions can be dealt with by scheduling more frequent but shorter sessions (Goldstein et al., 1986), and/or by dividing sessions into multiple miniactivities designed to keep the children engaged (La Greca et al., 1989; see also Chapter 12).

Group Leadership and Staffing

Most of the experimental coaching programs have utilized graduate students as therapeutic coaches, whereas most school-based social problem-solving programs train classroom teachers to deliver the intervention (Weissberg & Allen, 1986). Intervention personnel can include a range of professional and paraprofessional therapists, who have been trained specifically in coaching techniques (Bierman et al., 1996).

Although coach–child relationships have not been studied empirically, from a theoretical perspective the coach functions both as an instructor and as a source of social–emotional support. As important as the teaching a group leader does is the therapeutic relationship the leader is able to establish with the children in the group, supporting them in their attempts to change the way they are thinking about and engaging in social relationships. Children need to feel comfortable and secure with their coach. Their interpersonal growth during the coaching program may be substantially dependent on their ability to trust and learn from a leader who is sensitive, responsive, and accepting. In addition, the coach must be an instructor. Growth will be optimized when the coach is able to provide clear and consistent social guidance and contingent responding, in the context of a compassionate sensitivity for each child's learning struggles. Hence, from a conceptual standpoint, group leaders need several types of skills—including both general skills related to working effectively with vulnerable children in a group setting, and specific skills needed to implement the social skills training model with fidelity (Goldstein et al., 1986).

Effective group leaders must be able to relate to anxious and aggressive children warmly, supportively, and with interpersonal sensitivity and compassion, fostering the children's feelings of comfort in the group setting. In addition, effective group leadership requires good teaching and communication skills. Group leaders also need to be able to set and maintain clear limits and group order, and to remain resilient and calm in the face of frustration; they must be able to work under pressure with a resourceful problem-solving orientation.

In addition to these general skills for working effectively with children in groups, the capacity to implement the coaching model with fidelity requires specific knowledge and experience in several key areas, including (1) a good working knowledge of the coaching model and its mechanisms of action; (2) the ability to present and discuss skill concepts in an engaging way; (3) the ability to adjust skill practice opportunities in ways that maintain an optimal learning window for the children; and (4) the ability to reflect, ask questions, and provide feedback during ongoing practice sessions in a way that fosters social learning.

Although single trainers have been effective in coaching individual children and small groups (dyads and triads), it is difficult for one trainer to manage the multiple leadership tasks alone in a larger group. Group sessions involving four or more children typically require a team of two trainers. Although one adult may serve as the group leader and the other as group assistant, it is important that both group coaches become confident in their understanding of and ability to carry out program objectives.

Rules and Routines

In addition to the skill training curriculum, coaching programs need to give careful consideration to behavioral management issues, particularly when groups include children with aggressive acting-out difficulties or ADHD (Guevremont, 1990). One of the goals of a coaching program is to foster a child's sense of efficacy in social interactions, which is predicated on a feeling of predictability and control. That is, competence entails the capacity to act in ways that produce positive outcomes and avoid negative outcomes. Perceived competence reflects a belief structure in which the child feels both that he/she understands how positive outcomes can be produced and how negative outcomes can be avoided (means–end or cause–effect understanding), and that he/she has the capability to behave in ways that can control social outcomes (Skinner, 1995). Coaching programs are designed to facilitate perceived efficacy in several ways. First, by focusing on specific skills, coaching programs seek to clarify for children the means–end relations in social interactions—the kinds of behaviors that are linked with positive outcomes or negative outcomes. Second, by providing carefully graduated experiences for skill practice, coaching programs seek to provide children with mastery experiences, in which their skill performance does lead predictably to positive social outcomes. Third, performance feedback serves not only to shape behavior, but also to help clarify for children the cause–effect relations in social interactions and to reinforce their capacity to control their social experiences by regulating their own behavior.

In order to "demystify" social interaction, and to promote the development of control beliefs that support the use of positive self-regulatory and social skills, it is important to create a social context within group settings that involves predictable social response contingencies and supports the social behaviors the program is designed to promote. As described in earlier chapters, many problematic social behaviors emerge and become habitual aspects of children's social interaction styles because they have functional value—they promote some aspect of control over interpersonal experiences. To encourage a child to give up some of those habitual response styles and replace them with others requires more than adult recommendation; it requires that the new styles of interaction demonstrate value in terms of providing self-protection with greater predictability and control over interpersonal outcomes. Hence it is important to create a therapeutic group context in which social interaction patterns are predictable. During initial sessions, the interpersonal contingencies supporting skill performance need to be quite high to encourage skill production. Rules and routine structures in group sessions help to accomplish this goal.

Group rules should be clearly stated, kept to a minimum, and phrased whenever possible in positive terms (e.g., positive standards of behavior). For example, four rules are used in the Fast Track first-grade Friendship Group program: (1) "Listen to the coaches," (2) "Take care of our place," (3) "No fighting," and (4) "No put-downs" (e.g., calling names, saying mean things). During initial sessions, the rationale for each rule should be stated clearly, and children should be offered a chance to contribute to this rule discussion. The warning system and set of consequences that accompany rule infractions need to be prespecified, clearly stated, and consistently followed. In some cases, token or point systems may be used to encourage children to comply with rules. As discussed in Chapter 12, however, there are costs as well as benefits associated with highly structured behavioral management systems such as token and point systems. Although they increase the predictability of the social interaction context by making desired and undesired behaviors highly salient to children, they can draw children's attention away from the more subtle interpersonal cues that signal the interpersonal impact of their behavior in naturally occurring settings. Hence group sessions that regulate social interaction with tokens and points differ from naturally occurring peer interaction settings in marked ways, and these increase the challenge for generalization of intervention effects.

In addition to the provision of rules, established routines provide a predictable order to intervention sessions, give children a sense of the agenda for each session, and support anticipatory planning. Particularly when coaching programs involve larger groups and longer sessions, Rose and Edleson (1987) recommend that the agenda for each session be posted in a visible location or distributed to members as a handout, identifying the planned activities for each session. (Typically, this structure is not needed in shorter-term programs that utilize the same agenda through each session.)

For first and second graders in the Fast Track program, in coaching groups that contain four to six children with conduct problems and are scheduled outside the school day for 60- to 90-minute sessions, agenda pictures are used to help children identify the session routine. These pictures describe the sequence of activities planned for the group—for example, (1) "We will meet in our friendship circle and watch a video about sharing," (2) "We will put on a play about sharing," (3) "We will make a sharing snack together," (4) "We will share markers and stickers to make a friendship poster," and (5) "We will have a compliment circle." These agenda pictures are posted in a visible location, so that children can look at them as they enter the group session; this helps them to identify the routines in the sessions and to build anticipatory planning skills.

Working with older grade school children, Guevremont (1990) describes the routine followed in his training sessions:

1. Review of group rules and behavioral management system.
2. Introduction of a social skill with instructions, rationale, and group discussion.
3. Discussion of the step-by-step components of the skill, which are posted on a blackboard or sign.
4. Modeling of the skill by therapists.
5. Role playing between a therapist and one participant.

6. Coaching and feedback in response to the role play.
7. Child-to-child role playing, with group feedback.
8. Videotaping of child-to-child role plays with feedback.
9. Summary of the skills focused on during the session.
10. Assignment of homework.
11. Delivery of rewards.

SUMMARY

This chapter has focused on the organization, design, and content of social competence coaching interventions. Drawing upon past research, I have emphasized the importance of an instructional approach, with a variety of presentation strategies and practice activities to train skills selected on the basis of their established correlations with social competence. I have advocated the selection of skills from seven general domains (i.e., social participation, emotional understanding, prosocial behavior, self-control, communication skills, fair-play skills, and social problem-solving skills), while also recognizing that the specific content of a coaching intervention should reflect the assessed needs of the participating children.

In addition to the selected skills and the programmed steps of skill presentation, practice, and performance feedback, I have postulated that a child's learning is affected by his/her interpersonal experiences within the intervention group context. Although little empirical research is available to guide decisions about group size and composition, the number and length of sessions, the number and characteristics of group leaders, and the rules and routines established for sessions, these are all important aspects of program design that may influence the effectiveness of the program. One of the goals of coaching programs is to foster children's sense of efficacy in social interactions; this is done by clarifying means–end relations in social interactions, by providing children with mastery experiences in which their skill performance leads predictably to positive social outcomes, and by strengthening their belief that they can control their social experiences by regulating their own behavior. This goal requires careful attention to the interpersonal processes and behavior management strategies used in coaching interventions—a topic discussed in further detail in the next chapter.

Chapter 12

Intervention Process and the Promotion of Self-System Change

Based upon the premise that a child's behavior toward others is a major determinant of the social responses he/she receives, the social skills training approach targets behavior change (Ladd & Mize, 1983). The goal of such training is to give children the social-cognitive and behavioral performance skills that will enable them to change their habitual patterns of social responding (those that have alienated peers), and to replace them with social interaction patterns that are effective for themselves and appealing to their social partners.

However, habitual patterns of social responding are not easy to change, particularly when they have served adaptive functions in the past and have become an established part of a child's affective, cognitive, and behavioral orientation toward his/her social world and sense of self. Unfortunately, we know relatively little about how children reconstruct perceptual and interpretive systems, particularly those that serve self-protective functions. Social competence coaching interventions continue to rely heavily on the provision of information and encouragement to enhance children's social knowledge and change their social beliefs. The hope is that if children are introduced to and reinforced for new ways of thinking and behaving during intervention sessions, they will begin to behave more appropriately in their interactions with peers outside those sessions. Correspondingly, it is hoped that they will elicit positive peer responding, which, along with their improved social knowledge, will provide social experiences that reinforce positive changes in the children's broader self-system development (including emotional, motivational, and self-evaluative features).

For the reasons reviewed in Chapter 4, adult instruction, exhortation, and reinforcement may have limited power to change children's social behavior or corresponding self-system processes outside the settings that adults control. Research is needed to examine the impact of different strategies designed to promote the reworking of "internal models" and conceptions of the self in the context of peer relations. These may include new kinds of instructional or coaching strategies that place more emphasis on emotions and motivations in the skills targeted in interventions; however, attention is probably also required to the noncognitive features of coaching session processes that influence children's emotional experiences with peers during those sessions. That is, although lessons in skill domains such as emotional understanding and self-control may be helpful, such lessons still depend on changes in children's "cold cognition" (their ability to think about and talk about feelings outside a problem situation) to bring about changes in the underlying feelings and motivations that influence their functioning under "hot-cognition" conditions in real-life interactions. As an addition to "cold-cognition" lessons, graduated experiences that allow for commentary, questions, and support during actual emotion-charged social interactions may provide critical learning opportunities (Selman & Schultz, 1990). In addition, greater attention to peer experiences outside coaching sessions may be needed, as changes induced during intervention sessions may be sustained only if naturalistic interpersonal experiences validate the functional value of new attitudes, affect, and behavior (Price & Dodge, 1989; Selman & Schultz, 1990).

This chapter addresses the challenges associated with promoting sustained changes in children's relational schemas and self-system processes. Due to the lack of direct empirical research, the ideas presented here are based upon theory and my colleagues' and my own observations, which emphasize the need to focus more attention on the motivational and emotional aspects of children's peer interactions—chiefly by monitoring the interpersonal dynamics and responding to the affective experiences children have during their "online" peer interactions in coaching sessions.

Specifically, in this chapter, I suggest that the manner in which coaches deal with the ongoing processes of social interaction during coaching sessions represents a critically important, yet unexplored, feature of coaching sessions. In particular, the ways coaches choose to elicit and respond to interpersonal affect and dynamic interpersonal exchanges during sessions may affect the impact of those interpersonal experiences on children's working models of peer relations and their corresponding affect-charged orientation toward others and toward themselves. First, I provide a brief review of the conceptualization of relational schemas, including their functional value and corresponding resistance to change. Then I discuss the rationale for focusing on coaching session processes as a potential mechanism for promoting positive changes in children's relational schemas, including their social self-conceptions. I also identify a set of coaching strategies that, based upon theory and our experience, may be useful in strengthening children's feelings of security and connectedness in their peer relations; their capacity to balance autonomy striving with interpersonal sensitivity and accommodation to others; and their understanding of cause–effect social transactions, as well as their perceived competence to predict and control their own social outcomes.

THE FUNCTIONAL VALUE OF RELATIONAL SCHEMAS AND THEIR RESISTANCE TO CHANGE

As discussed in Chapter 4, the relational schemas that children develop have important functional value, helping them to make sense out of their social world (Baldwin, 1992; Skinner, 1995). Conceptions of their relations with others, intertwined with conceptions of themselves, enable children to act strategically—predicting and controlling their social world, maximizing their opportunities for social support, and reducing the anxiety and distress associated with social exclusion or rejection (Bowlby, 1969; Cairns, 1991; Epstein, 1991).

Relational schemas influence a child's affective experiences in social interaction, as well as his/her perceptions, interpretations, and recall regarding interpersonal interactions (Baldwin, 1992; Crick & Dodge, 1994). Relationship histories can support the development of social-cognitive frames or biases promoting social behaviors that, although sometimes self-protective in the immediate setting, are detrimental to the development of positive peer relations in the long run (Crick & Dodge, 1994). In theory, a child's relationship experiences contribute to the development of an emotion-laden informational database that influences social information processing at various levels—social perception and appraisal, cause–effect interpretations, and decision making about social responses. This influence works unconsciously, shaping an affective bias that influences the child's sensitivity and reactions to particular social cues (Baldwin, 1992; Crick & Dodge, 1994). As a heuristic that can guide the intervention approach, it is useful to think of relational patterns of dysfunction as representative of three types of sensitivity and self-protective activity, corresponding to the three themes around which relational schemas are organized developmentally (Connell & Wellborn, 1991; Skinner, 1995).

First is the desire to experience a sense of relatedness or connectedness to others—to form relationships that are supportive and responsive (Connell & Wellborn, 1991). Friendships with these qualities promote feelings of security and well-being, are characterized by shared positive affect, and provide an opportunity for intimacy and self–other integration (Selman & Schultz, 1990). The desire for connectedness is threatened for children when they are unable to identify relationships that will provide them with predictable opportunities for responsive support. This inability contributes both to felt anxiety in interpersonal settings and to limited experience of (in some cases, limited capacity to experience) positive affect or intimacy in friendships (Bandmaster & Leary, 1995). Hence children with low levels of perceived security may approach peer relations with hesitation, anxiety, and/or anger; they remain vigilant and emotionally reactive to signs of perceived rejection or loss of support. To protect themselves against anxiety, children may avoid social interactions, behaving with hostile isolation or anxious withdrawal. Alternatively, children who are anxious about their interpersonal connections may behave in socially intrusive or disruptive ways, in which they force others to attend to them on their terms (Jacobvitz & Sroufe, 1987).

The second universal desire around which relational schemas are organized involves autonomy—the capacity to make choices about one's actions and to direct one's behavior toward chosen goals (Deci & Ryan, 1985). Balancing the desire to connect intimately with others with the desire for autonomous self-direction, and being able to succeed with both goals in social relations, are important facets of social effectiveness (Selman & Schultz, 1990). Many children who have experienced a history of coercive control in relationships develop a high level of vigilance and sensitivity to situations in which others may be thwarting their goals or restricting their autonomy. One common response to frequent autonomy threats is to become adept at the rapid escalation of countercontrol strategies, which often involve aggressive, domineering, and coercive behaviors that function to reduce aversive constraints.

Relational schemas are also constructed to support the desire to attain competence, including understanding cause–effect relations and acquisition of the means that allow a child to produce desired and prevent undesired events in particular action domains (Patrick, Skinner, & Connell, 1993; Skinner, 1995). Perceived social competence motivates engagement and confidence in social interactions, and promotes adaptive coping and social problem-solving attempts. Perceived incompetence is linked with feelings of helplessness and anxiety, and contributes to disengagement, passivity, or disorganized reactions in the face of social challenges.

Many of the behavior problems that emerge in the context of social skill training sessions reflect emotions associated with threats to connectedness, autonomy, or competence. For example, consider the following two examples of disruptive behavior that have emerged in the context of our social skill training groups: A boy routinely puts his face up against another person's face, trying to press his forehead against the other's forehead; and a girl repeatedly grabs and hangs onto the arms of adults and peers, letting her weight drag on them. These behaviors reflect both children's desire to connect with others. In a third case, a child reacts repeatedly to adult requests with noncompliance and alternative attention-getting behavior. When a coach requests that the group members meet at the table for a snack, for example, this child runs away and climbs on a chair. This sort of oppositional behavior reflects a habitual defense of autonomy. Yet another boy uses silly and provocative language in conversations, making serious communication difficult. For example, when children are trying to decide what game to play, he barks like a dog rather than stating his preference. By thus controlling the discourse, he avoids entry into games or other peer interactions in which he lacks competence. In each of these cases, understanding the feelings associated with the problem behavior can assist coaches in selecting responses that both redirect the problematic behavior and support alternative coping strategies to enhance the child's feelings of interpersonal security, autonomy, and competence. Children are often unaware of the impact their relational schemas and associated control beliefs have on their social behavior; hence this impact must be inferred by coaches from the coaches' observation of the children's social behavior and apparent affect.

PROMOTING CHANGE IN SELF-SYSTEM PROCESSES

As discussed, the self-system processes associated with interpersonal relations are affectively charged belief systems that reflect past experiences and influence emotion regulation and information processing (including social perceptions, interpretations and attributions, response generation, and response evaluation), as well as social behavior. As such, these processes involve the interactions (and transactions) of affective, cognitive, behavioral, and interpersonal experiences (Greenberg, Speltz, & DeKlyen, 1993).

Theoretically, change in any one of these dimensions of functioning can facilitate change in the others. For example, cognitive-behavioral interventions for anxiety or depression often focus on changing the cognitions associated with learned helplessness (including self-perceptions, attributions, and behavioral intentions), with the assumption that changes in these cognitions will improve mood and motivate new behavioral coping, which will elicit more positive responses from the environment. Coaching programs for disliked children typically target social cognitions and behavior changes, with the assumption that affect and self-perceptions regarding interpersonal relations will improve as a function of the increased positive peer responding and social acceptance that accompany improved social behavior.

On the one hand, then, the interdependence of cognitive, affective, behavioral, and experiential dimensions of social functioning may create multiple opportunities for intervention, as change in any one of these dimensions may trigger changes in the other. On the other hand, given the tendency for self-system processes to maintain synchrony (Cairns, 1991), the interdependence of these functional dimensions may also create resistance to change, particularly if change efforts are directed toward only one or two of these dimensions (Price & Dodge, 1989). Sustained and internalized change may occur more readily if interventions are designed to target multiple aspects of the self-system simultaneously—including cognitive, affective, and behavioral experiences, particularly when those interventions also promote "corrective" interpersonal experiences that support the functional value of reconstructed beliefs.

In Chapter 11, I have described the ways in which the instructional strategies used in coaching programs can be expanded to include target skill domains such as emotional understanding and self-control. For example, coaching sessions can include presentation strategies (modeling, discussion), practice, and support for skills such as recognizing the feelings of others, labeling one's own feelings, inhibiting impulsive reactivity under conditions of emotional arousal, and coping effectively with feelings of anger.

In addition to addressing emotions and motivations by targeting them as instructional skill domains (designed to influence children's social-cognitive processes and behavior change), leaders can also design group coaching sessions in ways that provide high levels of interpersonal support and positive peer responsivity; low levels of threat and coercion; and high levels of causal explanation, commentary, and reasoning. Theoretically, an emotionally and socially supportive context will increase children's feelings of interpersonal security—allowing them to reduce their reliance on self-protective strategies learned in the context of past relationships, and providing a safe context in which to "try out" new ways of behaving, thinking, and feelings in peer relationships. The use of "inductive" behavior management strategies, in contrast to power-assertive strategies, may minimize perceived threats to autonomy and encourage children to self-regulate in appropriate ways; ideally, this will foster internalized attributions to support generalized behavior change. In addition, by providing commentary and eliciting feedback from others, coaches can increase the predictability of children's social experiences. Making more explicit for the children the cause–effect relations between their behaviors and the interpersonal responses they receive should increase their perceived control and perceived competence in peer relations.

In the next sections, each of the following three aspects of group coaching is explored more fully, with a discussion of processing techniques that may enhance the power of coaching interventions to influence cognitive, affective, and behavioral dimensions of experience simultaneously: (1) creating a supportive and nonthreatening context for change; (2) providing autonomy support to promote internalized self-regulation and social regulation; and (3) increasing causal understanding and perceived competence in interpersonal relationships.

CREATING A SUPPORTIVE CONTEXT FOR CHANGE

In an interesting study conducted by Rabiner and Coie (1989), rejected boys were observed as they entered a room to initiate play with children they did not know. Some of the boys were informed by the experimenter that the peers they were going to play with liked them and were looking forward to the opportunity to play with them. When they were compared with children who were given no information prior to group entry, the rejected children who believed the unfamiliar peers wanted to play with them received more positive sociometric ratings from those peers after the play sessions (peers who, in fact, had not expressed prior play preferences and who had no knowledge of the experimental manipulation). Observers could not detect differences in the behaviors exhibited by rejected children who did or did not have information about the peers, but the investigators believed that the confidence and optimism created by the expectation that peers would like them increased the social approach of the rejected children in subtle ways that increased their actual likability. Relatedly, Dodge (1983) found that rejecting behavior by peers led to disengagement by target children, who withdrew and became more negative in their social behavior. These studies suggest that creating a warm and accepting intervention group will foster child participation and positive affect—engagement that may be critical for program impact. In addition, Izard (2002) suggests that positive mood facilitates learning; hence children who feel comfortable and happy in the coaching context may process information more effectively.

Strategies designed to foster feelings of inclusion and connectedness within the group may also foster increases in positive peer responding that support social skill acquisition. When I (Bierman, 1986a) conducted sequential analyses of peer interactions during social skills training sessions, I found that the contingent responding of peers (i.e., peers' responding positively when a target child initiated conversation, asked a question, or made a suggestion) predicted gains in target child conversational skills at posttreatment and follow-up assessments.

For each of these reasons, strategies designed to enhance positive affect and intergroup support and cohesion may strengthen the impact of coaching sessions. In addition, coaches should be sensitive to behavior problems that can emerge in groups, fueled by feelings of alienation or anxieties about acceptance. Two problematic interaction patterns in particular often appear associated with a child's affective concerns about his/her connection to and acceptance by group members: (1) the child's avoidance or refusal to join group activities; and (2) intrusive, attention-demanding behavior that disrupts the group and calls attention to the child. In either of these cases, coach interventions that support feelings of connectedness can help the child reorganize him-/herself and rejoin the group. The following strategies both foster a positive group climate and increase the positive social support available to children who display problematic social behaviors during group sessions, by increasing their feelings of relatedness and their positive engagement in the intervention: (1) friendly, warm coach involvement; (2) identification of common ground; (3) use of cooperative tasks and superordinate goals; (4) provision of physical proximity and supportive contact; (5) supportive social referencing; (6) use of frequent praise; (7) statements of positive expectations; and (8) cuing with positive redirection. Each of these strategies is described briefly.

The adult–child relationships set a tone for the group. One critically important support strategy is to provide a high rate of warm, friendly comments, and positive feedback, in order to promote each child's feelings of acceptance and security. Displays of affection, such as a pat on the shoulder, smiles, and welcoming comments, reinforce the message that the children are accepted and liked in the group. Frequent praise of positive social behavior promotes both prosocial behavior and feelings of inclusion.

Coaches can also use social reflection and comments to foster feelings of connectedness among children. For example, some ongoing narration that includes reflections about the activities of group members, along with conversational questions and comments, can be used to model social chat and to help children attend to each other. Active listening (in which an adult restates or emphasizes a child's comments) can provide a useful scaffold, validating the child's viewpoint or feelings and helping him/her feel supported by the group. Pointing out similarities among children particularly fosters connectedness.

Examples of this kind of social chat designed to foster intergroup connections include comments such as these: "Oh, here's Mike. It's good to see you, Mike. We were hoping you'd be able to make it this week," "I see Sam chose the red paper again. Jim likes red best, too, and so do I," and "Jason had an interesting idea. I think you guys might like his idea about how we could play this game."

In addition, positive interactions in the group can be encouraged by choosing tasks that emphasize common ground and cooperative interaction. Tasks that involve "superordinate goals"—goals that can be obtained only when group members work together—can enhance feelings of group connectedness. Superordinate goals create a structure that encourages inclusion, provides a social niche for all group members, and rewards group members for collaborative support. Cooperative activities with group rewards create a superordinate goal structure and represent practice activities with opportunities to elicit and support skill acquisition. For superordinate goals to be effective, however, it is essential that group members have the skills and structure needed to be successful at goal attainment. Hence the specific tasks chosen need to be within the capability level of the group.

When children show signs of disengagement from the group, supportive nonverbal and physical contact by an adult often helps settle, organize, and reassure children—particularly when it is used proactively, before a child's behavior has deteriorated (or escalated) into an oppositional or avoidant stance. For example, coaches can strategically place themselves in a position that allows them to maintain proximity to children who have particular difficulty in certain group settings. Frequent social referencing toward a child—including frequent eye contact and warm smiles, a pat on the shoulder, mentioning the child's name in a positive way, and commenting on his/her positive actions—can all reassure the child that he/she is accepted by the group, and can reinforce the child's attendance to and participation in the group activities.

Praising other children in the group can also help to elicit more positive behavior among children who are disrupting or resisting group participation. Such praise provides a cue for appropriate ways to achieve group connection, and reinforces a positive affective valence among group members. In the face of one child's inappropriate behavior, this strategy involves looking for children who are displaying the behavior the coaches would like to see, and praising those children specifically. Examples include "Jim has his hand up—he has an idea to share with us," and "Sue and Jill have joined the circle. It's great to have you with us."

Praising positive models can be combined with a strategy in which the coaches express hopes and positive expectations about the behavior they would like to see among other group members. This kind of expression cues children in a positive way and provides them with an explicit invitation to join in. This strategy can also be used in the face of disruptive or avoidant behavior, and in this case it involves labeling hopes for the kind of behavior the coaches would like to see. Here are some examples: "I see that John and Eric are sitting at the table ready for their snack. I'm hoping Steve can join us, because we're hungry," and "It would be nice if Laura could join us for our compliment circle; I have a compliment I'd like to share with her today."

Positive redirection can have a similar function. In positive redirection, a coach provides guidance to a child by directing his/her attention to a constructive task to be done, particularly when there are natural rewards—for example, "Zachary, I could use a helper to carry the tray so we can start our snack."

Particularly when a particular child behaves in intrusive or insensitive ways that elicit negative reactions from other group members, it is important to look for opportunities to elicit and reinforce prosocial behavior from that child. This should both prevent peers in the group from developing negative reputational biases against that child, and allow that child to reconnect in positive ways with other group members. (See Table 12.1 for a summary of strategies to foster feelings of connectedness.)

PROVIDING AUTONOMY SUPPORT TO PROMOTE SELF-CONTROL

In addition to promoting positive connections among group members, it is important to prevent negative interpersonal escalations within the group (e.g., the exchange of aggressive or hostile behavior). Negative peer exchanges may trigger self-protective escalation and extended chains of coercive attempts to dominate the interaction on the part of aggression-prone target children (Asarnow, 1983), fostering distrust and vigilance, interpersonal animosity, and withdrawal. Here it is important to distinguish interpersonal conflict or disagreement (which represents an important and inevitable part of any close relationships) from fighting or hostile exchanges (which represent an unnecessary escalation of anger and aggression) (Shantz & Shantz, 1985). Whereas coaching programs recognize the value of helping children learn to discuss their own viewpoints and listen to others in conflict situations— both of which are core components of effective social problem solving—

TABLE 12.1. Process Techniques to Induce Self-Regulation and Enhance Positive Control Beliefs

Increase positive support

Friendly, warm involvement: Show positive affect; engage children in conversation.

Identify common ground: Identify contributions to the group; note areas of common interest.

Cooperative tasks, superordinate goals: Use activities that foster collaboration.

Physical proximity/contact: Sit or stand by a child; pat him/her on the shoulder.

Supportive social referencing: Look at the child; nod toward the child; use his/her name.

Frequent praise: Praise the behaviors of positive models.

Positive expectations: Express positive expectations for child behavior.

Positive redirection: Identify constructive tasks and appropriate actions or roles.

Reduce threats to autonomy

Ignore minor infractions: Refrain from unnecessary prohibitions; use induction instead.

Give choices: Provide choices that indicate the appropriate behavioral options.

Focus on consequences that matter for the child: Emphasize the child's potential gains or losses associated with different behavioral choices.

Use a soft voice tone to deescalate conflicts: Intervene in a low, neutral tone.

Increase understanding of cause and effect in interpersonal relations

Use active listening and reflect feelings: Help children recognize and express verbally their feelings in interpersonal situations.

Elicit peer feedback: Elicit information about the interpersonal impact of child actions.

Use I-statements: Describe the interpersonal and group impact of particular behaviors.

they also focus on helping children to inhibit and control impulses to fight or aggress.

Children who engage in high rates of oppositional and aggressive behavior also often elicit high rates of commands and prohibitions from coaches in the group coaching context (Guevremont, 1990). Paradoxically, commands and prohibitions may increase the children's resistant and aggressive behaviors, as they seek to "escape" from or terminate these control attempts (Patterson, 1986). The affective dynamic associated with these kinds of coercive exchanges often involves anger and frustration, as children respond emotionally to the perceived threats to their autonomy. Some children become sensitized and overreactive to perceived autonomy threats, responding with impulsive resistance to commands (including adult and peer directives) and with defiance to goal blocking (including such events as not going first, not getting their choice in an activity, or losing at a game).

Establishing clear rule structures with consistent consequences provides an important foundation for the creation and maintenance of an accepting and nonthreatening group. The behaviors that merit time out or other response cost consequences should be specified clearly in the first session, and should be posted in a visible location.

However, in addition to needing clear external constraints to control aggressive and destructive behaviors, children with aggressive/oppositional social problems often show "low-grade" behavior problems. These are behaviors that do not break the rules of the group and are not destructive to the group, but are distracting and bothersome (such as squirming, nonparticipation, interrupting, making strange noises, or rough play). It is important to resist the temptation to correct these behaviors with "stop" commands (e.g., "Don't push in line," "Don't rock the chairs," "Don't do karate kicks in here"), and instead to use more inductive behavior management strategies, which are less likely to incite reactive resistance. "Inductive" strategies cue children to consider the impact of their problematic behaviors and suggest alternative behaviors, but do not involve commands or power-oriented constraints that directly threaten a child's self-determination (Hoffman, 1967). These strategies are designed to minimize adult/external control of children's behavior, and to encourage children's self-regulation in appropriate ways. Inductive strategies include (1) ignoring minor infractions; (2) giving alternative choices in the face of inappropriate behavior; (3) focusing on consequences that matter to a child; and (4) using a soft voice tone that deescalates affect and connotes support for the child, rather than vocal attempts to overpower and dominate the child.

To the extent that children's behaviors are inappropriate or annoying, but not directly destructive or damaging to the intervention or group members, it is best for coaches to avoid reprimands, ignore the minor infractions or misbehaviors, and use the positive support strategies mentioned earlier in this chapter to encourage reengagement by the children. For instance, the coaches can praise other children who are modeling desired behaviors ("Great, Julie has come over to the table"), can make statements about positive expectations ("I'm hoping that we'll have everyone over at the table soon, so I can show you this game"), or can identify constructive tasks ("John, maybe you'd like to carry this game to the table for us").

When behavior cannot be ignored, giving children choices that indicate the possible appropriate behavioral options open to them provides guidance without direct prohibition. Faced with undesirable behavior, a coach might say something like this: "You can join the group at the table, or you can sit in a chair and just watch until you feel ready to join us," or "I'm worried that someone will get hurt if there is kicking in the circle. You can sit on the chair there and kick, or stay in the circle sitting cross-legged like this."

To support a child's sense of self-protective autonomy, it is helpful for an adult to focus on consequences that matter for the child when pointing out the desirable and undesirable consequences of various behavioral choices (rather than focusing on the adult's own displeasure). For example, the coach might explain, "I'm worried that other children won't want to play with you if you push them during the game" (rather than "Pushing isn't nice"), or "I'm afraid you won't know how to play the game if you don't listen to the directions" (rather than "I need you to listen now"). By stating cues as concerns, the adult "stays on the child's side." This prevents a power play and provides the child with information the child can use to make more effective interactional choices.

Importantly, coaches can use their voice tone, as well as words, to deescalate conflicts and associated negative behaviors. For example, if children are getting loud (excited or angry), coaches should avoid attempts to overpower them by shouting (which is likely to encourage further escalation), and instead should use a soft, stage-whisper voice tone to help deescalate the noise level. Some adults feel that reprimands must be given in a negative voice tone to be effective—to show a child that an adult is displeased and means business. However, research suggests that reprimands given in a neutral voice tone are just as effective as those given in a negative tone (Rosen et al., 1984). We recommend avoidance of angry, bossy, or displeased voice tones, as any of these can serve to escalate the child's own angry and upset mood. (See the summary of strategies to support autonomy in Table 12.1.)

INCREASING CAUSAL UNDERSTANDING AND PERCEIVED COMPETENCE IN INTERPERSONAL RELATIONS

When a child is able to use social behaviors to elicit positive social outcomes, those behaviors are likely to be repeated. Unfortunately, some behaviors produce highly salient and immediate gains, whereas their longer-term and more subtle negative social consequences go unnoticed by the child actor (but not by the peer group). For example, by grabbing a game, taking the dice, and pushing a partner out of the way, a child can be first at the game of his/her choice. In terms of this salient outcome, a domineering strategy is more effective than a prosocial one, since behaviors such as taking turns or throwing the dice result in only a 50/50 chance of going first. Children who are not tracking the responses of their social partners can easily miss the negative consequences (e.g., alienating playmates) of strategies that appear effective. Hence an important goal of coaching is to help children identify their feelings, inhibit their immediate self-serving reactions, consider the impact of their behaviors on the feelings of their partners, and choose behaviors that will elicit positive peer responding.

A coach can help children understand and express verbally their mixed feelings in social situations in which relational and instrumental goals collide (Denham, 1998). For example, in the example of grabbing dice used above, the group leader can, in a calm and supportive voice, intercede in the action and help the perpetrator identify his/her own motives (e.g., "You're worried that you won't get a turn," or "You want to go first") and label the problem (e.g., "Our problem is to think of a fair way to decide who goes first—so you both get a chance to go first today and you both have fun").

Eliciting peer feedback is a particularly useful method of drawing a child's attention to the interpersonal consequences of his/her behavior. For example, if a child grabs the dice, the coach might stop the action and cue the children to discuss the conflict, using a prompt such as "Oh, just a minute. I wonder how Jimmy feels about you taking the dice like that," or "Hmm, I think we might have a problem to solve here. Jimmy, can you say how you feel about Jane taking the dice?" This method of guidance allows the perpetrator of an insensitive social behavior to get immediate feedback about the effects of his/her behavior on another and to take corrective action before the conflict escalates. Similarly, if a child appears to be annoying another, the coach can respond by eliciting feedback from that peer: "Jason, I wonder how John feels about you leaning on him like that. John, can you tell Jason how you feel about that?" Coaches can also encourage children to elicit peer feedback directly: "Susan, I wonder how Amy feels about you coloring on her paper. Maybe you can ask her if that's OK with her."

When a child is disturbing the coach, I-statements provide a useful way of describing to that child how his/her behavior is affecting others. This strategy can help children understand the cause–effect impact of their behavior, and can serve as a cue for behavioral redirection. For example, a coach might say, "I don't like it when you put your face against mine. It's just not comfortable for me," or "I'm afraid that our posters will get torn and ruined if you kick at them."

In these examples, conflicts that arise in the course of group interaction are viewed as learning opportunities that, with appropriate adult guidance, can help children gain an understanding of and competence in the skills needed to maintain mutually rewarding relationships (Selman et al., 1992). By slowing down the action, encouraging children to reflect on their behavior, and facilitating constructive peer feedback, coaches can help children understand their own feelings better, monitor the impact of their behavior on others, and make more informed and thoughtful behavioral choices (Selman & Schultz, 1990).

The use of social problem-solving steps in group processing can also support children's development of positive control beliefs. For example, before an activity or game, coaches can lead children in planning sessions to help them anticipate and negotiate how they will work together toward their goal (e.g., "What would be a fair way to divide the snack?", "How shall we decide which game to play?"). These group discussion exercises help children develop confidence in their ability to influence others with verbal expression, and provide a foundation of experiences linking negotiation and cooperation with exciting and rewarding interactions. (See the summary of strategies to support causal understanding in Table 12.1.)

BEHAVIORAL MANAGEMENT: TO TOKEN OR NOT TO TOKEN?

In thinking about coaching strategies designed to increase child self-regulation and positive control beliefs, it is important to consider the impact of the behavioral management system used in the group. Particularly when coaching interventions target children with problems involving aggression, disruptiveness, or inattention, clear methods for behavioral management are needed within the group setting. A token system is often recommended as a straightforward and noncoercive method of reducing problem behaviors and enhancing compliance during coaching sessions (Bierman, Miller, & Stabb, 1987; Dumas, Prinz, Smith, & Laughlin, 1999; Guevremont, 1990). In this kind of system, group rules and expectations for behavior are established early and are typically posted in a visible location, along with a clear specification of how tokens can be earned and redeemed. During training sessions, feedback is delivered frequently, with points or tokens distributed to participants who are participating and following rules. At the end of the session, the tokens are exchanged for specific rewards, such as a special snack, privileges, or small prizes.

When well specified, token systems function effectively to reduce problematic behavior and improve compliance and participation. Yet, paradoxically, they may not support the development of self-regulatory skills, and in certain cases may even undermine the development of self-control. First, children who are focusing their attention on getting points or rewards from adults may be less aware of and less focused on the impact of their behavior on their peer social partners. Hence a token program may distract children from attending to peer social cues and responses. Second, when highly salient external rewards are used to maintain certain behaviors, the development of an internalized motivation to display those behaviors may be inhibited. That is, children may attribute their good behavior to the external contingencies controlled by adults, rather than to their personal disposition and desire to be more friendly and rewarding playmates for peers. Price and Dodge (1989) make a similar point about peers, suggesting that under conditions of salient token rewards, peers who respond in a positive way to rejected children during group sessions may attribute the positive behaviors of the target children and themselves to external constraints (e.g., "They shared so they could earn a point"), rather than adjusting their opinion of the target children in a positive direction (e.g., "They shared because they are nice"). Third, external rewards will not be available when children are interacting with peers in naturalistic settings; hence reliance on this control strategy may limit the generalizability of behaviors developed in the group setting to naturalistic peer contexts.

Given these limitations, it is worthwhile to consider alternatives to the use of token reinforcement systems in running social competence coaching interventions, or at least to limit reliance on such systems when possible. For example, making careful choices about the composition and characteristics of children assigned to a particular group, along with limiting the size of the group, can reduce the potential for escalating behavior problems. Program design, including the selection of structured, fast-paced activities that elicit active participant involvement, can also reduce management problems. The availability of adult support and the way in which materials and space are organized and used can all affect the extent to which children can sustain their positive engagement and avoid oppositional or disruptive behavior.

SUMMARY

In addition to promoting behavior change, group coaching interventions may foster changes in children's self-system processes, including feelings of interpersonal security, capacities for self-regulation, and control beliefs and perceived competence regarding peer relations. Developmental theory suggests that the strategies coaches use to support and discuss interpersonal interactions during group sessions may influence children's perceptions and constructions regarding the meaning of those interpersonal experiences. Of particular importance are coach behaviors that support positive affect and group cohesion, foster children's self-regulation, and process conflicts in a way that helps children gain perceived competence through their improved understanding of cause–effect relations in their peer interactions. These coach behaviors increase the likelihood that children will begin to (1) notice and understand the ways in which their behaviors affect the feelings of their peers; (2) experience positive responses to their skillful behaviors; (3) inhibit reactive, self-serving behaviors; and (4) believe in and demonstrate their capability to regulate their social behavior in a way that promotes positive peer responding and avoids rejection. "Inductive" behavior management strategies, in contrast to power-assertive or external constraint (token system) strategies, are designed to minimize adult/external control of children's behavior, to encourage appropriate self-regulation, and (ideally) to foster internalized attributions that will support generalized behavior change.

At the same time, attaining effective generalization from social competence coaching sessions to "real-world" peer interaction settings is not an easy task. Even with extensive effort during coaching sessions, it is difficult to prepare children to sustain skillful behavior in naturalistic peer settings that provide relatively low levels of contingent positive peer responding. Even worse, some children face well-established reputational biases, making it difficult for them to change negative peer expectations and to achieve entry into positive peer networks. For these reasons, in addition to preparing a child for generalizing positive behaviors to naturalistic peer settings, it is also useful to consider strategies that focus on preparing the naturalistic peer environment to provide niches of social opportunity and positive responding to sustain the target child's behavioral gains in naturalistic contexts. The next chapter considers these kinds of collateral social competence training interventions; it examines school-based interventions that focus on improving the quality of peer relations in school contexts, strategies that parents can use to increase social leaning opportunities at home, and multicomponent programs in which social competence coaching is combined with classroom-level and/or parent-focused intervention strategies.

Chapter 13

Collateral Interventions
Providing Support at School and Home

Since the 1970s, researchers have emphasized the need to attend carefully to issues of generalization in social competence interventions, arguing that effective generalization will occur only if reinforcement contingencies support new behaviors in the natural environment (see Stokes & Osnes, 1989). For this reason, Baer (1989) and others have called for designs that actively include a child's natural social environment in the intervention. For the most part, social competence coaching programs have tried to enhance generalization by giving homework assignments, designing intervention sessions to include more naturalistic peer interaction practice opportunities, and including selected peer partners in coaching sessions. This chapter discusses additional strategies designed to increase peer involvement in social competence programs, in ways that might have a stronger impact on peer attraction and positive peer treatment of rejected children. I examine classroom-based social competence education and cooperative learning programs designed to increase overall levels of positive peer interaction (and reduce levels of negative peer interaction) in the classroom, and I also consider the potential value of different kinds of peer-pairing techniques, designed to enhance peer support opportunities for identified target children. In addition, I discuss the role that parents may play in supporting the development of child social competence and friendships at home.

The chapter begins with a discussion of the feasibility of multi-component interventions that combine social competence coaching with teacher-focused, classroom-focused, and parent-focused components. The implications of two recent large-scale intervention trials for the design of effective social competence programs are considered.

MULTICOMPONENT INTERVENTIONS FOR CHILDREN WITH EXTERNALIZING BEHAVIOR PROBLEMS

During the past 15 years, several large prevention and intervention trials have been mounted to test the effectiveness of multifaceted programs that include teacher-, classroom-, and parent-focused components along with social competence coaching for children with externalizing behavior problems (Conduct Problems Prevention Research Group [CPPRG], 1992; Dumas, Lynch, Laughlin, Smith, & Prinz, 2001; MTA Cooperative Group, 1999a, 1999b; Tremblay et al., 1992). Some researchers have suggested that these programs represent the future for social competence training (McFadyen-Ketchum & Dodge, 1998), but this optimism is not fully warranted. Certainly each of these programs has made critical contributions to our understanding of interventions for children with externalizing problems—an important subgroup of rejected children. However, these programs were designed with the central intervention goal of reducing problematic behaviors in home and school settings for children with clinically significant externalizing disorders or risk levels for such disorders. As such, their focus was complementary to, but somewhat different from, that of research directed toward understanding how best to promote child social competence and positive peer relations.

Externalizing behaviors are an important correlate of rejected status, but not all children with externalizing problems are rejected by peers, nor do all rejected children have externalizing problems. Hence multicomponent programs targeting children with significant externalizing problems can inform, but not replace, research focused on developing and evaluating intervention technology for improving peer relations. Many questions remain for social competence interventions serving rejected children—including strategies for influencing peer involvement and attraction, improving school-based friendships, decreasing victimization, and fostering parental support for positive peer relations, in addition to issues regarding effective coaching procedures (described in Chapters 11 and 12). In this section, I provide a brief description of two of the larger-scale multicomponent studies, and discuss their potential implications for social competence programs targeting peer rejection. Then I move on to describe other models for school- and home-based intervention components that may hold promise for strengthening social competence interventions.

The six-site Collaborative Multisite Multimodal Treatment Study of Children with Attention Deficit Hyperactivity Disorder (the MTA Study; MTA Cooperative Group, 1999a, 1999b) compared the effectiveness of psychosocial treatments and medication, alone and in combination, for children aged 7–10, with primary diagnoses of attention-deficit/hyperactivity disorder (ADHD), combined type. In the psychosocial conditions, an intensive summer treatment program was designed to enhance child social competence and positive peer relations. The program included daily social skills training using modeling, coaching, role playing, and practice opportunities with feedback and reinforcement to facilitate the acquisition of social problem-solving skills, fair-play skills/good sportsmanship, and following rules. Cooperative tasks, superordinate goals, and nonproblematic peer buddies were used to create a positive peer learning environment. In addition, school-based teacher consultation and a structured behavioral management plan (i.e., a point system, time out, and contingency management) were designed to reduce school off-task and disruptive/aggressive behavior problems.

In general, the study demonstrated that a combined treatment—medication plus the various psychosocial treatment components (parent training, teacher consultation, and the summer treatment program)—produced better child outcomes (including higher levels of teacher-rated social skills) than the psychosocial treatment alone or a community treatment comparison condition (MTA Cooperative Group, 1999a). These findings highlight the utility of carefully monitored medication for children with properly diagnosed ADHD, in combination with a multicomponent psychosocial support program. Clouding the interpretation of effects of the psychosocial treatment alone was the fact that the community treatment comparison group included children on medication (whereas children receiving the psychosocial treatment alone were not medicated), and that the posttreatment assessment occurred 6 months after the intensive phase of the psychosocial treatment, when social and behavioral support had been faded out. Interestingly, the model of social competence intervention used in this study incorporated a number of theoretically salient design features, such as the addition of nonproblematic peer buddies and multiple opportunities for naturalistic play practice in the summer camp context. In addition, the teacher consultation component of the program was designed to foster the generalization of intervention gains in the school setting. However, teacher consultation focused on effective behavioral management at school and did not address the promotion of positive peer relations per se. In addition, a comparative study examining the impact of different delivery contexts on coaching effectiveness would have been worthwhile. Possibly the intensity of the summer program, the density of behavior problems represented in the camp peer group (half of these children had ADHD), and its separation from school-based peer groups may have limited opportunities for the consolidation of skills and generalization to school peer relations. Given the purpose and design of the study, it is not possible to evaluate how characteristics of the coaching program and additional parent or teacher components might have affected the impact on children's peer relations, or how this kind of program might work for rejected children without ADHD. However, the program does provide a model for intervention delivery that is worth further comparative evaluation.

A second large-scale trial was initiated in 1990—the Fast Track project, designed to prevent adolescent conduct disorder. At the elementary school level, the program utilized a classroom-based prevention program taught by the teacher (i.e., the Providing Alternative Thinking Strategies [PATHS] curriculum; Greenberg, Kusche, Cook, & Quamma, 1995; Kusche & Greenberg, 1995). In addition, the families of at-risk children (those who scored in the top 10% of the school population on a combined teacher–parent rating screen of behavior problems) were offered separate extracurricular parent training groups, social skill training groups (Friendship Groups), parent–child relationship support sessions, peer pairing, academic tutoring, and home visiting. Of these, three components (PATHS, the Friendship Groups, and peer pairing) were focused specifically on the promotion of social competence and positive peer relations. PATHS was designed to promote a positive peer climate at the classroom level, targeting skills of emotional understanding, positive play and communication, self-control, and social problem solving. The Friendship Groups provided target children with additional coaching in the same skill domains, using a comprehensive coaching method with cooperative practice activities. The peer-pairing program was used to enhance skill generalization from extracurricular group sessions to peer relations within the school setting, by giving high-risk children supportive play opportunities with rotating classroom partners (see Bierman, Greenberg, & CPPRG, 1996, for more details on program design). At the end of the first 3 years of prevention services, high-risk children in the intervention group, compared to those in the nontreated comparison group, showed improved social-cognitive skills (reflected in their responses to structured child interviews), reduced levels of aggressive/oppositional behaviors at home (by parent report) and at school (by teacher report), and a reduced need for special education services (indicated in school records)

(CPPRG, 1992, 1999a, 1999b). At the end of first grade, direct observations of peer interactions in playground and classroom settings revealed higher rates of positive peer exchange for children in the intervention group than for those in the control condition. In addition, children in the intervention group had higher social preference scores based on peer sociometric nominations than children in the control group did. However, although reduced aggression was still evident at the end of third grade on child social-cognitive interviews and teacher ratings of aggressive/disruptive behavior, peer sociometric nominations did not show sustained effects (CPPRG, 2002). The Friendship Groups were provided intensively in grades 1 (weekly) and 2 (biweekly), and faded to monthly in grade 3. In addition, after grade 1, peer pairing was conducted only with children who were rejected by peers. Possibly reductions in the degree of social support offered these children in the intervention accounted for the weakening of peer relation effects over time.

The MTA and Fast Track studies (and others of their kind) are critically important in order to address questions about the overall efficacy of multicomponent intervention programs to prevent or treat serious child social–emotional and behavioral disorders, such as conduct problems and ADHD. They represent attempts to adapt interventions to meet the needs of high-risk children with significant behavioral or emotional difficulties, for whom single-component programs (social competence coaching, parenting, or classroom management) are insufficient (La Greca, 1993). At the same time, they have not been designed specifically to test variations in the impact on children's peer relations of different types of social competence program packages. As we in this field move forward in examining the impact of multicomponent programs for very high-risk children, it is also important that we continue developing and evaluating the intervention technology for improving social competence and peer relations. The behavioral characteristics of rejected children (e.g., aggressive behaviors, inattentive/hyperactive behaviors) may (or may not) moderate the impact of various intervention components designed to promote social competence and positive peer relations. This issue warrants close examination.

In targeting ADHD and conduct problems, the MTA and Fast Track studies have included teacher training and parent training components focusing on the effective management of problem behaviors. In addition to those components, which may be particularly appropriate for children who are rejected because of their acting-out behaviors, the next sections of this chapter consider teacher-focused, classroom-focused, and parent-focused components designed specifically to enhance child social competence and positive peer involvement.

"UNIVERSAL" SCHOOL-BASED SOCIAL
COMPETENCE INTERVENTIONS

Within the school context, two levels of support activities can foster positive peer relations—those designed for the classroom as a whole ("universal" programs), and those designed to support identified children who are experiencing peer difficulties ("indicated" programs). Universal interventions, once termed "primary prevention" strategies, are directed at an entire population (e.g., all students in a particular classroom or school) and are designed to build aspects of competence that will support successful adaptation to school, thus preventing the emergence of school adjustment difficulties and associated mental health problems (Mrazek & Haggerty, 1994). Indicated interventions are aimed at children with existing adjustment difficulties, for whom competence-building support may remediate those difficulties and prevent the development of negative consequences (Mrazek & Haggerty, 1994). Increasingly, these two levels of support are being integrated, as schools and communities design multifaceted programs that both promote positive social development for all students and offer additional, indicated support for students experiencing significant social difficulties (Weissberg & Allen, 1986; Weissberg & Greenberg, 1998). In this section and the next, I consider universal school-based intervention approaches as a method for enhancing the effects of social competence coaching by increasing the positive receptivity of the classroom peer group. Later, I consider indicated approaches applied in the school setting to increase positive peer involvement with and responding toward targeted children.

The idea that formal classroom-level curricula could be implemented by teachers to promote the social competence of all children in the classroom was introduced by Spivack and Shure (1974), who used classroom instructional techniques to promote children's social problem-solving skills. The premise underlying this approach was that children's cognitive capacities to recognize and assess social problems, to generate and evaluate multiple potential responses, to set goals, and to self-monitor their behavioral performance in light of those goals provide the critical building blocks for flexible, socially responsive, and adaptive behaviors (Allen, Chinsky, Larcen, Lochman, & Selinger, 1976; Weissberg & Greenberg, 1998).

The Spivack and Shure (1974) curriculum emphasized the acquisition of these cognitive skills. Approximately 8 weeks of daily lessons were devoted to teaching prerequisite skills, such as listening to others, observing social cues, identifying emotions, and understanding cause–effect relations. The next 4 weeks focused on recognizing problems, generating alternative solutions, and anticipating consequences. Teachers provided multiple examples and gave children evaluative feedback on their responses. Participating socioeconomically disadvantaged children showed posttreatment gains in their capacity to generate alternative solutions and consequences to hypothetical social problems, and teachers rated them more positively on a measure of adaptive classroom behavior (compared with untrained children in comparison classrooms). Although encouraging, the Spivack and Shure trial did not examine the impact on peer ratings; nor were teacher ratings free from the biased knowledge of student participation in the program.

A later trial conducted by Allen and colleagues (1976) focused on third- and fourth-grade children, and also emphasized teacher-led instructional sessions (a 24-session curriculum, including lessons on identifying problems, generating alternative solutions, considering consequences, and selecting solutions). Like Spivack and Shure (1974), Allen and colleagues demonstrated that children who received intervention could generate more solutions to hypothetical problems than nontrained children could. However, these gains were not maintained at a 4-month follow-up, and trained children did not show improvements relative to untrained children on teacher or peer ratings of social behavior (Allen et al., 1976; McClure, Chinsky, & Larcen, 1978).

Weissberg and colleagues (1981) found that the effectiveness of classroom-based social problem-solving curricula could be enhanced with several changes: (1) increasing the breadth of instructional strategies used to teach adaptive conflict resolution strategies, including greater use of teacher and videotaped modeling, class discussion, and role playing; (2) limiting the discussion of aggressive solutions and focusing more time on prosocial alternatives; (3) placing an increased emphasis on the generalized use of the social problem-solving steps by teachers in their day-to-day interactions with students as they mediated peer conflicts; and (4) extending the amount of program time focused on applying the social problem-solving steps in an integrated way to real-life problems. With this expanded focus, Weissberg and colleagues documented increases among children in intervention classes (compared to those in control classrooms) in areas of perceived social competence and teacher ratings of shy/anxious behaviors, general school adjustment, and global ratings of likability. However, sociometric scores showed no intervention effects.

More recently, classroom-based social competence curricula have been expanded to focus on a broad range of positive social–emotional skills, in addition to social problem solving. For example, the PATHS curriculum (CPPRG, 1999b; Greenberg & Kusche, 1993; Kusche & Greenberg, 1995) targets multiple types of skills, including emotional understanding, self-regulation, communication skills, friendship skills, and problem-solving skills. PATHS lessons, which are 20–30 minutes in length, are taught by teachers two or three times each week. Skill concepts are typically presented via instruction, discussion, modeling stories, and/or video presentations. Discussion and role-playing activities follow, giving children a chance to practice each skill. In addition to these formal lessons, teachers are instructed in how to generalize their use of PATHS concepts across the school day and to other settings of the school outside the classroom. For example, teachers are encouraged to help children identify their feelings; to communicate clearly with others; and, as interpersonal problems emerge, to use self-control strategies and apply the three "traffic light" steps of problem solving (see Chapter 11 for a description of these). Each classroom also has a mailbox where students can write down and submit problems or concerns for discussion in classroom problem-solving meetings. The curriculum also includes frequent parent updates on curriculum content, along with home activities and tips for parents, designed to foster support for the social competence skills at home. Moreover, PATHS provides teachers with suggestions and consultation in the area of effective classroom management of disruptive behavior (e.g., establishing clear rules and directions; providing positive and corrective feedback for appropriate behavior; and applying reprimands, time out, or response cost procedures contingent upon the occurrence of problematic behavior).

The PATHS curriculum has been evaluated in several randomized controlled field trials, which have included students in regular education, students with special needs, and students with hearing impairments (Greenberg & Kusche, 1993; Greenberg et al., 1995). Across these groups, PATHS has produced significant increases in the targeted skills, as reflected both in child assessments (e.g., of emotion recognition and social problem-solving skills) and in teacher ratings (e.g., of student self-control, emotional understanding, and conflict resolution). In addition, students in special education who received PATHS reported lower levels of sadness and depression, and their teachers rated them as improved in social competence (e.g., frustration tolerance and positive peer relations) relative to students in comparison classes. PATHS has also been evaluated in the context of the Fast Track prevention program. At the end of first grade, observers (who were naive concerning classroom conditions) rated PATHS classrooms higher than control classrooms on overall rates of student on-task behavior and student enthusiasm and engagement. In addition, even when the high-risk children who received additional intervention were removed from the analysis, peer sociometrics revealed lower levels of peer-nominated aggressive and disruptive behavior in PATHS than in non-PATHS classrooms, as well as higher classroom mean levels of positive peer nominations (CPPRG, 1999b).

These findings suggest that classroom curricula that focus on a broad range of social competencies, use multiple instructional strategies, and provide children with guided opportunities for practice and feedback along with positive classroom management practices can improve child social competence, classroom behavior, and peer relations at the classroom level. For a more comprehensive overview of school-based approaches to promoting social competence, including a description of other exemplar programs, the reader is referred to Elias and colleagues (1997).

In addition, recent years have witnessed the development of school-based programs designed specifically to reduce bullying in school (Olweus, 1991). For example, the program designed by Olweus (1993) includes several basic steps: (1) the development of a school supervision plan to monitor unstructured settings (recess, lunch, restrooms) where bullying takes place; (2) the development of school-wide policies against bullying, including a clear statement of intolerance of bullying written into classroom rules; (3) the empowerment of teachers to intervene quickly and decisively, to put a stop to any bullying incidents; (4) the establishment of sanctions for bullying; and (5) collaboration with parents, including informing parents of the school-wide bullying plan and about any bullying incidents involving their children.

Universal school-based programs, such as the social competence programs and bullying prevention programs described above, are not replacements for indicated social competence coaching programs designed for peer-rejected children. Focused on the entire classroom, teacher-led programs are unlikely to provide the intensity of instructional support, guided practice, and feedback needed to remediate the substantial behavioral, affective, and social-cognitive difficulties that characterize most rejected children. However, universal school-based programs may complement indicated social competence coaching programs in important ways, by enhancing positive peer responding in the classroom, creating more opportunities for positive peer support, and thus enhancing the generalization of coaching program effects (Weissberg & Greenberg, 1998). The next section describes another approach to improving positive peer relations at the classroom level, which involves the use of cooperative learning activities.

SCHOOL-BASED APPROACHES UTILIZING COOPERATIVE LEARNING

Whereas classroom curricula focus on direct instruction for the development of social competence, a second type of universal school-based program involves the use of cooperative learning activities to support positive social development. In these activities, small groups of students work together on academic material, in a context that promotes and rewards interpersonal sharing, helping, and collaborative goal attainment (Furman & Gavin, 1989). Cooperative learning programs are built upon the premise that as children work toward common goals, they will gain in their abilities to cooperate, communicate, and collaborate with others; these changes should foster heightened levels of interpersonal understanding, and reduce prejudice and social isolation. A number of different models for cooperative learning have been developed and evaluated empirically (Bridgeman, 1981; Johnson & Johnson, 1994; Slavin, 1983).

Two of the evaluated programs, Learning Together (Johnson & Johnson, 1994) and the Group Investigations Method (Sharan, 1980), involve the assignment of topics to small groups of two to six students. In the former program, teachers and students discuss the goals and expected outcomes of the group, and the group members work together on an assignment, which they then submit to the teacher. In the Group Investigations Method, each student in the group takes responsibility for a different task associated with the group project. The group combines the pieces developed by different members and puts them together to present to the class. In both of these programs, students are graded as a group on their projects, to provide an incentive to support active efforts to collaborate. Evaluation studies suggest that these kinds of small-group cooperative learning experiences promote self-esteem and intrinsic motivation, along with more positive attitudes toward peers, increased altruism, and perceptions of greater peer support in the classroom (Hertz-Lazarowitz, Sharan, & Steinberg, 1980; Johnson & Johnson, 1994).

One method of systematically incorporating cooperative learning into classrooms has involved the establishment of student learning teams (DeVries & Slavin, 1978; Slavin, 1983). In one version of this method, the Student Teams–Achievement Divisions (STAD), students meet in four- or five-member teams to review and study material that has been presented by teachers. Teams are constructed to be heterogeneous according to ability and to reflect the ethnic/racial mix of the classroom. Students in each team work together to complete worksheets and help each other master the material. Students then take individual tests, and they bring back points to the team for their improvements over past quiz performance. A similar team learning structure is utilized in the Teams–Games–Tournament (TGT) model, but the testing process differs. In TGT, students from different teams compete at tournament tables (organized according to difficulty level of the subject matter), where children compete with others who are working at similar levels of material difficulty. The purpose is to allow each child an equal opportunity to bring back points to his/her team by achieving at a tournament table. Compared to students in control classrooms, students in classrooms utilizing student teams (STAD or TGT) reduced rejection of academically handicapped children (Madden & Slavin, 1982) and developed more cross-race friendships (DeVries & Edwards, 1973).

In a descriptive review of the effects of cooperative learning across studies, Slavin (1983) found that the majority of the studies that collected peer ratings (14 out of 19) found improvements in liking among classmates. Positive effects on academic achievement were also common, with 29 of the 46 studies that evaluated achievement showing greater academic gains in the cooperative learning classrooms than in control comparison classrooms. Summarizing across studies, Slavin reported that the combination of group study and group reward for individual learning appeared most effective.

The value of cooperative learning for peer-rejected children has not been examined empirically. To the extent that the skill deficits of rejected children make it difficult for them to contribute in positive ways to the group goal attainment, cooperative learning programs could potentially exacerbate their peer difficulties. That is, research suggests that working together on cooperative tasks and superordinate goals enhances peer liking only when the group members are able to achieve their goals together; the same level of interdependence could increase disliking for any group member who impairs group goal attainment. Hence cooperative learning should probably not be used as a method for promoting the peer relations of rejected children without careful consideration for the nature and timing of the cooperative activities, so that these permit the rejected child to contribute in positive ways to the group's goals. However, under those conditions, cooperative learning activities may foster niches of opportunity for positive interaction with classroom peers.

In general, universal classroom programs, including both instructional social-competence-building curricula and cooperative learning programs, appear effective in building more positive social climates in the classrooms. These programs have not been evaluated specifically for their effectiveness with peer-rejected children, but it would be useful to determine whether, by promoting positive peer responding, they facilitate the impact and generalization of indicated interventions that provide social competence training to rejected children. The next section describes indicated programs designed specifically to enhance the social inclusion of disliked or withdrawn children in the classroom setting.

"INDICATED" PROGRAMS TO ENHANCE THE ACCEPTANCE
OF TARGET CHILDREN: CREATING NICHES

A number of programs have been designed to enhance the acceptance of target children by restructuring the peer environment in ways that create new niches of social opportunity through play or cooperative activities. Most of these programs were developed for socially withdrawn children or children with developmental delays, and have not been tested specifically as mechanisms to foster the generalization of social competence coaching programs for peer-rejected target children. Nonetheless, they warrant consideration as strategies that may give rejected children who have developed new social skills in coaching programs the opportunity to demonstrate these skills in supported interactions with classroom peers, and thereby to improve their peer acceptance. The following approaches represent possible structures for strategic peer pairing, in which target rejected children are paired with peer partners who represent good models and potential friends.

Sociodramatic Play

At the preschool level, investigators have found that sociodramatic play, which involves structured interactions among peers, can elicit increased social involvement in socially withdrawn peers. For example, Strain and his colleagues (Strain, 1977; Strain & Wiegerink, 1976) introduced sociodramatic play in preschool classrooms, having children act out common nursery stories or fairy tales (e.g., "Little Red Riding Hood"). This play increased rates of social interaction between classroom peers and socially withdrawn children with developmental delays. The activity provided affordances for positive social interaction, setting up a scaffold for reciprocal social interchanges between participants. Teachers supported the social interaction with prompts, modeling of responses, and social praise.

Play with Younger Peers

Also working with preschool children, Furman, Rahe, and Hartup (1979) assigned socially withdrawn preschool children to dyadic play sessions with younger peers. Their hope was that when paired with less sophisticated playmates, the withdrawn children would have the opportunity to take an assertive, leadership role in play. Indeed, this intervention produced marked increases in the rates of positive interaction that the socially withdrawn children exhibited with peers, in comparison to untreated children or children paired with agemates.

Providing Target Children with a Leadership Role

In order to improve the peer status of children with developmental delays, Aloia, Beaver, and Pettus (1978) first taught them a new game. They then let these children teach this game to their nondelayed peers. They found that enhancing the competence of the target children in a game-playing task increased the likelihood that peers would be select them as play partners in subsequent play sessions.

Using Cooperative Tasks

Just as they have been used to improve classroom peer relations in universal programs, cooperative tasks have also been used in more selective ways to promote positive peer interactions for targeted children. In several studies, cooperative tasks were evaluated for their capacity to enhance the peer acceptance of children with developmental delays. In one of the first of these studies, Chennault (1967) formed small groups that included junior high school students with developmental delays and their popular peers. These groups, which met twice a week for 5 weeks, were charged with developing and performing dramatic skits. This program led to significant improvements in the sociometric ratings received by the students with developmental delays. In 1970, Rucker and Vincenzo replicated the positive findings of Chennault, but also found that the gains in peer acceptance made by the children with developmental delays were not sustained 1 month following treatment. Using a slightly different cooperative activity, Lilly (1971) created groups that paired low-achieving, poorly accepted children with well-accepted classmates, and gave them 5 weeks to create a movie together. Similar to the effects of Chennault's dramatic activities, the cooperative movie making led to increased peer status for the poorly accepted children. However, as Rucker and Vincenzo (1970) did, Lilly found that the improved acceptance was not sustained over time.

In general, these studies suggest that involvement in small cooperative activities with peer-accepted classmates can improve the peer status of disliked children. Such improvements do not tend to last when cooperative activities are used alone. However, when combined with social competence coaching, peer involvement and cooperative activities may extend the impact, generalization, and maintenance of gains (Bierman & Furman, 1984). Further exploration and evaluation of these kinds of cooperative activities or other peer-pairing strategies as mechanisms to improve the generalization of social competence coaching programs for rejected children, and to increase positive peer responding, are certainly warranted. In addition to school-based interventions that target positive peer responding, parent-focused programs may provide useful supplements to social competence coaching programs. These are discussed next.

PROMOTING POSITIVE SOCIAL DEVELOPMENT AT HOME: PARENT CONTRIBUTIONS

Parents play an important role in fostering their children's positive social development. In general, developmental researchers have found three key ways in which parents affect their children's peer relations: through (1) their discipline practices, (2) the quality of parent–child relationships, and (3) their service as "gatekeepers" of their children's access to opportunities for positive peer interaction. Each of these models of influence is reviewed briefly (for more details, see Parke & Ladd, 1992; Pettit & Mize, 1993; Putallaz & Heflin, 1990).

Discipline Strategies

As described previously, disruptive behavior problems are often associated with problematic peer relationships, and discipline practices are linked in important ways with the development or exacerbation of noncompliant and aggressive child behaviors (Patterson, 1986). For this reason, discipline practices have been a central focus of the multicomponent programs described earlier, which were designed to reduce child aggressive/disruptive behavior problems. Research has documented associations between punitive parental discipline and peer rejection, via the mediating link of elevated levels of child aggressive behavior (Bierman & Smoot, 1991; Dodge, Bates, & Pettit, 1990). Coercive discipline strategies may also contribute to elevated levels of conflict among siblings, which in turn can foster child aggression (Stormshak, Bierman, McMahon, Lengua, & CPPRG, 2000). In addition to their discipline practices, parents affect their children's social development through the quality of the relationships they establish with them.

Parent–Child Relationships

As described in earlier chapters, children with poor peer relations often show deficits in social competence and emotion regulation capabilities. Developmental researchers have postulated that a child's capacity to regulate emotions in the context of interpersonal relationships derives largely from early experiences with his/her parents, which serve as prototypes for the child's later interpersonal expectancies and affect (Greenberg, Kusche, & Speltz, 1991). Research with infants and toddlers suggests that when caregivers respond to children's distress with consistency and sensitivity, children are less irritable, less anxious, and better emotionally regulated (Ainsworth, Blehar, Waters, & Wall, 1978), possibly as a result of greater feelings of security and of the modeling and internalization of calming behaviors. In addition, caregivers can foster the development of social competence by helping their children to develop the cognitive and verbal skills for recognizing and discussing their feelings, and thereby to develop greater flexibility in coping adaptively and regulating their emotional arousal (Greenberg et al., 1991; Kopp, 1982). Creating time for positive parent–child interactions, being available and responsive to a child's needs, and supporting a child's capacity to talk about feelings and relationships may all enhance the child's interpersonal security.

Parents as "Gatekeepers" and Coaches

Finally, parents may serve as important "gatekeepers," arranging opportunities for and monitoring the positive peer interactions of their children (Ladd & Hart, 1992). In addition, by providing sensitive supervision of peer interactions and by participating in discussions with their children about strategies for handling peer problems, parents serve as social competence coaches (Parker, Rubin, Price, & DeRosier, 1995). Parents may also promote the development of social competence by modeling positive social interaction styles and engaging in play interactions that foster the development of perspective taking and play skills (Putallaz & Heflin, 1990).

Intervention Implications

As described earlier in this chapter, a number of comprehensive prevention and intervention programs have documented the feasibility of coordinating parent-focused intervention components with child- and teacher-focused components. Given that child externalizing behaviors have been the target of these programs, the parent training programs have emphasized positive discipline strategies, parent–child relationship enhancement, and family communication and coping skills (CPPRG, 1992; Dumas et al., 2001). The provision of this kind of parent training, with a central focus on positive discipline strategies, may be particularly important for peer-rejected children who display high rates of noncompliant and aggressive behaviors in the home setting (CPPRG, 1992).

However, research is needed to examine the utility of parent components that focus on parents' other roles in social development (i.e., relationship enhancement and "gatekeeping" of peer interactions). As Guevremont (1990) suggests, parental involvement may be an important key to fostering the generalization of social competence coaching to children's interactions with siblings and peers in the neighborhood. Parents may benefit from support that helps them identify potential social niches for their children in the community. Parents may also benefit from discussions on coaching strategies they can use to help their children initiate and sustain positive peer interactions at home. However, systematic research is needed to determine the extent to which, and ways in which, parental involvement in social competence interventions fosters improved peer relations.

SUMMARY

This chapter has provided an overview of intervention strategies teachers can use to foster social competencies and positive peer relations in the classroom, including both "universal" programs (such as social competence curricula and cooperative learning structures) and "indicated" programs to promote the peer acceptance of identified target children. The chapter has also identified parenting strategies that promote positive child social development, and noted the critical need for research that addresses the utility of coaching parents in strategies to support their children's social development and positive peer relations. Multifaceted programs, which combine school-, parent-, and child-focused intervention components, have proven feasible and valuable in interventions targeting children with externalizing behavior disorders. The specific effects of these various components for rejected children with varying behavioral profiles require further research, however. Of critical importance are studies evaluating the impact of different approaches for improving the generalization of child gains acquired during social competence coaching programs; enhancing children's capacity to use prosocial skills in classroom and neighborhood peer interactions; and fostering improvements in positive peer responding, as well as peer reputation and status.

Chapter 14

Future Directions

The past four decades have witnessed tremendous growth in the understanding and treatment of social maladjustment and poor peer relations in children. During this time, developmental research has established the importance of positive peer relations as a context for socialization and emotional development. It has clarified the developmental vulnerability of peer-rejected children, who not only miss out on the benefits of peer acceptance, but also suffer hostility and ostracism. The research base offers substantial hope for these children, indicating the effectiveness of social competence coaching interventions, but it also reveals the limitations of these programs and the challenges for the future.

A major goal of this book has been to examine the implications of developmental research for the assessment and treatment of peer rejection. Several conclusions can be drawn. First, the assessment and treatment of problematic peer relations must recognize the range of child factors (including multiple dimensions of social behavior and associated cognitive–affective processes) and the dynamics of peer group–child interactions that contribute to peer rejection processes. Correspondingly, social competence coaching programs must promote prosocial skills and reduce problematic social behavior, and must do so in a way that supports self-system changes in child emotion regulation, social cognition, and interpersonal comfort and motivation. Second, interventions must account for the role of the peer group, recognizing and treating peer rejection as a dynamic interpersonal process rather than solely as a child characteristic. Third, interventions should address the niches of social opportunity available to a rejected child; this involves attending to social networks and focusing on building friendship skills, as well as improving peer acceptance, in both school and home contexts.

On the one hand, the advances in the technology of social competence interventions warrant celebration. Fueled by developmental research, interventions have become increasingly multifaceted, with corresponding refinements and extensions in the techniques used to promote child social competence. At the same time, there is still much work to be done. Interventions continue to show mixed patterns of effects across studies and limited generalization, creating a need for further research.

Three major areas of challenge for future social competence intervention research exist:

1. Further examination of program characteristics, including attention to the characteristics of the children being treated; the range of social–emotional, cognitive, and behavioral skills they need to attain positive peer relations; and intervention features associated with improvements in various types of outcomes for various types of children.
2. A better understanding of the mechanisms underlying effective treatment processes and the dynamics of change.
3. Further development of the technology for involving peers in interventions and promoting generalized improvements in peer relations.

Each of these three challenge areas is discussed briefly.

PROGRAM CHARACTERISTICS

As La Greca (1993) concluded, developmental research has clarified the complexity of children's social relations, and has identified the heterogeneity that exists within the group of children with poor peer relations. Accordingly, the challenge is to develop interventions of corresponding complexity and breadth. Coaching programs have already expanded beyond a focus on promoting positive interaction skills to incorporate skills associated with behavioral self-control, conflict resolution, and effective social problem solving. In addition, however, accumulating research suggests that producing the organizational capacity to sustain effective peer relations may require an even broader focus in interventions. In particular, this research suggests that emotions, motivation, and control beliefs may require more attention. Furthermore, intervention strategies are needed to help children move from the acquisition of skill components to capable engagement in social processes—that is, the ability to coordinate their cognitions, behaviors, and emotions in sensitive, responsive, and socially effective ways.

Promoting group acceptance and reducing rejection are critically important foci of coaching programs, given the strong evidence linking peer rejection with concurrent and future risk for behavioral and emotional difficulties. At the same time, other dimensions of peer relations warrant closer attention in interventions, including the facilitation of high-quality friendships, the control of victimization, and the promotion of niches of opportunity for positive affiliations in adaptive peer networks, along with reducing deviant peer partnerships. These various social goals may require some expansion in social competence coaching program targets and strategies (Asher, Parker, & Walker, 1996; La Greca, 1993).

Recent years have seen the emergence of valuable multicomponent programs that combine social competence coaching with parent training, school-based interventions, and/or academic tutoring to meet the needs of high-risk children with significant behavioral or emotional difficulties, for whom single-component programs (social competence coaching, parenting, or classroom management) are insufficient (Coie & Koeppl, 1990; La Greca, 1993). As noted in Chapter 13, however, further research is needed to examine the impact of multicomponent programs for children with various problem profiles. In this domain, it is important to base multicomponent interventions on a strong theoretical foundation. Rather than simply combining existing social competence, parenting, and academic support programs, multicomponent programs need to be based upon the developmental model of the targeted children's problems. Children may have problematic peer relations for a variety of reasons; hence the particular multicomponent packages that may be appropriate may differ for children who are rejected for various reasons.

Indeed, careful research is needed to understand the degree to which the behavioral (e.g., aggressive/disruptive behaviors, anxious/avoidant behaviors) and cognitive (e.g., inattention, learning disabilities) characteristics of rejected children moderate the impact of various intervention components and multicomponent packages designed to promote social competence and positive peer relations. In general, greater attention to the characteristics of the target children is needed in coaching research, so that investigators can understand variations in intervention impact and design interventions that are sensitive to such factors as the characteristics of the children, the nature and severity of their peer problems, their developmental level and gender, and the ethnic/cultural context of their social interactions. Careful evaluation of the utility of individualized or tailored interventions is warranted (Collins, Murphy, & Bierman, 2001).

MECHANISMS OF CHANGE

In general, we know relatively little about the mechanisms that account for effective intervention effects. For example, programs vary considerably in structure and content. It is unclear how length, skill content, intervention staff characteristics, group composition, and process dynamics are related to the outcomes of social competence interventions (Furman & Gavin, 1989). We also need to understand the impact of program intensity. For example, what are the comparative advantages of coaching programs that are intense (e.g., summer treatment programs; see MTA Cooperative Group, 1999a) versus programs that are dispersed over time (e.g., the weekly and biweekly Friendship Groups of the Fast Track program; Conduct Problems Prevention Research Group, 1992)? On the one hand, the more intense delivery system allows for sustained efforts and potential growth in a condensed period of time; on the other hand, the program dispersed over time may offer children more time between sessions for the practice and consolidation of skills. The potential benefits and disadvantages of different schedules and structures for social competence coaching remain empirical questions. Research on this topic will have practical utility (providing guidance in the optimal organization for social competence coaching programs), as well as theoretical significance (contributing to our understanding of the process of change in a child's social and relationship capacities).

In addition, process research is needed to clarify the active mechanisms underlying effective coaching programs. Children may benefit from social competence interventions via mechanisms other than the acquisition of specific social skills (Furman & Gavin, 1989; Schneider, 1992). For example, intervention experiences may lead to reductions in social anxiety, increased motivation for social interaction, or the opportunity to form relationships that provide children with a new social niche in the peer group. Some investigators have suggested that in addition to promoting skill acquisition, elements such as the child–coach relationship and peer influence/support may be critical to the success of coaching programs (McFadyen-Ketchum & Dodge, 1998). Certainly these studies suggest that our models for understanding social competence training need to be expanded, in order to better represent the complex influences that affect peer relations and the intervention experiences that are relevant to sustained change.

In addition, aspects of self-system processes, including control beliefs and self-perceptions (perceived control as well as feelings of psychological distress), warrant closer attention in social competence coaching programs—both in terms of program design (as noted above), and also in understanding change processes. We know relatively little about the kinds of intervention experiences that foster the reworking of "internal models" regarding peer relations, and corresponding self-conceptions and feelings of social anxiety and loneliness. Experiential, as well as instructional, aspects of coaching programs may be important influences in this regard. In particular, scaffolded experiences that allow for commentary, inquiry, and support during "online," emotion-charged social interactions may provide critical opportunities for the modification of working models and control beliefs. Specifically, the ways that coaches choose to elicit and respond to interpersonal affect and dynamic interpersonal exchanges during sessions may affect the impact of those interpersonal experiences on children's working models of peer relations and their corresponding affect-charged orientation toward others and toward themselves. Clearly, this is an area that warrants empirical examination.

PEER INVOLVEMENT

Several investigators have suggested that the limited impact of social skills interventions may be due in large part to a lack of attention to the social milieu in which peer relations exist (La Greca, 1993; Weissberg & Greenberg, 1998). Certainly developmental research suggests that peer rejection is a dynamic interpersonal process rather than simply a child characteristic, and that peers influence children's social behavior by the ways in which they initiate and respond to child behavior, the expectations they develop (which bias their initiations and responses), and the opportunities for social interaction they provide (or deny) to children.

Social competence coaching programs have frequently included nontarget peers as partners in coaching sessions (Bierman & Furman, 1984; Ladd, 1981; Oden & Asher, 1977). Conceptually, the inclusion of nonproblematic peers in intervention sessions creates a positive social learning environment for target children, in which their skill acquisition and performance is supported by the contingent positive responses of those peers. Including peers in interventions may change the peers as well as the target children—increasing their sensitivity and positive responsivity to skillful behaviors displayed by the disliked children, and fostering positive changes in their affect toward and liking of those children (Bierman, 1986a).

At the same time, more research is needed to understand the optimal strategies for involving peers in coaching programs and for enhancing positive peer responding. Price and Dodge (1989) have emphasized this point, noting that we know relatively little about how the social-cognitive processes and behavioral responding of peers contribute to rejection processes and are affected (or could be affected) by social competence interventions. This line of research should include inquiry into impression formation processes among peers, and the factors that influence stability and change in those perceptions. In addition, although there is reason to believe that groups composed of children who share aggressive/disruptive behavior problems may be iatrogenic in some cases (Dishion, Poulin, & Burraston, 2001), it is not clear which peers might make optimal peer partners. On the one hand, highly skilled and well-liked children might be good partners, providing outstanding models of socially skillful behavior and possibly providing entree into mainstream peer groups. On the other hand, popular children may have many friends and may thus be less likely than more "average" children to be open to new friendships. The relative impact on coaching success of different partner characteristics has yet to be studied.

The potential benefits of embedding social competence coaching programs for target children within classroom-based programs designed to promote a positive peer context (e.g., social–emotional learning curricula, cooperative learning strategies, bullying programs) also await empirical evaluation. Conceptually, classroom-based programs and associated increased opportunities for positive collaborative activities with peers may enhance interpersonal attraction and niche finding. Moreover, focusing with parents on niche finding in peer groups outside the school context is a strategy worth considering as an addition to social competence coaching.

Finally, the degree of malleability in children's attraction to different peers warrants exploration. Particularly among aggressive–rejected children, attraction to other aggressive children contributes to deviant partnerships that support problematic social behaviors and may buffer these children against a need or desire to change. Developing intervention strategies that prepare the naturalistic peer environment to provide alternative niches of social opportunity for rejected and aggressive youth, and increasing the attraction value of those niches to the target youth, are challenges for future program designs and research.

CONCLUSION

As we look to the future, it is instrumental to consider the "lessons learned" over the past four decades regarding the developmental nature of child peer relations, the determinants of peer rejection, and the intervention strategies associated with effective social competence promotion. This literature base provides a solid foundation for future discovery and innovation, highlighting both the "known" and the "unknown" in this important area of child development and social–emotional adjustment. Let us hope that the coming years will prove equally productive, providing new levels of understanding and increasingly effective interventions.

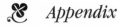 *Appendix*

Description of Exemplar
Session Activities

*T*his appendix provides an explanation of the exemplar session presentation activities and games that are identified in Chapter 11 (see especially Table 11.3).

DOMAIN OF SOCIAL PARTICIPATION

Naming Games

Name and Favorite Food Memory Game

Guevremont (1990) asks children to introduce themselves and name their favorite foods. Children are told to listen carefully and see how many names and favorite foods they can remember. In the game, children in the circle each have a chance to try to recall names and foods for all other group members, and participation is praised.

Friend, Friend, Chase

For younger children, the game Duck, Duck, Goose can be played as a naming game called Friend, Friend, Chase. Children sit in a circle. The person who is "it" walks around the outside of the circle. As "it" passes each other person, he/she taps that person lightly on the head and says the person's name. (The group leaders and other group members can also say the names aloud, in order to help the person who is "it" remember the names.) At some point in the circling, the person who is "it" adds the word "chase" (e.g., "Terry, Jimmy, Susie, chase"). The person who was tagged with "chase" stands up and chases "it" around the circle. When "it" reaches the chaser's seat, "it" sits down in the circle, and the chaser becomes "it."

Who Ate the Cookies?

Who Ate the Cookies? is another naming game for young elementary children. Children sit in a circle and follow the coach in clapping to a rhythm. In time with the rhythm, the coach says, "Who ate the cookies in the cookie jar?" "Jimmy ate the cookies in the cookie jar." Jimmy then answers, "Who, me?" and the entire group chants back, "Yes, you." Then Jimmy says, "Not me," and the entire group chants back, "Then who?" Then Jimmy picks the name of another child in the group, saying, "Susie ate the cookies in the cookie jar." Susie answers, "Who, me?" and the cycle goes on.

Self-Disclosure Activities

Hot-Potato Friendship Discovery

Children pass a potato around the circle to music. When the music stops, the person holding the potato has to say something about him-/herself. The game begins with a brief discussion about the kinds of things players can share with each other to help others get to know them better. Alternatively, questions can be listed on cards in the middle of the circle; the person holding the potato when the music stops draws a card and answers the question to tell about him-/herself. Question cards can include favorite movies, foods, colors, TV shows, number of sisters/brothers, pets, and so forth.

Discovery Posters

Each group is given a poster and told that the members must work together to fill in the blanks. The poster is divided into sections with questions listed at the top of each section, such as "What is the total number of pets that children in your group have?," "What is a musical or rap group that everyone in your group likes?," "What is a food no one in the group likes?," "What is a place everyone in the group would like to visit?," and "List a game everyone in the group likes to play." Group members work together to fill in answers to the questions on their poster.

Friendship Team Activities

Naming the Group

Group members work together to select a group name.

Designing a Group Logo; Painting Hats or T-Shirts

Group members work together to design a group logo, and use it to decorate group hats or T-shirts.

DOMAIN OF EMOTIONAL UNDERSTANDING

Recognizing and Labeling Feelings

Feelings Collage

Group members work together to create a collage showing different feeling expressions, using drawings along with pictures cut from magazines and written labels.

Feeling Paper Plate Masks

Children use markers and paper plates to design masks that illustrate different feeling expressions. For younger children, it is helpful to have some model examples of completed masks. By cutting out eye holes, and pasting the plates onto craft sticks, the children create masks that can be used in sociodramatic play or role plays.

Name That Feeling

Name That Feeling is a game used in the Fast Track program, in which children watch coaches portraying a peer interaction and raise their hands to label the feeling they see being expressed by a coach.

Role-Play Feelings Display

Feelings Charades

One child or team draws a feeling card and then mimes the feeling as the other children (or other team) try to guess which feeling is being presented.

Feelings Treasure Hunt

Children work in pairs to find "clues" hidden around the room, which describe different events that might elicit emotion. They move forward in the hunt by finding a clue, labeling the emotion correctly, displaying the feeling face themselves, and then describing a time they felt that way. After they complete one clue, they are allowed to move on to find their next clue, until they reach the end of the set of clues available.

Sociodramatic Play

Children act out familiar stories (e.g., "The Three Little Pigs," "Billy Goats Gruff," etc.). The coaches provide (or help the children generate) a list of the key events in each story. The children then act out each step, describing and showing the feelings of the story characters as they experience different events in the story.

Feelings Hot Potato

Children pass a potato around the circle to music. When the music stops, the person holding the potato has to choose a card from the middle that lists a feeling, show the feeling face, and see whether the others can guess the feeling. Then the person has to tell about a time when he/she felt that way.

DOMAIN OF PROSOCIAL BEHAVIORS

Cooperative Activities

Cooperative Art Projects

Cooperative activities are set up so that the group (or partners within the group) must share materials and coordinate their efforts to create a joint product). Topics for cooperative art projects can include banners, murals, signs, or collages on themes such as feelings or cooperation, or on shared interests to foster common ground (e.g., favorite sports, holidays). The degree of challenge and level of collaboration can be increased by limiting the materials to share (such as one pair of scissors, one glue stick, and a few attractive stickers) or increasing the size of the working group. Before and during the project, coaches should help the group members discuss their ideas and negotiate their plans.

Cooperative Play (e.g., with Play-Doh)

Cooperative play, such as Play-Doh play, can provide opportunities for practicing prosocial behavior when it is structured to require substantial sharing, turn taking, and negotiation. For example, playing with Play-Doh provides such opportunities when just one rolling pin, one cookie cutter, and one Play-Doh press are available to share.

Negotiation Activities

Sharing Snacks

Children are provided with different ingredients that need to be combined to make a snack. This activity requires group discussion, planning, and sharing.

For example, each child may be given a different ingredient for a trail mix, and then must talk with the others to divide up and share the ingredients so that each team member ends up with an equivalent amount of trail mix.

Cracker Stackers

Cracker Stackers is another version of Sharing Snacks, in which each child is given an ingredient for a snack—peanut butter, jelly, soda crackers, graham crackers, raisins, or sprinkles. Each child needs to ask each other team member whether that person would like some of the ingredients he/she has, and distributes them accordingly.

Partner Activities

Blindfold Partners

Children divide into pairs, and one child is blindfolded. His/her partner must help this child accomplish a task, such as completing a maze or moving through an obstacle course (e.g., going around a desk, over a low chair and under a table, etc.). After the partner has helped the blindfolded child safely through the course, the two switch roles and repeat the process.

Partner Interdependent Tasks

Children must complete a series of challenges that require working together. For example, each child in a pair puts one hand behind each other's back (i.e., the two stand arm in arm), and the children can use only their two outside hands to accomplish tasks such as putting a ring on a string, coiling a string and putting it on a hook, or taping a tail onto a bunny picture.

DOMAIN OF SELF-CONTROL

Role-Play Practice

Obstacle Course

Obstacle Course is a Fast Track program activity designed to engage children in role-playing the three self-control steps of the Red Light (i.e., "Tell yourself to stop," "Take a long, deep breath," and "Say the problem and how you feel"). Dyads or triads tackle an obstacle. At each station, they draw a card that describes a hypothetical problem situation. They describe and show how they would "go to the Red Light" to calm down in that situation. Then they have a chance to tackle the obstacle. Once they have all completed the obstacle challenge successfully, they move on to the next station, where they role-play their self-control response to a hypothetical problem and then tackle the next obstacle. Obstacle challenges are simple physical challenges (e.g., dropping a paper ball from a chair into a bowl, pitching a penny into a plate, blowing a piece of cotton across a table to land in a circle, etc.).

Fortune Noodle Hunt.

Fortune Noodle Hunt is another activity designed to engage children in the role-playing process. A line of newspaper is set down on the floor, with five rigatoni noodles in a row for each child. The rigatoni noodles have "fortunes" inside. The children stand in front of their first noodle and listen to a hypothetical problem read by the coach. They talk about and show how they could use the self-control steps of the Red Light to cope effectively with that problem. Then they each step on their rigatoni noodle and break it open to get their fortune. The process continues until they have role-played five problem situations and collected their five fortunes. The fortunes are typed messages that the coaches have prepared, rolled up, and placed into the rigatoni noodles, with messages such as "You share with others—you are a good friend," "You stick up for your friends and help them—you are a true-blue friend," and "You know how to keep your cool!"

Self-Control Games

Red Light, Green Light

The Red Light, Green Light game provides practice in inhibitory control and following game rules. The person (or pair) playing the role of "traffic controller" stands against a wall. The other children line up some distance away. When the traffic controller turns toward the wall and says "Green Light," children are allowed to move toward him/her. When the traffic controller turns back around to face the children and says "Red Light," the children must freeze. Anyone still moving who is seen by the traffic controller when he/she turns around must go back to the starting place. The first child (or pair) to reach the traffic controller safely takes over that role. This game can also be played with pairs holding hands, or with "three-legged" pairs who are working as a team to start and stop themselves.

Pass the Bell

Children sit in a circle, and the coach brings out a bell. The coach explains that the goal of the game is to see whether the children can pass the bell all the way around the circle without ringing it. Children practice a self-calming activity (going to the Red Light) before they start, and then try to stay calm enough to pass the bell without ringing it. If the bell rings, the game starts over.

DOMAIN OF COMMUNICATION SKILLS

Interview Games

TV Talk Show

Guevremont (1990) uses the TV Talk Show game to give children structured opportunities to practice basic communication skills. In this game, one child serves as a TV "host" whose job is to interview a "guest." The host's task is to make the guest feel welcome, learn something about the guests' interests, and provide the guest with information about his/her own interests. The mock interviews are videotaped, and the children and group review the tapes to identify positive communication behaviors and to brainstorm ways to make the interview show better.

Twenty Questions

One child draws a card that illustrates an item. The other children ask questions to see whether they can guess which item is on the card.

Partner Challenges

Partner Puzzles

The Partner Puzzles task involves referential communication, and requires careful attention to and responding to cues from one's partner. One child tries to solve a puzzle by placing objects into certain squares on a piece of paper. The partner, who knows the correct solution to the puzzle, can help by giving nonverbal cues about the correctness or incorrectness of the placement of various objects.

Partner Picture Challenge

Again, children work in pairs. Each child is given a blank "award" sheet, along with several stickers, ribbon, and glitter pens with which to decorate it. However, rather than decorating his/her own award sheet, each child decorates the partner's under the direction of the partner. Hence each child has to ask his/her partner which colors, stickers, and ribbons he/she (the partner) wants on the award sheet, and where they should go.

Partner Design Challenge

Once more, children work in pairs. Each child is given a set of colored shapes (e.g., a blue square, a red heart, a green triangle, a brown rectangle, a yellow circle, a black diamond). The children sit back to back. First, one child is the "leader." The leader puts together a design with the shapes, telling the partner where he/she is placing each shape. The partner tries to place his/her shapes in the same design. The partner can ask questions to make sure he/she knows where each shape goes, and the leader is encouraged to go slowly and try to make sure the partner is following him/her. Once the children are finished, they turn around and compare their designs to see how well the leader helped the partner make the same design. Then, each child is given a new set of shapes and the game is played again, this time with the roles of leader and partner reversed. Prizes or special celebration snacks can increase child engagement and enjoyment of this and the other partner games.

DOMAIN OF FAIR-PLAY SKILLS

Competitive Games

Carnival Games with Decision Wheel

Carnival games are useful for initial practice with competition, because they are fairly quick and allow children the opportunity to "try again," making it easier to cope with the disappointment of losing. Examples are pinning a tail on a donkey, tossing a pin into a pail, and throwing a paper ball through a hoop. At each carnival game station, children may use the Decision Wheel to practice good ways to decide who goes first, and may benefit from the cue sheets of "Good Things to Say When You Win" and "Good Things to Say When You Lose" to practice good sportsmanship.

Simple Board Games

Simple board games include Tic-Tac-Toe, Pig-in-a-Poke, Concentration, or Memory (with a relatively small set of cards). These games involve more sustained practice in competitive game playing, but are still brief enough to fit within coaching sessions and to provide multiple practice opportunities in winning and losing.

Coordinated Play

Rescue Squads

Rescue squad kits include firefighters, police officers, and other emergency vehicles and figures. They allow children to practice the equitable distribution of different play pieces (e.g., characters and vehicles), and require children to negotiate the terms of their play together (e.g., defining the themes of play and reciprocal roles). Coaches can support children in anticipatory planning, re-

sponding sensitively to each other during the play, and reviewing their performance.

DOMAIN OF SOCIAL PROBLEM-SOLVING SKILLS

Role Plays

Common Conflict Situations

Using problems from a "problem-solving mailbox" that children have generated, or drawing from examples that are common experiences for children in
the group, coaches can prepare short scenarios describing social conflict situations; these are written down on index cards. Coaches work with children to
role-play each problem and to apply the problem-solving steps (i.e., defining
the problem, generating alternatives, discussing potential consequences, and
planning a course of action) in finding a solution to one of the identified conflict situations. Role plays can be videotaped for later review and performance
feedback.

Team Challenges

Line Up

Engaging team challenges provide naturalistic opportunities for social problem
solving and group negotiation/collaboration. In the Line Up game, the coach
makes a line with masking tape on the floor, and gives the team the challenge
of getting the whole group lined up along the line in alphabetical order by the
first letter of each team member's middle name. Children are then encouraged
to work through the traffic light steps, in order to identify their problem, generate alternative problem solutions, and create and follow a problem-solving
plan. Following the completion of this group challenge, the coach encourages
children to reflect on their process ("Did you solve the problem?," "How did
you do it?," "How did you feel when you first started?," "How did you feel
when you got it?"). In a variation of this activity, children can be asked to line
up in order of their shoe size, but with the caveat that they cannot use talking
to communicate with each other.

Crossing the River

The coaches mark off a "river" with masking tape, and give each team a "log"
(made of cardboard or paper). The team's challenge is to get the entire group
across the river, under these conditions: (1) Only two people can ride on the
log at one time; (2) at least one person must ride on the log to move it across

the river; and (3) no person can cross the river more than three times. Again, the team members are led through the problem-solving steps in order to help them plan and execute a solution to this challenge.

Maze

The coaches tape colored pieces of construction paper on the floor to create a multicolored checkerboard. They then create a secret pathway through the maze by drawing a route on a piece of paper that includes a small replica of the checkerboard they have taped onto the floor. Children are told that their task as a group is to find the correct way through the maze. To do so, they each take turns trying out different pathways through the maze. One at a time, they step onto one block in the maze. If their choice is incorrect, a coach "beeps" them out of the maze. If their choice is correct, they continue and move onto a second block in the maze. The members of the group can learn from each other's trial-and-error mistakes to master the maze. This can be an affectively arousing game that challenges children to focus on the group, regulate their behavior, attend to the action, and support each other. Coaches can cue the group members prior to the activity to encourage them to think of ways they can help each other with the challenge, and can lead a postplay review with the group members to discuss positive features of their performance and areas for improvement.

References

Abelson, R. P. (1981). Psychological status of the script concept. *American Psychologist, 36*, 715–729.

Abramson, L. Y., Seligman, M. E. P., & Teasdale, J. D. (1978). Learned helplessness in humans. *Journal of Abnormal Psychology, 87*, 49–74.

Achenbach, T. M., McConaughy, S. H., & Howell, C. T. (1987). Child/adolescent behavioral and emotional problems: Implications of cross-informant correlations for situational specificity. *Psychological Bulletin, 101*, 213–232.

Ainsworth, M. D. S., Blehar, M. C., Waters, E., & Wall, S. (1978). *Patterns of attachment.* Hillsdale, NJ: Erlbaum.

Allen, G. J., Chinsky, J. M., Larcen, S. W., Lochman, J. E., & Selinger, H. V. (1976). *Community psychology and the schools: A behaviorally oriented multilevel preventive approach.* Hillsdale, NJ: Erlbaum.

Allen, K. E., Hart, B., Buell, J. B., Harris, R. W., & Wolf, M. M. (1964). Effects of social reinforcement of isolate behavior of a nursery school child. *Child Development, 34*, 511–518.

Aloia, G. F., Beaver, R. J., & Pettus, W. F. (1978). Increasing initial interactions among integrated EMR students and their nonretarded peers in a game-playing situation. *American Journal of Mental Deficiency, 82*, 573–579.

American Psychiatric Association. (1994). *Diagnostic and statistical manual of mental disorders* (4th ed.). Washington, DC: Author.

Ames, R., Ames, C., & Garrison, W. (1977). Children's causal ascriptions for positive and negative interpersonal outcomes. *Psychological Reports, 41*, 595–602.

Asarnow, J. R. (1983). Children with peer adjustment problems: Sequential and nonsequential analyses of school behaviors. *Journal of Consulting and Clinical Psychology, 51*, 709–717.

Asarnow, J. R., & Callan, J. W. (1985). Boys with peer adjustment problems: Social cognitive processes. *Journal of Consulting and Clinical Psychology, 53*, 80–87.

Asendorpf, J. B. (1993). Beyond temperament: A two-factorial coping model of the development of inhibition during childhood. In K. H. Rubin & J. B. Asendorpf (Eds.), *Social withdrawal, inhibition and shyness in childhood* (pp. 265–289). Hillsdale, NJ: Erlbaum.

Asher, S. R., & Dodge, K. A. (1986). Identifying children who are rejected by their peers. *Developmental Psychology, 22*, 444–449.

Asher, S. R., & Hymel, S. (1981). Children's social competence in peer relations: Socio-metric and behavioral assessment. In J. D. Wine, J. D. Smye, & M. D. Smye (Eds.), *Social competence* (pp. 125–157). New York: Guilford Press.

Asher, S. R., Hymel, S., & Renshaw, P. D. (1984). Loneliness in children. *Child Development, 55,* 1456–1464.

Asher, S. R., Markell, R. A., & Hymel, S. (1981). Identifying children at risk in peer relations: A critique of the rate-of-interaction approach to assessment. *Child Development, 52,* 1239–1245.

Asher, S. R., Oden, S. L., & Gottman, J. M. (1977). Children's friendships in school settings. In S. R. Asher & J. M. Gottman (Eds.), *The development of children's friendships* (pp. 273–296). New York: Cambridge University Press.

Asher, S. R., Parker, J. G., & Walker, D. L. (1996). Distinguishing friendship from accep-tance: Implications for intervention and assessment. In W. M. Bukowski, A. F. New-comb, & W. W. Hartup (Eds.), *The company they keep: Friendship during childhood and adolescence* (pp. 366–405). New York: Cambridge University Press.

Asher, S. R., Parkhurst, J. T., Hymel, S., & Williams, G. A. (1990). Peer rejection and loneli-ness in childhood. In S. R. Asher & J. D. Coie (Eds.), *Peer rejection in childhood* (pp. 253–273). Cambridge, England: Cambridge University Press.

Asher, S. R., & Renshaw, P. (1981). Children without friends: Social knowledge and social skill training. In S. R. Asher & J. M. Gottman (Eds.), *The development of children's friend-ships* (pp. 273–296). New York: Cambridge University Press.

Asher, S. R., Rose, A. J., & Gabriel, S. W. (2001). Peer rejection in everyday life. In M. R. Leary (Ed.), *Interpersonal rejection* (pp. 105–142). New York: Oxford University Press.

Asher, S. R., Singleton, L. C., Tinsley, B. R., & Hymel, S. (1979). A reliable sociometric mea-sure for preschool children. *Developmental Psychology, 15,* 443–444.

Asher, S. R., Zelis, K. M., Parker, J. G., & Bruene, C. M. (1991). *Self-referral for peer relations problems among aggressive and withdrawn low-accepted children.* Paper presented at the bi-ennial meeting of the Society for Research in Child Development, Seattle, WA.

Atlas, R. S., & Pepler, D. J. (1998). Observations of bullying in the classroom. *Journal of Edu-cational Research, 92,* 86–99.

Baer, R. A. (1989). Maintenance of child behavior change: What happens after the experi-menters leave? *Education and Treatment of Children, 12,* 190–199.

Baldwin, M. W. (1992). Relational schemas and the processing of social information. *Psycho-logical Bulletin, 112,* 461–484.

Bandura, A. (1969). *Principles of behavior modification.* New York: Holt, Rinehart & Winston.

Bandura, A. (1977). Self-efficacy: Toward a unified theory of behavioral change. *Psychologi-cal Review, 84,* 191–215.

Barkley, R. A. (1996). Attention-deficit/hyperactivity disorder. In E. J. Mash & R. A. Barkley (Eds.), *Child psychopathology* (pp. 63–112). New York: Guilford Press.

Bandmaster, R. F., & Leary, M. R. (1995). The need to belong: Desire for interpersonal at-tachments as a fundamental human motivation. *Psychological Bulletin, 117,* 497–529.

Beelmann, A., Pfingsten, U., & Losel, F. (1994). Effects of training social competence in children: A meta-analysis of recent evaluation studies. *Journal of Clinical Child Psychol-ogy, 23,* 260–271.

Bell-Dolan, D. J., & Allan, W. D. (1998). Assessing elementary school children's social skills: Evaluation of the parent version of the Matson Evaluation of Social Skills with Young-sters. *Psychological Assessment, 10,* 140–148.

Bell-Dolan, D. J., Foster, S. L., & Christopher, J. S. (1992). Children's reactions to participat-ing in a peer relations study: An example of cost-effective assessment. *Child Study Jour-nal, 22,* 137–155.

Bell-Dolan, D. J., Foster, S. L., & Sikora, D. M. (1989). Effects of sociometric testing on children's behavior and loneliness in school. *Developmental Psychology, 25*, 306–311.

Bell-Dolan, D. J., Foster, S. L., & Tishelman, A. (1989). An alternative to negative nomination sociometric measures. *Journal of Clinical Child Psychology, 18*, 153–157.

Bellack, A. S., & Hersen, M. (1979). *Research and practice in social skills training.* New York: Plenum Press.

Berndt, T. J. (1982). The features and effects of friendship in early adolescence. *Child Development, 53*, 1447–1460.

Bierman, K. L. (1986a). Process of change during social skills training with preadolescents and its relation to treatment outcome. *Child Development, 57*, 230–240.

Bierman, K. L. (1986b). The relationship between social aggression and peer rejection in middle childhood. In R. Prinz (Ed.), *Advances in behavioral assessment of children and families* (Vol. 2, pp. 151–178). Greenwich, CT: JAI Press.

Bierman, K. L. (1987). The clinical significance and assessment of poor peer relations: Peer neglect vs. peer rejection. *Journal of Developmental and Behavioral Pediatrics, 8*, 233–240.

Bierman, K. L. (1988). Children's conceptions of social relationships. In S. Shirk (Ed.), *Cognitive development and child psychotherapy* (pp. 247–272). New York: Plenum Press.

Bierman, K. L., & Furman, W. (1984). The effects of social skills training and peer involvement on the social adjustment of preadolescents. *Child Development, 55*, 151–162.

Bierman, K. L., Greenberg, M. T., & Conduct Problems Prevention Research Group (CPPRG). (1996). Social skill training in the Fast Track program. In R. D. Peters & R. J. McMahon (Eds.), *Preventing childhood disorders, substance abuse, and delinquency* (pp. 65–89). Thousand Oaks, CA: Sage.

Bierman, K. L., & McCauley, E. (1987). Children's descriptions of their peer interactions: Useful information for clinical child assessment. *Journal of Clinical Child Psychology, 16*, 9–18.

Bierman, K. L., Miller, C. M., & Stabb, S. (1987). Improving the social behavior and peer acceptance of rejected boys: Effects of social skill training with instructions and prohibitions. *Journal of Consulting and Clinical Psychology, 55*, 194–200.

Bierman, K. L., & Montminy, H. P. (1993). Developmental issues in social skills assessment and intervention with children and adolescents. *Behavior Modification, 17*, 229–254.

Bierman, K. L., & Smoot, D. L. (1991). Linking family characteristics with poor peer relations: The mediating role of conduct problems. *Journal of Abnormal Child Psychology, 19*, 341–356.

Bierman, K. L., Smoot, D. L., & Aumiller, K. (1993). Characteristics of aggressive–rejected, aggressive (nonrejected), and rejected (nonaggressive) boys. *Child Development, 64*, 139–151.

Bierman, K. L., & Wargo, J. (1995). Predicting the longitudinal course associated with aggressive–rejected, aggressive (non-rejected) and rejected (non-aggressive) status. *Development and Psychopathology, 7*, 669–682.

Bierman, K. L., & Welsh, J. A. (1997). Social relationship deficits. In E. J. Mash & L. G. Terdal (Eds.), *Assessment of childhood disorders* (3rd ed., pp. 328–365). New York: Guilford Press.

Bierman, K. L., & Welsh, J. A. (2000). Assessing social dysfunction: The contributions of laboratory and performance-based measures. *Journal of Clinical Child Psychology, 29*, 526–539.

Bijou, S. W., Peterson, R. F., & Ault, M. H. (1968). A method to integrate descriptive and experimental field studies at the level of data and empirical concepts. *Journal of Applied Behavior Analyses, 1*, 175–191.

Boivin, M., & Begin, G. (1989). Peer status and self-perceptions among early elementary school children: The case of the rejected child. *Child Development, 60,* 591–596.

Boivin, M., Dodge, K. A., & Coie, J. D. (1995). Individual–group behavioral similarity and peer status in experimental playgroups of boys: The social misfit revisited. *Journal of Personality and Social Psychology, 69,* 269–279.

Boivin, M., Hymel, S., & Bukowski, W. M. (1995). The roles of social withdrawal, peer rejection, and victimization by peers in predicting loneliness and depressed mood in childhood. *Development and Psychopathology, 7,* 765–785.

Boivin, M., Poulin, J., & Vitaro, F. (1994). Depressed mood and peer rejection in childhood. *Development and Psychopathology, 6,* 483–498.

Bornstein, M. R., Bellack, A. S., & Hersen, M. (1977). Social-skills training for unassertive children: A multiple-baseline analysis. *Journal of Applied Behavior Analysis, 10,* 183–195.

Bowlby, J. (1969). *Attachment and loss: Vol. 1. Attachment.* New York: Basic Books.

Brendgen, M., Vitaro, F., Bukowski, W. M., Doyle, A. B., & Markiewicz, D. (2001). Developmental profiles of peer social preference over the course of elementary school: Associations with trajectories of externalizing and internalizing behavior. *Developmental Psychology, 37,* 308–319.

Bretherton, I. (1995). Attachment theory and developmental psychopathology. In D. Cicchetti & S. L. Toth (Eds.), *Rochester Symposium on Developmental Psychopathology: Vol. 6. Emotion, cognition, and representation.* Rochester, NY: University of Rochester Press.

Bridgeman, D. L. (1981). Enhanced role taking through cooperative interdependence: A field study. *Child Development, 52,* 1231–1238.

Bronfenbrenner, U. (1970). *Two worlds of childhood: U.S. and U.S.S.R.* New York: Russell Sage Foundation.

Brown, B. B. (1990). Peer groups and peer cultures. In S. S. Feldman & G. R. Elliot (Eds.), *At the threshold: The developing adolescent* (pp. 171–196). Cambridge, MA: Harvard University Press.

Brown, P., & Elliott, R. (1965). Control of aggression in a nursery school class. *Journal of Experimental Child Psychology, 2,* 103–107.

Bryan, J. H. (1975). Children's cooperation and helping behavior. In E. M. Hetherington (Ed.), *Review of child development research* (Vol. 5, pp. 127–181). Chicago: University of Chicago Press.

Bukowski, W. M., & Hoza, B. (1989). Popularity and friendship: Issues in theory, measurement, and outcome. In T. J. Berndt & G. W. Ladd (Eds.), *Peer relationships in child development* (pp. 15–45). Oxford, UK: Wiley.

Bukowski, W., Hoza, B., & Boivin, M. (1994). Measuring friendship quality during pre- and early adolescence: The development and psychometric properties of the Friendship Qualities Scale. *Journal of Social and Personal Relationships, 11,* 471–484.

Burks, V. S., Dodge, K. A., & Price, J. M. (1995). Models of internalizing outcomes of early rejection. *Development and Psychopathology, 7,* 683–695.

Cairns, R. B. (1991). Developmental epistemology and self-knowledge: Towards a reinterpretation of self esteem. In G. Greenberg & E. Tobach (Eds.), *Theories of the evolution of knowing* (pp. 69–86). Hillsdale, NJ: Erlbaum.

Cairns, R. B., & Cairns, B. D. (1991). Social cognition and social networks: A developmental perspective. In D. J. Pepler & K. H. Rubin (Eds.), *The development and treatment of childhood aggression* (pp. 249–276). Hillsdale, NJ: Erlbaum.

Cairns, R. B., Cairns, B. D., Neckerman, H., Ferguson, L., & Gariepy, J. L. (1989). Growth and aggression: 1. Childhood to early adolescence. *Developmental Psychology, 25,* 320–330.

Cairns, R. B., Cairns, B. D., Neckerman, H. J., Gest, S. D., & Gariepy, J. L. (1988). Social networks and aggressive behavior: Peer support or peer rejection? *Developmental Psychology, 24*, 815–823.

Cairns, R. B., Neckerman, H. J., & Cairns, B. D. (1989). Social networks and the shadows of synchrony. In G. R. Adams, T. P. Gulotta, & R. Montemayor (Eds.), *Advances in adolescent development* (Vol. 1, pp. 275–305). Beverly Hills, CA: Sage.

Cairns, R. B., Perrin, J. E., & Cairns, B. D. (1985). Social structure and social cognition in early adolescence: Affiliative patterns. *Journal of Early Adolescence, 5*, 339–355.

Calkins, S. D. (1994). Origins and outcomes of individual differences in emotion regulation. In N. A. Fox (Ed.), The development of emotion regulation: Biological and behavioral considerations. *Monographs of the Society for Research in Child Development, 59*(2–3, Serial No. 240), 53–72.

Cartledge, G., & Milburn, J. F. (1986). *Teaching social skills to children: Innovative approaches.* New York: Pergamon Press.

Caspi, A., Elder, G. H., & Bem, D. J. (1988). Moving away from the world: Life-course patterns of shy children. *Developmental Psychology, 24*, 824–831.

Cassidy, J., & Asher, S. R. (1992). Loneliness and peer relations in young children. *Child Development, 63*, 350–365.

Chen, X., Rubin, K. H., & Sun, Y. (1992). Social reputation and peer relationships in Chinese and Canadian children: A cross-cultural study. *Child Development, 63*, 1336–1343.

Chennault, M. (1967). Improving the social acceptance of unpopular educable mentally retarded pupils in special classes. *American Journal of Mental Deficiency, 72*, 455–458.

Chittenden, G. F. (1942). An experimental study in measuring and modifying assertive behavior in young children. *Monographs of the Society for Research in Child Development, 7*(1, Serial No. 31).

Cillessen, A. H. N., van IJzendoorn, H. W., van Lieshout, C. F. M., & Hartup, W. W. (1992). Heterogeneity of peer rejected boys. *Child Development, 63*, 893–905.

Clark, L., Gresham, F. M., & Elliott, S. N. (1985). Development and validation of a social skills assessment measure: The TROSS-C. *Journal of Psychoeducational Assessment, 3*, 347–356.

Coie, J. D. (1990). Toward a theory of peer rejection. In S. R. Asher & J. D. Coie (Eds.), *Peer rejection in childhood* (pp. 365–401). Cambridge, England: Cambridge University Press.

Coie, J. D., & Dodge, K. A. (1983). Continuities and changes in children's social status: A five-year longitudinal study. *Merrill–Palmer Quarterly, 29*, 261–282.

Coie, J. D., & Dodge, K. A. (1988). Multiple sources of data on social behavior and social status in the school: A cross-age comparison. *Child Development, 59*, 815–829.

Coie, J. D., & Dodge, K. A. (1998). Aggression and antisocial behavior. In W. Damon (Series Ed.) & N. Eisenberg (Vol. Ed.), *Handbook of child psychology: Vol. 3. Social, emotional, and personality development* (5th ed., pp. 779–862). New York: Wiley.

Coie, J. D., Dodge, K. A., & Coppotelli, H. (1982). Dimensions and types of status: A cross-age perspective. *Developmental Psychology, 18*, 557–570.

Coie, J. D., Dodge, K. A., & Kupersmidt, J. G. (1990). Peer group behavior and social status. In S. R. Asher & J. D. Coie (Eds.), *Peer rejection in childhood* (pp. 17–59). Cambridge, England: Cambridge University Press.

Coie, J. D., Dodge, K. A., Terry, R., & Wright, V. (1991). The role of aggression in peer relations: An analysis of aggression episodes in boys' play groups. *Child Development, 62*, 812–826.

Coie, J. D., & Koeppl, G. K. (1990). Adapting intervention to the problems of aggressive and disruptive rejected children. In S. R. Asher & J. D. Coie (Eds.), *Peer rejection in childhood* (pp. 309–337). Cambridge, England: Cambridge University Press.

Coie, J. D., & Krehbiel, G. (1984). Effects of academic tutoring on the social status of low-achieving, socially rejected children. *Child Development, 55*, 1465–1478.

Coie, J. D., & Kupersmidt, J. B. (1983). A behavior analysis of emerging social status in boys' groups. *Child Development, 54*, 1400–1416.

Cole, P. M., Michel, M. K., & Teti, L. O. (1994). The development of emotion regulation and dysregulation: A clinical perspective. In N. A. Fox (Ed.), The development of emotion regulation: Biological and behavioral considerations. *Monographs of the Society for Research in Child Development, 59*(2–3, Serial No. 240), 53–72.

Collins, L. M., Murphy, S. A., & Bierman, K. L. (2001). *Design and evaluation of adaptive preventive interventions* (Technical Report No. 01–49). University Park: Pennsylvania State University.

Combs, M. L., & Slaby, D. A. (1977). Social skill training with children. In B. B. Lahey & A. E. Kazdin (Eds.), *Advances in clinical child psychology* (Vol. 1, pp. 161–201). New York: Plenum Press.

Conduct Problems Prevention Research Group (CPPRG). (1992). A developmental and clinical model for the prevention of conduct disorder: The Fast Track program. *Development and Psychopathology, 4*, 509–528.

Conduct Problems Prevention Research Group (CPPRG). (1998). *Social Health Profile and TOCA-R: Technical Report*. [Online]. Available: http://www.fasttrackproject.org

Conduct Problems Prevention Research Group (CPPRG). (1999a). Initial impact of the Fast Track prevention trial for conduct problems: I. Child and parent effects. *Journal of Consulting and Clinical Psychology, 67*, 631–647.

Conduct Problems Prevention Research Group (CPPRG). (1999b). Initial impact of the Fast Track prevention trial for conduct problems: II. Classroom effects. *Journal of Consulting and Clinical Psychology, 67*, 648–657.

Conduct Problems Prevention Research Group (CPPRG). (2002). Evaluation of the first three years of the Fast Track prevention trial with children at high risk for adolescent conduct problems. *Journal of Abnormal Child Psychology, 30*, 19–35.

Connell, J. P., & Wellborn, J. G. (1991). Competence, autonomy and relatedness: A motivational analysis of self-system processes. In M. R. Gunnar & L. A. Sroufe (Eds.), *Minnesota Symposia on Child Psychology: Vol. 23. Self processes and development* (pp. 43–77). Hillsdale, NJ: Erlbaum.

Connelly, J., & Doyle, A. (1981). Assessment of social competence in preschoolers: Teachers versus peers. *Developmental Psychology, 17*, 454–462.

Connelly, J., Geller, S., Marton, P., & Kutcher, S. (1992). Peer responses to social interaction with depressed adolescents. *Journal of Clinical Child Psychology, 21*, 365–370.

Cooley, C. H. (1902). *Human nature and the social order*. New York: Schocken.

Cooke, T. P., & Apolloni, T. (1976). Developing positive social–emotional behaviors: A study of training and generalization effects. *Journal of Applied Behavior Analysis, 19*, 65–78.

Crick, N. R. (1996). The role of relational aggression, overt aggression, and prosocial behavior in the prediction of children's future social adjustment. *Child Development, 67*, 2317–2327.

Crick, N. R., & Bigbee, M. A. (1998). Relational and overt forms of peer victimization: A multiinformant approach. *Journal of Consulting and Clinical Psychology, 66*, 337–347.

Crick, N. R., Casas, J. F., & Mosher, M. (1997). Relational and overt aggression in preschool. *Developmental Psychology, 33*, 597–588.

Crick, N. R., & Dodge, K. A. (1994). A review and reformulation of social information-processing mechanisms in children's social adjustment. *Psychological Bulletin, 115*, 74–101.

Crick, N. R., & Grotpeter, J. K. (1995). Relational aggression, gender, and social-psychological aggression. *Child Development, 66*, 710–722.

Crick, N. R., & Ladd, G. W. (1990). Children's perceptions of the outcomes of social strategies: Do the ends justify being mean? *Developmental Psychology, 26*, 612–620.

Crick, N. R., Werner, N. E., Casas, J. F., O'Brien, K. M., Nelson, D. A., Grotpeter, J. K., &
Markon, K. (1999). Childhood aggression and gender: A new look at an old problem.
In D. Bernstein (Ed.), *Nebraska Symposium on Motivation* (Vol. 45, pp. 75–141). Lin-
coln: University of Nebraska Press.

de Castro, B. O., Veerman, J. W., Koops, W., Bosch, J. D., & Monshouwer, H. J. (2002). Hostile attribution of intent and aggressive behavior: A meta-analysis. *Child Development,
73*, 916–934.

Deci, E. L., & Ryan, R. M. (1985). *Intrinsic motivation and self-determination in human behavior.*
New York: Plenum Press.

Denham, S. A. (1998). *Emotional development in young children.* New York: Guilford Press.

DeRosier, M. E., Cillessen, A. H. N., Coie, J. D., & Dodge, K. A. (1994). Group social context
and children's aggressive behavior. *Child Development, 65*, 1068–1079.

DeVries, D. L., & Edwards, K. J. (1973). Learning games and student teams: Their effects on
classroom process. *American Educational Research Journal, 10*, 307–318.

DeVries, D. L., & Slavin, R. E. (1978). Teams–Games–Tournament (TGT): Review of ten
classroom experiments. *Journal of Research and Development in Education, 12*, 28–38.

Dishion, T. J., Andrews, D. W., & Crosby, L. (1995). Antisocial boys and their friends in
early adolescence: Relationship characteristics, quality and interactional process.
Child Development, 66, 139–151.

Dishion, T. J., Duncan, T. E., Eddy, J. M., Fagot, B. I., & Fetrow, R. (1994). The world of parents and peers: Coercive exchanges and children's social adaptation. *Social Development, 3*, 255–268.

Dishion, T. J., Poulin, F., & Burraston, B. (2001). Peer group dynamics associated with iatro-
genic effects in group interventions with high-risk young adolescents. In D. W. Nangle
& C. Erdley (Eds.), *The role of friendship in psychological adjustment.* (New Directions for
Child and Adolescent Development, Vol. 91, pp. 79–91). San Francisco: Jossey-Bass.

Dishion, T. J., Spracklen, K. M., Andrews, D. W., & Patterson, G. W. (1996). Deviancy training in male adolescent friendships. *Behavior Therapy, 27*, 373–390.

Dodge, K. A. (1980). Social cognition and children's aggressive behavior. *Child Development,
51*, 162–170.

Dodge, K. A. (1983). Behavioral antecedents of peer status. *Child Development, 51*, 162–170.

Dodge, K. A. (1986). A social information processing model of social competence in children. In M. Perlmutter (Ed.), *Cognitive perspectives on children's social and behavioral development.* Hillsdale, NJ: Erlbaum.

Dodge, K. A. (1989). Problems in social relationships. In E. J. Mash & R. A. Barkley (Eds.),
Treatment of childhood disorders (pp. 222–244). New York: Guilford Press.

Dodge, K. A., Asher, S. R., & Parkhurst, J. T. (1989). Social life as a goal coordination task. In
C. Ames & R. Ames (Eds.), *Research on motivation in education* (Vol. 3, pp. 107–135).
San Diego, CA: Academic Press.

Dodge, K. A., Bates, J. E., & Pettit, G. S. (1990). Mechanisms in the cycle of violence. *Science,
250*, 1678–1683.

Dodge, K. A., & Coie, J. D. (1987). Social information-processing factors in reactive and
proactive aggression in children's playgroups. *Journal of Personality and Social Psychology, 53*, 1146–1158.

Dodge, K. A., Coie, J. D., Pettit, G. S., & Price, J. M. (1990). Peer status and aggression in
boys' groups: Developmental and contextual analyses. *Child Development, 61*, 1289–
1309.

Dodge, K. A., McClaskey, C. L., & Feldman, E. (1985). A situational approach to assessment
of social competence in children. *Journal of Consulting and Clinical Psychology, 53*, 344–
353.

Dodge, K. A., & Murphy, R. R. (1984). The assessment of social competence in adolescents. *Advances in Child Behavior Analysis and Therapy, 3*, 61–96.

Dodge, K. A., Murphy, R. R., & Buchsbaum, K. (1984). The assessment of intention-cue detection skills in children: Implications for developmental psychopathology. *Child Development, 55*, 163–173.

Dodge, K. A., & Newman, J. P. (1981). Biased decision making processes in aggressive boys. *Journal of Abnormal Psychology, 90*, 375–379.

Dodge, K. A., Pettit, G. S., McClaskey, C. G., & Brown, M. M. (1986). Social competence in children. *Monographs of the Society for Research in Child Development, 51*(2, Serial No. 213).

Dodge, K. A., Schlundt, D., Schocken, I., & Delugach, J. (1983). Social competence and children's sociometric status: The role of peer group entry strategies. *Merrill–Palmer Quarterly, 29*, 309–336.

Dumas, J. E., Lynch, A. M., Laughlin, J. E., Smith, E. P., & Prinz, R. J. (2001). Promoting intervention fidelity: Conceptual issues, methods, and preliminary results from the EARLY ALLIANCE prevention trial. *American Journal of Preventive Medicine, 20*, 38–47.

Dumas, J. E., Prinz, R. J., Smith, E. P., & Laughlin, J. (1999). The EARLY ALLIANCE Prevention Trial: An integrated set of interventions to promote competence and reduce risk for conduct disorder, substance abuse, and school failure. *Clinical Child and Family Psychology Review, 2*, 37–53.

Dweck, C. S., & Elliott, E. S. (1983). Achievement motivation. In P. H. Mussen (Series Ed.) & E. M. Hetherington (Vol. Ed.), *Handbook of child psychology: Vol. 4. Socialization, personality, and social development* (4th ed., pp. 643–691). New York: Wiley.

Eder, D. (1985). The cycle of popularity: Interpersonal relations among female adolescents. *Sociology of Education, 58*, 154–165.

Eder, D., & Hallinan, M. T. (1978). Sex differences in children's friendships. *American Sociological Review, 43*, 237–250.

Egan, S. K., & Perry, D. G. (1998). Does low self-regard invite victimization? *Developmental Psychology, 34*, 299–309.

Eisenberg, N., & Fabes, R. A. (1992). Emotion, regulation, and the development of social competence. In M. S. Clark (Ed.), *Review of personality and social psychology: Vol. 14. Emotion and social behavior* (pp. 119–150). Newbury Park, CA: Sage.

Eisler, R. M., Hersen, M., Miller, P. M., & Blanchard, E. B. (1975). Situational determinants of assertive behaviors. *Journal of Consulting and Clinical Psychology, 43*, 330–340.

Elias, M. J., Zins, J. E., Weissberg, R. P., Frey, K. S., Greenberg, M. T., Haynes, N. M., Kessler, R., Schwab-Stone, M. E., & Shriver, T. P. (1997). *Promoting social and emotional learning: Guidelines for educators*. Danvers, MA: Association for Supervision and Curriculum Development.

Elliott, S. N., & Gresham, F. M. (1993). Social skills interventions for children. *Behavior Modification, 17*, 287–313.

Englund, M. M., Levy A. K., Hyson, D. M., & Sroufe, L. A. (2000). Adolescent social competence: Effectiveness in a Group Setting. *Child Development, 71*, 1049–1060.

Epstein, S. (1991). Cognitive–experiential self theory: Implications for developmental psychology. In M. R. Gunnar & L. A. Sroufe (Eds.), *Minnesota Symposia on Child Psychology: Vol. 23. Self-processes and development* (pp. 79–123). Hillsdale, NJ: Erlbaum.

Eron, L. D., & Huesmann, L. R. (1986). The role of television in the development of prosocial and antisocial behavior. In D. Olweus, J. Block, & M. Radke-Yarrow (Eds.), *Development of antisocial and prosocial behavior: Research, theories, and issues* (pp. 285–314). New York: Academic Press.

Evers, W. L., & Schwarz, J. C. (1973). Modifying social withdrawal in preschoolers: The effects of filmed modeling and teacher praise. *Journal of Abnormal Child Psychology, 1,* 248–256.

Evers-Pasquale, W., & Sherman, M. (1975). The reward value of peers: A variable influencing the efficacy of filmed modeling in modifying social isolation in preschoolers. *Journal of Abnormal Child Psychology, 3,* 179–189.

Farmer, T. W., Pearl, R., & Van Acker, R. M. (1996). Expanding the social skills deficit framework: A developmental synthesis perspective, classroom social networks, and implications for the social growth of students with disabilities. *Journal of Special Education, 30,* 232–256.

Fiske, S. T., & Taylor, S. E. (1984). *Social cognition.* New York: Random House.

Flanagan, K. S., Bierman, K. L., Kam, C., & the Conduct Problems Prevention Research Group (CPPRG). (in press). Identifying at-risk children at school entry: The usefulness of multibehavioral problem profiles. *Journal of Clinical Child and Adolescent Psychology.*

Fonzi, A., Schneider, B. H., Tani, F., & Tomada, G. (1997). Predicting children's friendship status from their dyadic interaction in structured situations of potential conflict. *Child Development, 68,* 496–506.

Foster, S. L., Bell-Dolan, D., & Berler, E. S. (1986). Methodological issues in the use of sociometrics for selecting children for social skills research training. *Advances in Behavioral Assessment of Children and Families, 2,* 227–248.

Foster, S. L., Inderbitzen, H., & Nangle, D. W. (1993). Assessing acceptance and social skills with peers in childhood: Current issues. *Behavior Modification, 17,* 255–286.

Foster, S. L., & Ritchey, W. (1985). Behavioral correlates of sociometric status of fourth, fifth and sixth grade children in two classroom situations. *Behavioral Assessment, 7,* 79–93.

French, D. C. (1988). Heterogeneity of peer rejected boys: Aggressive and nonaggressive subtypes. *Child Development, 59,* 976–985.

French, D. C., & Waas, G. A. (1985). Behavior problems of peer-neglected and peer-rejected elementary-age children: Parent and teacher perspectives. *Child Development, 56,* 246–252.

Furman, W. (1996). The measurement of friendship perceptions: Conceptual and methodological issues. In W. M. Bukowski, A. F. Newcomb, & W. W. Hartup (Eds.), *The company they keep: Friendship in childhood and adolescence* (pp. 41–65). New York: Cambridge University Press.

Furman, W., & Buhrmester, D. (1992). Age and sex differences in perceptions of networks of personal relationships. *Child Development, 63,* 103–115.

Furman, W., & Gavin, L. A. (1989). Peers' influence on adjustment and development. In T. J. Berndt & G. W. Ladd (Eds.), *Peer relationships in child development* (pp. 319–340). New York: Wiley.

Furman, W., Rahe, D. F., & Hartup, W. W. (1979). Rehabilitation of socially withdrawn children through mixed-aged and same-aged socialization. *Child Development, 50,* 915–922.

Furman, W., & Robbins, P. (1985). What's the point?: Selection of treatment objectives. In B. Schneider, K. H. Rubin, & J. E. Ledingham (Eds.), *Children's peer relations: Issues in assessment and intervention* (pp. 41–54). New York: Springer-Verlag.

Glow, R. A., & Glow, P. H. (1980). Peer and self-rating: Children's perception of behavior relevant to hyperkinetic impulse disorder. *Journal of Abnormal Child Psychology, 8,* 397–404.

Goetz, T., & Dweck, C. (1980). Learned helplessness in social situations. *Journal of Personality and Social Psychology, 39,* 246–255.

Goldstein, A. P., Sprafkin, R. P., Gershaw, N. J., & Klein, P. (1986). The adolescent: Social skills training through structured learning. In G. Cartledge & J. F. Milburn (Eds.), *Teaching social skills to children: Innovative approaches* (2nd ed., pp. 303–336). New York: Pergamon Press.

Gottman, J. M. (1983). How children become friends. *Monographs of the Society for Research in Child Development, 48*(2, Serial No. 201).

Gottman, J. M., Gonso, J., & Rasmussen, B. (1975). Social interaction, social competence, and friendship in children. *Child Development, 46,* 709–718.

Gottman, J. M., Gonso, J., & Schuler, P. (1976). Teaching social skills to isolated children. *Journal of Abnormal Child Psychology, 4,* 179–197.

Gouze, K. R. (1987). Attention and social problem solving as correlates of aggression in preschool males. *Journal of Abnormal Child Psychology, 15,* 181–197.

Graham, S., & Juvonen, J. (1998). Self-blame and peer victimization in middle school: An attributional analysis. *Developmental Psychology, 34,* 587–599.

Graham, P., & Rutter, M. (1968). The reliability and validity of the psychiatric assessment of the child: II. Interview with the parent. *British Journal of Psychiatry, 114,* 581–592.

Greenberg, M. T., & Kusche, C. A. (1993). *Promoting social and emotional development in deaf children: The PATHS project.* Seattle: University of Washington Press.

Greenberg, M. T., Kusche, C. A., Cook, E. T., & Quamma, J. P. (1995). Promoting emotional competence in school-aged deaf children: The effects of the PATHS curriculum. *Development and Psychopathology, 7,* 117–136.

Greenberg, M. T., Kusche, C. A., & Speltz, M. (1991). Emotional regulation, self control, and psychopathology: The role of relationships in early childhood. In D. Cicchetti & S. L. Toth (Eds.), *Rochester Symposium on Developmental Psychopathology: Vol. 2. Internalizing and externalizing expressions of dysfunction* (pp. 21–66). Hillsdale, NJ: Erlbaum.

Greenberg, M. T., & Speltz, M. L. (1988). Attachment and the ontogeny of conduct problems. In J. Belsky & T. Nezworski (Eds.), *Clinical implications of attachment* (pp. 177–218.) Hillsdale, NJ: Erlbaum.

Greenberg, M. T., Speltz, M. L., & DeKlyen, M. (1993). Toward a conceptual model for understanding the early development of disruptive behavior problems. *Development and Psychopathology, 5,* 191–213.

Gresham, F. M. (1985). Utility of cognitive-behavioral procedures for social skills training with children: A critical review. *Journal of Abnormal Child Psychology, 13,* 411–423.

Gresham, F. M. (1981). Social skills training with handicapped children: A review. *Review of Educational Research, 51,* 139–176.

Gresham, F. M. (1994). Generalization of social skills: Risks of choosing form over function. *School Psychology Quarterly, 9,* 142–144.

Gresham, F. M., & Elliott, S. N. (1984). Assessment and classification of children's social skills: A review of methods and issues. *School Psychology Review, 13,* 292–301.

Gresham, F. M., & Nagle, R. J. (1980). Social skills training with children: Responsiveness to modeling and coaching as a function of peer orientation. *Journal of Consulting and Clinical Psychology, 48,* 718–729.

Guevremont, D. (1990). Social skills and peer relationship training. In R. A. Barkley, *Attention-deficit hyperactivity disorder: A handbook for diagnosis and treatment* (pp. 540–572). New York: Guilford Press.

Guralnick, M. J., Connor, R., Hammond, M., Gottman, J. M., & Kinnish, K. (1996). The peer relations of preschool children with communication disorders. *Child Development, 67,* 471–489.

Guralnick, M. J., Gottman, J. M., & Hammond, M. A. (1996). Effects of social setting on the friendship formation of young children differing in developmental status. *Journal of Applied Developmental Psychology, 17,* 625–651.

Guralnick, M. J., & Weinhouse, E. (1983). Child–child social interactions: An analysis of assessment instruments for young children. *Exceptional Children, 50,* 268–271.

Hansen, D. J., St. Lawrence, J. S., & Christoff, K. A. (1988). Conversational skills of inpatient conduct-disordered youths: Social validation of component behaviors and implications for skills training. *Behavior Modification, 12*, 424–444.

Hart, B. M., Reynolds, N. J., Baer, D. M., Brawley, E. R., & Harris, F. R. (1968). Effects of contingent and noncontingent social reinforcement on the cooperative play of a preschool child. *Journal of Applied Behavior Analysis, 1*, 73–76.

Harter, S. (1982). The Perceived Competence Scale for Children. *Child Development, 53*, 87–97.

Harter, S. (1998). The development of self-representations. In W. Damon (Series Ed.) & N. Eisenberg (Vol. Ed.), *Handbook of child psychology: Vol. 3. Social, emotional, and personality development* (5th ed., pp. 553–618). New York: Wiley.

Hartup, W. W. (1979). The social worlds of childhood. *American Psychologist, 34*, 944–950.

Hartup, W. W. (1983). The peer system. In P. H. Mussen (Series Ed.) & E. M. Hetherington (Vol. Ed.), *Handbook of child psychology: Vol. 4. Socialization, personality, and social development* (4th ed., pp. 102–196). New York: Wiley.

Hartup, W. W. (1989). Social relationships and their developmental significance. *American Psychologist, 44*(2), 120–126.

Hartup, W. W., French, D. C., Laursen, B., Johnston, M. K., & Ogawa, J. R. (1993). Conflict and friendship relations in middle childhood: Behavior in a closed-field situation. *Child Development, 64*, 445–454.

Hawkins, L., Pepler, D., & Craig, W. (2001). Naturalistic observations of peer interventions in bullying. *Social Development, 10*, 512–527.

Hayvren, M., & Hymel, S. (1984). Ethical issues in sociometric testing: The impact of sociometric measures on interaction behavior. *Developmental Psychology, 20*, 844–849.

Hertz-Lazarowitz, R., Sharan, S., & Steinberg, R. (1980). Classroom learning style and cooperative behavior of elementary school children. *Journal of Educational Psychology, 72*, 99–106.

Hightower, A. D., Work, W. C., Cowen, E. L., Lotyczewski, B. S., Spinell, A. P., Guare, J. C., & Rohrbeck, C. A. (1986). The Teacher–Child Rating Scale: A brief objective measure of elementary school children's school problem behaviors and competencies. *School Psychology Review, 15*, 393–409.

Hinshaw, S. P., & Anderson, C. A. (1996). Conduct and oppositional defiant disorders. In E. J. Mash & R. A. Barkley (Eds.), *Child psychopathology* (pp. 113–149). New York: Guilford Press.

Hinshaw, S. P., Henker, B., & Whalen, C. (1984). Self-control in hyperactive boys in anger-inducing situations: Effects of cognitive-behavioral training and of methylphenidate. *Journal of Abnormal Child Psychology, 12*, 55–77.

Hodges, E. V. E., Malone, M. J., & Perry, D. G. (1995, March). *Behavioral and social antecedents and consequences of victimization by peers*. Paper presented at the biennial meeting of the Society for Research in Child Development, Indianapolis, IN.

Hodges, E. V. E., & Perry, D. G. (1996). Victims of peer abuse: An overview. *Journal of Emotional and Behavioral Problems, 5*, 23–28.

Hoffman, M. L. (1967). Parent discipline and the child's moral development. *Journal of Personality and Social Psychology, 5*, 45–57.

Hops, H., Alpert, A., & Davis, B. (1997). The development of same- and opposite-sex social relations among adolescents: An analogue study. *Social Development, 6*, 165–183.

Hops, H., & Stevens, T. (1987). *Peer Interaction Recording System V (PIRS V)*. Eugene: Oregon Research Institute.

Hops, H., & Walker, H. M. (1988). *Contingencies for Learning Academic and Social Skills (CLASS)*. Delray, FL: Educational Achievement Systems.

Hoza, B., Molina, B. S. G., Bukowski, W. M., & Sippola, L. R. (1995). Peer variables as predictors of later childhood adjustment. *Development and Psychopathology, 7*, 782–802.

Hughes, J. N., Cavell, T. A., & Grossman, P. B. (1997). A positive view of self: Risk or protection for aggressive children? *Development and Psychopathology, 9*, 75–94.

Hymel, S. (1983). Preschool children's peer relations: Issues in sociometric assessment. *Merrill–Palmer Quarterly, 29*, 237–260.

Hymel, S. (1986). Interpretations of peer behavior: Affective bias in childhood and adolescence. *Child Development, 57*, 431–445.

Hymel, S., & Asher, S. R. (1977, April). *Assessment and training of isolated children's social skills.* Paper presented at the biennial meeting of the Society for Research in Child Development, New Orleans, LA. (ERIC Document Reproduction Service No. ED 136 930)

Hymel, S., Bowker, A., & Woody, E. (1993). Aggressive versus withdrawn unpopular children: Variations in peer and self-perceptions in multiple domains. *Child Development, 64*, 879–896.

Hymel, S., & Franke, S. (1985). Children's peer relations: Assessing self-perceptions. In B. H. Schneider, K. H. Rubin, & J. E. Ledingham (Eds.), *Children's peer relations: Issues in assessment and intervention* (pp. 75–91). New York: Springer-Verlag.

Hymel, S., Franke, S., & Freigang, R. (1985). Peer relationships and their dysfunction: Considering the child's perspective. *Journal of Social and Clinical Psychology, 3*, 405–415.

Hymel, S., Wagner, E., & Butler, L. J. (1990). Reputational bias: View from the peer group. In S. R. Asher & J. D. Coie (Eds.), *Peer rejection in childhood* (pp. 156–186). Cambridge, England: Cambridge University Press.

Izard, C. (2002). Translating emotion theory and research into preventive interventions. *Psychological Bulletin, 128*, 796–824.

Izard, C. E., & Youngstrom, E. A. (1996). The activation and regulation of fear and anxiety. In D. A. Hope (Ed.), *Nebraska Symposium on Motivation, 1995: Perspectives on anxiety, panic, and fear. Current theory and research in motivation* (Vol. 43, pp. 1 59). Lincoln: University of Nebraska Press.

Jacobvitz, D., & Sroufe, L. A. (1987). The early caregiver–child relationship and attention deficit disorder with hyperactivity in kindergarten: A prospective study. *Child Development, 58*, 1496–1504.

Johnson, D. W., & Johnson, R. T. (1994). *Learning together and alone: Cooperative, competitive, and individualistic learning* (4th ed.). Needham Heights, MA: Allyn & Bacon.

Jones, E. E., & Harris, V. A. (1967). The attribution of attitudes. *Journal of Experimental Social Psychology, 3*, 1–24.

Jones, E. E., & Nisbett, R. E. (1972). The actor and the observer: Divergent perceptions of the causes of behavior. In E. E. Jones, D. E. Kanouse, H. H. Kelley, R. E. Nisbett, S. Valins, & B. Weiner (Eds.), *Attribution: Perceiving the causes of behavior* (pp. 79–94). Morristown, NJ: General Learning Press.

Kellam, S. G., Werthamer-Larsson, L., Dolan, L. J., Brown, C. H., Mayer, L. S., Rebok, G. W., Anthony, J. C., Laudolff, J., Edelsohn, G., & Wheeler, L. (1991). Developmental epidemiology based preventive trials: Baseline modeling of early target behaviors and depressive symptoms. *American Journal of Community Psychology, 19*, 563–584.

Kirby, F. D., & Toler, H. C. (1970). Modification of preschool isolate behavior: A case study. *Journal of Applied Behavior Analysis, 5*, 343–372.

Kistner, J., Metzler, A., Gatlin, D., & Risi, S. (1993). Classroom racial proportions and children's peer relations: Race and gender effects. *Journal of Educational Psychology, 85*, 446–452.

Klein, A. R., & Young, R. D. (1979). Hyperactive boys in their classroom: Assessment of teacher and peer perceptions, interactions, and classroom behaviors. *Journal of Abnormal Child Psychology, 7*, 425–442.

Kochenderfer, B., & Ladd, G. (1996). Peer victimization: Causes or consequences of school maladjustment? *Child Development, 67*, 1305–1317.

Kopp, C. (1982). Antecedents of self-regulation: A developmental perspective. *Developmental Psychology, 18*, 199–214.

Koslin, B. L., Haarlow, R. N., Karlins, M., & Pargament, R. (1968). Predicting group status from members' cognitions. *Sociometry, 31*, 64–75.

Kupersmidt, J. B., Burchinal, M., & Patterson, C. J. (1995). Developmental patterns of childhood peer relations as predictors of externalizing behavior problems. *Development and Psychopathology, 7*, 825–843.

Kupersmidt, J., & Coie, J. D. (1990). Preadolescent peer status, aggression, and school adjustment as predictors of externalizing problems in adolescence. *Child Development, 61*, 1350–1362.

Kusche, C. A., & Greenberg, M. T. (1995). *The PATHS curriculum*. Seattle, WA: Developmental Research & Programs.

Ladd, G. W. (1981). Effectiveness of a social learning method for enhancing children's social interaction and peer acceptance. *Child Development, 52*, 171–178.

Ladd, G. W. (1983). Social networks of popular, average and rejected children in school settings. *Merrill–Palmer Quarterly, 29*, 282–307.

Ladd, G. W. (1990). Having friends, keeping friends, making friends, and being liked by peers in the classroom: Predictors of children's early school adjustment? *Child Development, 61*, 1061–1100.

Ladd, G. W., & Asher, S. R. (1985). Social skill training and children's peer relations: Current issues in research and practice. In L. L'Abate & M. Milan (Eds.), *Handbook of social skill training* (pp. 219–244). New York: Wiley.

Ladd, G. W., & Hart, C. H. (1992). Creating informal play opportunities: Are parents' and preschoolers' initiations related to children's competence with peers? *Developmental Psychology, 28*, 1179–1187.

Ladd, G. W., & Kochenderfer-Ladd, B. (2002). Identifying victims of peer aggression from early to middle childhood: Analysis of cross-informant data for concordance, estimation of relational adjustment, prevalence of victimization, and characteristics of identified victims. *Psychological Assessment, 14*, 74–96.

Ladd, G. W., & Mars, K. T. (1986). Reliability and validity of preschoolers' perceptions of peer behavior. *Journal of Clinical Psychology, 15*, 16–25.

Ladd, G. W., & Mize, J. (1983). A cognitive-social learning model of social skill training. *Psychological Review, 90*, 127–157.

Ladd, G. W., & Oden, S. (1979). The relationship between peer acceptance and children's ideas about helpfulness. *Child Development, 50*, 402–408.

Ladd, G. W., & Profilet, S. M. (1996). The Child Behavior Scale: A teacher report measure of young children's aggressive, withdrawn, and prosocial behaviors. *Developmental Psychology, 32*, 1008–1024.

La Greca, A. M. (1993). Social skills training with children: Where do we go from here? *Journal of Clinical Child Psychology, 22*, 288–298.

La Greca, A. M., Dandes, S. K., Wick, P., Shaw, K., & Stone, W. L. (1988). Development of the Social Anxiety Scale for Children: Reliability and concurrent validity. *Journal of Clinical Child Psychology, 17*, 84–91.

La Greca, A. M., & Santogrossi, D. S. (1980). Social skills training with elementary school students: A behavioral group approach. *Journal of Consulting and Clinical Psychology, 48*, 220–227.

La Greca, A. M., Stone, W. L., & Noriega-Garcia, A. (1989). Social skills intervention: A case example with a learning disabled boy. In M. C. Roberts & C. E. Walker (Eds.), *Casebook of child and pediatric psychology* (pp. 139–160). New York: Guilford Press.

Landau, S., Milich, R., & Whitten, P. (1984). A comparison of teacher and peer assessment of social status. *Journal of Clinical Child Psychology, 13*, 44–49.

Ledingham, J. E. (1981). Developmental patterns of aggressive and withdrawn behavior in childhood: A possible method for identifying preschizophrenics. *Journal of Abnormal Child Psychology, 9,* 1–22.

Ledingham, J. E., & Schwartzman, A. E. (1984). A 3-year follow-up of aggressive and withdrawn behavior in childhood: Preliminary findings. *Journal of Abnormal Child Psychology, 9,* 1–22.

Ledingham, J. E., Younger, A. S., Schwartzman, A. E., & Bergeron, G. (1982). Agreement among teacher, peer, and self ratings of children's aggression, withdrawal, and likability. *Journal of Abnormal Child Psychology, 10,* 363–372.

Lewin, L. M., Davis, B., & Hops, H. (1999). Childhood social predictors of adolescent antisocial behavior: Gender differences in predictive accuracy and efficacy. *Journal of Abnormal Child Psychology, 27,* 277–292.

Lilly, M. S. (1971). Improving social acceptance of low sociometric status, low achieving students. *Exceptional Children, 37,* 341–348.

Lochman, J. E., Burch, P. R., Curry, J. F., & Lampron, L. B. (1984). Treatment and generalization effects of cognitive-behavioral and goal setting interventions with aggressive boys. *Journal of Consulting and Clinical Psychology, 52,* 915–916.

Lochman, J. E., Coie, J. D., Underwood, M. K., & Terry, R. (1993). Effectiveness of a social relations intervention program for aggressive and nonaggressive, rejected children. *Journal of Consulting and Clinical Psychology, 61,* 1053–1058.

Lochman, J. E., & Curry, J. J. (1986). Effects of social problem-solving training and self-instruction with aggressive boys. *Journal of Clinical Child Psychology, 15,* 159–164.

Lochman, J. E., & Dodge, K. A. (1994). Social-cognitive processes of severely violent, moderately aggressive and nonaggressive boys. *Journal of Consulting and Clinical Psychology, 62,* 366–374.

Lochman, J. E., & Lenhart, L. A. (1993). Anger coping intervention for aggressive children: Conceptual models and outcome effects. *Clinical Psychology Review, 13,* 785–805.

Madden, N. A., & Slavin, R. E. (1982). *Effects of cooperative learning on the social acceptance of mainstreamed academically handicapped students.* Baltimore: Johns Hopkins University Center for the Social Organization of Schools.

Markus, H., & Wurf, E. (1987). The dynamic self-concept: A social psychological perspective. *Annual Review of Psychology, 38,* 299–337.

Martin, C. S., Earleywine, M., Blackson, T. C., Vanyukov, M. M., Moss, H. B., & Tartar, R. (1994). Aggressivity, inattention, hyperactivity, and impulsivity in boys at high and low risk for substance abuse. *Journal of Abnormal Child Psychology, 22,* 177–203.

Masten, A. S., Morison, P., & Pellegrini, D. S. (1985). A revised class play method of peer assessment. *Developmental Psychology, 21,* 523–533.

Matson, J. L., Rotatori, A. F., & Helsel, W. J. (1983). Development of a rating scale to measure social skills in children: The Matson Evaluation of Social Skills with Youngsters (MESSY). *Behaviour Research and Therapy, 21,* 335–340.

McClure, L. F., Chinsky, J. M., & Larcen, S. W. (1978). Enhancing social problem-solving performance in an elementary school setting. *Journal of Educational Psychology, 70,* 504–513.

McFadyen-Ketchum, S. A., & Dodge, K. A. (1998). Problems in social relationships. In E. J. Mash & R. A. Barkley (Eds.). *Treatment of childhood disorders* (2nd ed., pp. 338–365). New York: Guilford Press.

McFall, R. M. (1982). A review and reformulation of the concept of social skills. *Behavioral Assessment, 4,* 1–33.

McKim, B. J., & Cowen, E. L. (1987). Multiperspective assessment of young children's school adjustment. *School Psychology Review, 16,* 370–381.

McMahon, R. J., & Wells, K. C. (1998). Conduct problems. In E. J. Mash & R. A. Barkley

(Eds.), *Treatment of childhood disorders* (2nd ed., pp. 111–207). New York: Guilford Press.

Milich, R., & Dodge, K. A. (1984). Social information processing patterns in child psychiatric populations. *Journal of Abnormal Child Psychology, 12,* 471–490.

Miller-Johnson, S., Coie, J. D., Maumary-Gremaud, A., Bierman, K., & Conduct Problems Prevention Research Group (CPPRG). (2002). Peer rejection and aggression and early starter models of conduct disorder. *Journal of Abnormal Child Psychology, 30,* 217–230.

Mize, J., & Ladd, G. W. (1990). Toward the development of successful social skills training for preschool children. In S. R. Asher & J. D. Coie (Eds.), *Peer rejection in childhood* (pp. 274–308). Cambridge, England: Cambridge University Press.

Morrison, P., & Masten, A. S. (1991). Peer reputation in middle childhood as a predictor of adaptation in adolescence: A seven-year follow up. *Child Development, 62,* 991–1007.

Mrazek, P. J., & Haggerty, R. J. (Eds.). (1994). *Reducing risks for mental disorders: Frontiers for preventive intervention research.* Washington, DC: National Academy Press.

MTA Cooperative Group. (1999a). A 14–month randomized clinical trial of treatment strategies for attention deficit hyperactivity disorder (ADHD). *Archives of General Psychiatry, 56,* 1073–1086.

MTA Cooperative Group. (1999b). Moderators and mediators of treatment response for children with attention-deficit/hyperactivity disorder. *Archives of General Psychiatry, 56,* 1088–1096.

Newcomb, A. F., & Bagwell, C. L. (1995). Children's friendship relations: A meta-analytic review. *Psychological Bulletin, 117,* 306–347.

Newcomb, A. F., Bukowski, W. M., & Pattee, L. (1993). Children's peer relations: A meta-analytic review of popular, rejected, neglected, controversial, and average sociometric status. *Psychological Bulletin, 1113,* 99–128.

Nolen-Hoeksema, S., Girgus, J. S., & Seligman, M. E. P. (1986). Learned helplessness in children: A longitudinal study of depression, achievement, and explanatory style. *Journal of Personality and Social Psychology, 51,* 435–442.

O'Connor, R. D. (1972). Relative efficacy of modeling, shaping, and the combined procedures for modification of social withdrawal. *Journal of Abnormal Psychology, 79,* 327–334.

Oden, S. L., & Asher, S. R. (1977). Coaching children in social skills for friendship making. *Child Development, 48,* 495–506.

Olweus, D. (1991). Bully/victim problems among school children: Basic facts and effects of a school based intervention program. In D. Pepler & K. Rubin (Eds.), *The development and treatment of childhood aggression* (pp. 411–488). Hillsdale, NJ: Erlbaum.

Olweus, D. (1993). *Bullying in school: What we know and what we can do.* Oxford: Blackwell.

O'Neil, R., Welsh, M., Parke, R. D., Wang, S., & Strand, C. (1997). A longitudinal assessment of the academic correlates of early peer acceptance and rejection. *Journal of Clinical Child Psychology, 26,* 290–303.

Osterweil, Z., & Nagano-Nakamura, K. (1992). Maternal views on aggression: Japan and Israel. *Aggressive Behavior, 18,* 263–270.

Parke, R. D., & Ladd, G. W. (1992). *Family–peer relationships: Modes of linkage.* Hillsdale, NJ: Erlbaum.

Parker, J. G., & Asher, S. R. (1987). Peer acceptance and later personal adjustment: Are low-accepted children at risk? *Psychological Bulletin, 102,* 357–389.

Parker, J. G., & Asher, S. R. (1993a). Beyond group acceptance: Friendship adjustment and friendship quality as distinct dimensions of children's peer adjustment. In D. Perlman & W. H. Jones (Eds.), *Advances in personal relationships* (Vol. 4, pp. 261–294). London: Kingsley.

Parker, J. G., & Asher, S. R. (1993b). Friendship and friendship quality in middle childhood: Links with peer group acceptance and feelings of loneliness and social dissatisfaction. *Developmental Psychology, 29,* 611–621.

Parker, J. G., & Herrera, C. (1996). Interpersonal processes in friendship: A comparison of abused and nonabused children's experiences. *Developmental Psychology, 32,* 1025–1038.

Parker, J. G., Rubin, K. H., Price, J. M., & DeRosier, M. E. (1995). Peer relationships, child development and adjustment: A developmental psychopathological perspective. In D. Cicchetti & D. Cohen (Eds.), *Developmental psychopathology: Vol. 2. Risk, disorder, and adaptation* (pp. 96–161). New York: Wiley.

Parkhurst, J. T., & Asher, S. R. (1992). Peer rejection in middle school: Subgroup differences in behavior, loneliness, and interpersonal concerns. *Developmental Psychology, 28,* 231–241.

Patterson, G. R. (1982). *Coercive family processes.* Eugene, OR: Castalia.

Patterson, G. R. (1986). Performance models for antisocial boys. *American Psychologist, 41*(4), 432–444.

Patterson, G. R., Littman, R. A., & Bricker, D. (1967). Assertive behavior in children: A step toward a theory of aggression. *Monographs of the Society for Research in Child Development, 32*(5, Serial No. 113).

Patrick, B. C., Skinner, E. A., & Connell, J. P. (1993). What motivates children's behavior and emotion?: The joint effects of perceived control and autonomy in the academic domain. *Journal of Personality and Social Psychology, 65,* 781–791.

Peery, J. C. (1979). Popular, amiable, isolated, rejected: A reconceptualization of sociometric status in preschool children. *Child Development, 50,* 1231–1234.

Pekarik, E. G., Prinz, R. J., Liebert, D. E., Weintraub, S., & Neale, J. M. (1976). The Pupil Evaluation Inventory: A sociometric technique for assessing children's social behavior. *Journal of Abnormal Child Psychology, 14,* 83–97.

Pepler, D. J., & Craig, W. M. (1998). Assessing children's peer relationships. *Child Psychology and Psychiatry Review, 3,* 176–182.

Perry, D. G., Kusel, S. J., & Perry, L. C. (1988). Victims of peer aggression. *Developmental Psychology, 27,* 663–671.

Perry, D. G., Perry, L. C., & Kennedy, E. (1992). Conflict and the development of antisocial behavior. In C. Shantz & W. Hartup (Eds.), *Conflict in child and adolescent development* (pp. 301–329). Cambridge, England: Cambridge University Press.

Perry, D. G., Perry, L. C., & Rasmussen, P. (1986). Cognitive social learning mediators of aggression. *Child Development, 57,* 700–711.

Perry, D. G., Williard, J. C., & Perry, L. C. (1990). Peers' perceptions of the consequences that victimized children provide aggressors. *Child Development, 61,* 1310–1325.

Pettit, G. S., & Mize, J. (1993). Substance and style: Understanding the ways in which parents teach children about social relationships. In S. Duck (Ed.), *Learning about relationships* (pp. 118–151). Newbury Park, CA: Sage.

Pianta, R. C. (1999). *Enhancing relationships between children and teachers.* Washington, DC: American Psychological Association.

Pinkston, E. M., Reese, N. M., LeBlanc, J. M., & Baer, D. M. (1973). Independent control of a preschool child's aggression and peer interaction by contingent teacher attention. *Journal of Applied Behavior Analysis, 6,* 115–124.

Plienis, A. H., Hansen, D. J., Ford, F., Smith, S., Jr., Stark, L. J., & Kelly, J. A. (1987). Behavioral small group training to improve the social skills of emotionally-disordered adolescents. *Behavior Therapy, 18,* 17–32.

Pope, A. W., & Bierman, K. L. (1999). Predicting adolescent peer problems and antisocial activities: The relative roles of aggression and dysregulation. *Developmental Psychology, 35,* 335–346.

Pope, A. W., Bierman, K. L., & Mumma, G. H. (1991). Aggression, hyperactivity, and inattention–immaturity: Behavior dimensions associated with peer rejection in elementary school boys. *Developmental Psychology, 27,* 663–671.

Price, J. M., & Dodge, K. A. (1989). Peers' contributions to children's social maladjustment. In T. J. Berndt & G. W. Ladd (Eds.), *Peer relationships in child development* (pp. 341–370). New York: Wiley.

Price, J. M., & Ladd, G. W. (1986). Assessment of children's friendships: Implications for social competence and social adjustment. In R. J. Prinz (Ed.), *Advances in behavioral assessment of children and families* (Vol. 2, pp. 121–149). Greenwich, CT: JAI Press.

Putallaz, M. (1983). Predicting children's sociometric status from their behavior. *Child Development, 54,* 1417–1426.

Putallaz, M., & Gottman, J. M. (1981). An interactional model of children's entry into peer groups. *Child Development, 52,* 986–994.

Putallaz, M., & Heflin, A. H. (1990). Parent–child interaction. In S. R. Asher & J. D. Coie (Eds.), *Peer rejection in childhood* (pp. 189–216). Cambridge, England: Cambridge University Press.

Quiggle, N., Garber, J., Panak, W., & Dodge, K. A. (1992). Social-information processing in aggressive and depressed children. *Child Development, 63,* 1305–1320.

Rabiner, D., & Coie, J. (1989). Effect of expectancy inductions on rejected children's acceptance by unfamiliar peers. *Developmental Psychology, 25,* 450–457.

Rabiner, D. L., Lenhart, L., & Lochman, J. E. (1990). Automatic versus reflective social problem solving in relation to children's sociometric status. *Developmental Psychology, 26,* 1010–1016.

Reid, M., Landesman, S., Treder, R., & Jaccard, J. (1989). "My Family and Friends": Six- to twelve-year-old children's perceptions of social support. *Child Development, 60,* 896–910.

Renshaw, P. D. (1981). The roots of current peer interaction research: A historical analysis of the 1930s. In S. R. Asher & J. M. Gottman (Eds.), *The development of children's friendships* (pp. 1–28). New York: Cambridge University Press.

Renshaw, P. D., & Asher, S. R. (1983). Children's goals and strategies for social interaction. *Merrill–Palmer Quarterly, 29,* 353–374.

Renshaw, P. D., & Brown, P. J. (1993). Loneliness in middle childhood: Concurrent and longitudinal predictors. *Child Development, 64,* 1271–1284.

Richard, B., & Dodge, K. (1982). Social maladjustment and problem solving among school aged children. *Journal of Consulting and Clinical Psychology, 50,* 226–233.

Richters, J. E., Arnold, L. E., Jensen, P. S., Abikoff, H., Conners, C. K., Greenhill, L. L., Hechtman, L., Hinshaw, S. P., Pelham, W. E., & Swanson, J. M. (1995). NIMH collaborative multisite multimodal treatment study of children with ADHD: I. Background and rationale. *Journal of the American Academy of Child and Adolescent Psychiatry, 34,* 987–1000.

Robin, A. L., Schneider, M., & Dolnick, M. (1976). The turtle technique: An extended case study of self control in the classroom. *Psychology in the Schools, 13,* 449–453.

Roistacher, R. C. (1974). A microeconomic model of sociometric choice. *Sociometry, 37,* 219–238.

Rose, S. D., & Edleson, J. L. (1987). *Working with children and adolescents in groups: A multimethod approach.* San Francisco: Jossey-Bass.

Rosen, L. A., O'Leary, S. G., Joyce, S. A., Conway, G., & Pfiffner, L. J. (1984). The importance of prudent negative consequences for maintaining the appropriate behavior of hyperactive students. *Journal of Abnormal Child Psychology, 12,* 581–604.

Rubin, K. H. (1985). *Play Observation Schedule.* Unpublished manuscript.

Rubin, K. H., Bukowski, W., & Parker, J. G. (1998). Peer interactions, relationships, and groups. In W. Damon (Series Ed.) & N. Eisenberg (Vol. Ed.), *Handbook of child psychol-*

ogy: Vol. 3. Social, emotional, and personality development (5th ed., pp. 619–700). New York: Wiley.

Rubin, K. H., Daniel-Beirness, T., & Bream, L. (1984). Social isolation and social problem-solving: A longitudinal study. *Journal of Consulting and Clinical Psychology, 52*, 17–25.

Rubin, K. H., & Stewart, S. L. (1996). Social withdrawal. In E. J. Mash & R. A. Barkley (Eds.), *Child psychopathology* (pp. 277–307). New York: Guilford Press.

Ruble, D. N., & Frey, K. S. (1991). Changing patterns of comparative behavior as skills are acquired: A functional model of self-evaluation. In J. Suls & T. A. Wills (Eds.), *Social comparison: Contemporary theory and research* (pp. 70–112). Hillsdale, NJ: Erlbaum.

Rucker, C. N., & Vincenzo, F. M. (1970). Maintaining social acceptance gains made by mentally retarded children. *Exceptional Children, 36*, 679–680.

Rudolph, K. D., & Clark, A. G. (2001). Conceptions of relationships in children with depressive and aggressive symptoms: Social-cognitive distortion or reality? *Journal of Abnormal Child Psychology, 29*, 41–56.

Rudolph, K. D., Hammond, C., & Burge, D. (1997). A cognitive-interpersonal approach to depressive symptoms in preadolescent children. *Journal of Abnormal Child Psychology, 25*, 33–45.

Russell, R. L., & van den Broek, P. (1988). A cognitive-developmental account of storytelling in child psychotherapy. In S. Shirk (Ed.), *Cognitive development and child psychotherapy* (pp. 247–272). New York: Plenum Press.

Rutter, M., Maughan, B., Mortimore, P., & Ousten, J. (1979). *Fifteen thousand hours: Secondary schools and their effects on children.* Cambridge, MA: Harvard University Press.

Rys, G. S., & Bear, G. G. (1997). Relational aggression and peer relations: Gender and developmental issues. *Merrill–Palmer Quarterly, 43*, 87–106.

Salmivalli, C., Lagerspetz, K., Bjorkqvist, K., Osterman, K., & Kaukianen, A. (1996). Bullying as a group process: Participant roles and their relations to social status within the group. *Aggressive Behavior, 22*, 1–15.

Saltz, E., & Medow, M. L. (1971). Concept conservation in children: The dependence of belief systems on semantic representation. *Child Development, 42*, 1533–1542.

Saunders, B., & Chambers, S. M. (1996). A review of the literature on attention-deficit hyperactivity disorder children: Peer interactions and collaborative learning. *Psychology in the Schools, 33*, 333–340.

Schneider, B. H. (1992). Didactic methods for enhancing children's peer relations: A quantitative review. *Clinical Psychology Review, 12*, 363–382.

Schneider, B. H., & Byrne, B. M. (1987). Individualizing social skills training for behavior-disordered children. *Journal of Consulting and Clinical Psychology, 55*, 444–445.

Schwartz, D., Dodge, K. A., & Coie, J. D. (1993). The emergence of chronic peer victimization in boys' play groups. *Child Development, 64*, 1755–1772.

Schwartz, D., McFadyen-Ketchum, S., Dodge, K. A., Pettit, G. S., & Bates, J. E. (1999). Early behavior problems as a predictor of later peer group victimization: Moderators and mediators in the pathways of social risk. *Journal of Abnormal Child Psychology, 27*, 191–201.

Seligman, M. E. P. (1975). *Helplessness: On depression, development, and death.* San Francisco: Freeman.

Selman, R. L., & Schultz, L. H. (1990). *Making a friend in youth: Developmental theory and pair therapy.* Chicago: University of Chicago Press.

Selman, R. L, Schultz, L. H., Nakkula, M., Barr, D., Watts, C., & Richmond, J. B. (1992). Friendship and fighting: A developmental approach to the study of risk and prevention of violence. *Development and Psychopathology, 4*, 529–558.

Shantz, C. U., & Shantz, D. W. (1985). Conflict between children: Social-cognitive and sociometric correlates. *New Directions for Child Development, 20*, 3–21.

Sharabany, R. (1994). Intimate Friendship Scale: Conceptual underpinnings, psychometric properties, and construct validity. *Journal of Social and Personal Relationships, 11*, 449–469.

Sharan, S. (1980). Cooperative learning in small groups: Recent methods and effects on achievement, attitudes, and ethnic relations. *Review of Educational Research, 50*, 241–271.

Sherif, M., Harvey, O. J., White, B. J., Hood, W. R., & Sherif, C. W. (1961). *Inter-group conflict and cooperation: The Robbers Cave experiment.* Norman: University of Oklahoma Press.

Skinner, E. A. (1995). *Perceived control, motivation, and coping.* Thousand Oaks, CA: Sage.

Slavin, R. E. (1983). *Cooperative learning.* New York: Longman.

Sobol, M. P., Earn, B. M., Bennett, D., & Humphries, T (1983). A categorical analysis of the social attributions of learning-disabled children. *Journal of Abnormal Child Psychology, 11*, 217–228.

Solomon, R. W., & Wahler, R. G. (1973). Peer reinforcement control of classroom problem behavior. *Journal of Applied Behavior Analysis, 6*, 49–56.

Speltz, M. L., Greenberg, M. T., & DeKlyen, M. (1990). Attachment in preschoolers with disruptive behavior: A comparison of clinic-referred and nonproblem children. *Development and Psychopathology, 2*, 31–46.

Spivack, G., & Shure, M. B. (1974). *Social adjustment of young children: A cognitive approach to solving real-life problems.* San Francisco: Jossey-Bass.

Sroufe, L. A. (1990). An organizational perspective on the self. In D. Cicchetti & M. Beeghly (Eds.), *The self in transition: Infancy to childhood* (pp. 281–307). Chicago: University of Chicago Press.

Sroufe, L. A. (1996). *Emotional development: The organization of emotional life in the early years.* Cambridge, England: Cambridge University Press.

Sroufe, L. A., & Egeland, B. (1989, April). *Early predictors of psychopathology.* Symposium presented at the biennial meeting of the Society for Research in Child Development, Kansas City, MO.

Stanger, C., & Lewis, M. (1993). Agreement among parents, teachers, and children on internalizing and externalizing behavior problems. *Journal of Clinical Child Psychology, 22*, 107–115.

Steinberg, L., & Silverberg, S. (1986). The vicissitudes of autonomy in adolescence. *Child Development, 57*, 841–851.

Stephens, T. M. (1977). *Teaching skills to children with learning and behavior disorders.* Columbus, OH: Merrill.

Stokes, T., & Osnes, P. (1989). An operant pursuit of generalization. *Behavior Therapy, 20*, 337–355.

Stormshak, E. A., Bierman, K. L., Bruschi, C., Dodge, K. A., Coie, J. D., & Conduct Problems Prevention Research Group (CPPRG). (1999). The relation between behavior problems and peer preference in different classroom contexts. *Child Development, 70*, 169–182.

Stormshak, E. A., Bierman, K. L., McMahon, R. J., Lengua, L. J., & Conduct Problems Prevention Research Group. (2000). Parenting practices and child disruptive behavior problems in early elementary school. *Journal of Clinical Child Psychology, 29*, 17–29.

Strain, P. S. (1977). An experimental analysis of peer social initiations on the behavior of withdrawn preschool children: Some training and generalization effects. *Journal of Abnormal Child Psychology, 5*, 445–455.

Strain, P. S., Lambert, D. L., Kerr, M. M., Stagg, V., & Lenkner, D. A. (1983). Naturalistic assessment of children's compliance to teacher's requests and consequences for compliance. *Journal of Applied Behavior Analysis, 16*, 243–249.

Strain, P. S., Shores, R. E., & Kerr, M. M. (1976). An experimental analysis of "spillover" effects on the social interaction of behaviorally handicapped preschool children. *Journal of Applied Behavior Analysis, 9*, 31–40.

Strain, P. S., Steele, P., Ellis, T., & Timm, M. A. (1982). Long-term effects of oppositional child treatment with mothers as therapists and therapist trainers. Journal of Applied Behavior Analysis, 15, 163 169.

Strain, P. S., & Weigerink, R. (1976). The effects of sociodramatic activities on social interaction among behaviorally handicapped preschool children. *Journal of Special Education, 10*, 71–75.

Sullivan, H. S. (1953). *The interpersonal theory of psychiatry.* New York: Norton.

Taylor, A. R., & Trickett, P. K. (1989). Teacher preference and children's sociometric status in the classroom. *Merrill–Palmer Quarterly, 35*, 343–361.

Taylor, S. E., & Brown, J. (1988). Illusion and well-being: A social psychological perspective on mental health. *Psychological Bulletin, 103*, 193–210.

Terry, R., & Coie, J. D. (1991). A comparison of methods for defining sociometric status among children. *Developmental Psychology, 27*, 867–880.

Tiffen, K., & Spence, S. H. (1986). Responsiveness of isolated versus rejected children to social skills training. *Journal of Child Psychology and Psychiatry, 27*, 343–355.

Tomada, G., & Schneider, B. H. (1997). Relational aggression, gender, and peer acceptance: Invariance across culture, stability over time, and concordance among informants. *Developmental Psychology, 33*, 601–609.

Tremblay, R. E., Loeber, R., Gagnon, C., Charlebois, P., Larivee, S., & LeBlanc, M. (1991). Disruptive boys with stable and unstable high fighting behavior patterns during junior elementary school. *Journal of Abnormal Child Psychology, 19*, 285–300.

Tremblay, R. E., Masse, L. C., Vitaro, F., & Dobkin, P. L. (1995). The impact of friends' deviant behavior on early onset of delinquency: Longitudinal data from 6 to 13 years of age. *Development and Psychopathology, 7*, 649–667.

Tremblay, R. E., Pihl, R. O., Vitary, F., & Dobkin, P. L. (1994). Predicting early onset of male antisocial behavior from preschool behavior. *Archives of General Psychiatry, 51*, 732–739.

Tremblay, R. E., Vitaro, F., Bertrand, L., LeBlanc, M., Beauchesne, H., Boileau, H., & David, L. (1992). Parent and child training to prevent early onset of delinquency: The Montreal longitudinal study. In J. McCord & R. E. Tremblay (Eds.), *Preventing antisocial behavior: Interventions from birth through adolescence* (pp. 117–138). New York: Guilford Press.

Trower, P. (1980). Situational analyses of the components and processes of behavior of social skilled and unskilled patients. *Journal of Consulting and Clinical Psychology, 3*, 327–339.

Underwood, M. K. (2003). *Social aggression among girls.* New York: Guilford Press.

Vaughn, B. E., Azria, M. R., Krzysik, L., Caya, L. R., Bost, K. K., Newell, W., & Kazura, K. L. (2000). Friendship and social competence in a sample of preschool children attending Head Start. *Developmental Psychology, 36*, 326–338.

Vitaro, F., Tremblay, R. E., Gagnon, D., & Boivin, M. (1992). Peer rejection from kindergarten to grade 2: Outcomes, correlates, and prediction. *Merrill–Palmer Quarterly, 38*, 382–400.

Vitaro, F., Tremblay, R. E., Kerr, M., Pagani, L., & Bukowski, W. M. (1997). Disruptiveness, friends' characteristics, and delinquency in early adolescence: A test of two competing models of development. *Child Development, 68*, 676–689.

Volling, B. L., MacKinnon-Lewis, C., Rabiner, D., & Baradaran, L. P. (1993). Children's social competence and sociometric status: Further exploration of aggression, social withdrawal, and peer rejection. *Development and Psychopathology, 5*, 459–483.

Waas, G. A., & Honer, S. A. (1990). Situational attributions and dispositional inferences: The development of peer reputations. *Merrill–Palmer Quarterly, 36*, 239–260.

Walker, H. M. (1983). *Walker Problem Behavior Identification Checklist: Test and manual* (2nd ed.). Los Angeles: Western Psychological Services.

Walker, H. M., & McConnell, S. R., (1988). *Walker–McConnell Scale of Social Competence and School Adjustment*. Austin, TX: Pro-Ed.

Waters, E., & Sroufe, L. A. (1983). Social competence as a developmental construct. *Developmental Review, 3,* 79–97.

Weiner, B. (1985). An attributional theory of achievement motivation and emotion. *Psychological Review, 92,* 548–573.

Weissberg, R. P., Gesten, E. L., Carnrike, C. L., Toro, P. A., Rapkin, B. D., Davidson, E., & Cowen, E. L. (1981). Social problem-solving skills training: A competence building intervention with second- to fourth-grade children. *American Journal of Community Psychology, 9,* 411–423.

Weissberg, R. P., & Greenberg, M. T. (1998). Prevention science and collaborative community action research: Combining the best from both perspectives. *Journal of Mental Health, 7,* 479–492.

Werthamer-Larsson, L., Kellam, S., & Wheeler, L. (1991). Effects of first-grade classroom environment on shy behavior, aggressive behavior, and concentration problems. *American Journal of Community Psychology, 19,* 585–602.

Whalen, C. K., Henker, B., Collins, B. E., McAuliffe, S., & Vaux, A. (1979). Peer interaction in a structured communication task: Comparisons of normal and hyperactive boys and of methylphenidate (Ritalin) and placebo effects. *Child Development, 50,* 388–401.

Wheeler, V. A., & Ladd, G. (1982). Assessment of children's self-efficacy for social interactions with peers. *Developmental Psychology, 18,* 795–805.

Wiggins, J. S., & Winder, C. L. (1961). The Peer Nomination Inventory: An empirically derived sociometric measure of adjustment in preadolescent boys. *Psychological Reports, 9,* 643–677.

Williams, G. A., & Asher, S. R. (1987, April). *Peer and self perceptions of peer rejected children: Issues in classification and subgrouping.* Paper presented at the biennial meeting of the Society for Research in Child Development, Baltimore.

Work, W. C., Hightower, A. D., Fantuzzo, K. W., & Rohrbeck, C. A. (1987). Replication and extension of the Teachers Self-Control Rating Scale. *Journal of Consulting and Clinical Psychology, 55,* 115–116.

Wright, J. C., Giammarino, M., & Parad, H. W. (1986). Social status in small groups: Individual–group similarity and the social misfit. *Journal of Personality and Social Psychology, 50,* 523–536.

Younger, A. J., Schwartzman, A. E., & Ledingham, J. E. (1986). Age-related differences in children's perceptions of social deviance: Changes in behavior or in perspective? *Developmental Psychology, 22,* 531–542.

Zakriski, A. L., & Coie, J. D. (1996). A comparison of aggressive–rejected and nonaggressive-rejected children's interpretations of self-directed and other-directed rejection. *Child Development, 67,* 1048–1070.

Index